Orthopaedics
in Primary Care

Orthopaedics in Primary Care

Chinni Pennathur Ramamurti,

M.D., F.R.C.S., F.A.A.O.S.

Chief of Orthopaedics
Group Health Cooperative of Puget Sound
Clinical Associate Professor of Orthopaedics
University of Washington School of Medicine

edited by
Richard Vernon Tinker, M.D.

Associate Director, Family Practice Residency Program
Group Health Cooperative of Puget Sound
Clinical Associate Professor of Family Medicine
University of Washington School of Medicine

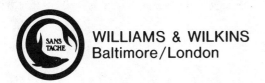

WILLIAMS & WILKINS
Baltimore/London

Library of Congress Cataloging in Publication Data

Ramamurti, Chinni Pennathur.
    Orthopaedics in primary care.

    Includes bibliographical references and index.
    1. Orthopedia. I. Tinker, Richard V. II. Title. [DNLM: 1. Orthopedics. 2. Primary health care. WE168 R165o]
RD731.R25   617'.3   78-4497
ISBN 0-683-07150-5

Composed and printed at the
Waverly Press, Inc.
Mt. Royal and Guilford Aves.
Baltimore, Md. 21202, U.S.A.

DEDICATION

Carol Ramamurti and her daughter Kanti wish to dedicate this book to the Medical Staff of Group Health Cooperative of Puget Sound, in appreciation for the challenge and fulfillment Doctor Ramamurti attained during his 16 years at Group Health. They also wish to express their gratitude to all those whose labor and support brought Doctor Ramamurti's book to publication.

In Memory of the Author

The foundation for this book was laid by Chinni Pennathur Ramamurti during his 16 years as an orthopaedic surgeon with the Medical Staff of Group Health Cooperative of Puget Sound. During those years, he had done much of the teaching of orthopaedics to the members of the Family Practice Section and was, of course, one of their consultants. From those labors, he gleaned an understanding of the generalist's need and a method of didactic organization and presentation that seemed to meet that need. When the opportunity arose for him to prepare a chapter on musculoskeletal problems for a primary care textbook, he jumped at the opportunity, but poured out the first draft of this book instead. Dictating evenings, weekends, and when ideas wakened him in the small hours of the morning, he completed the first draft during the winter of 1975–1976. When it was clear that the large manuscript was hardly what the editor had in mind, he quickly produced a succinct chapter regarding the common soft tissue musculoskeletal pain syndromes, and then began to seek a publisher for what now had become his dream book. He was persuaded that his conception could make a unique contribution to the didactic orthopaedic literature. He could find no text that in his opinion dealt adequately with the primary care problem. When Williams and Wilkins offered a contract, he was overjoyed, and incorrectly but quite soberly he told some of his friends this book was his "only claim to fame." He had already begun to rewrite the text in more polished, efficient form. His intention was to complete it during the winter of 1976–1977, but he desired to visit his childhood home and family in Madras, India, before beginning the final labor. He never reached home, and he never returned to his book. The airplane from Bombay to Madras exploded in flight.

Doctor Ramamurti wrote like he spoke, repetitively and emphatically. He would make a point three times and then summarize it. The style was utterly characteristic and immutable, and it made his spoken teaching remarkably effective. In writing, however, it became redundant and threatened to be overlong. While the editor's efforts to avoid that danger may have given the book a certain efficiency, it took from it a charm unique to the author's style, which the editor could under no circumstance reproduce.

Doctor Ramamurti was born a Brahmin in Madras, India, September 30, 1922. His father was a physician and professor of medicine at Madras Medical College. Fearing unemployment, which was and still is the fate of many young Brahmins, Doctor Ramamurti was at first reluctant to begin the long training that would lead him in his father's path and vowed to take the first job he could find. Ultimately, he did endure the extended dependency, performing with great energy and considerable talent, and finished his general surgical training in Madras in 1950. Upon completing the Honorary Senior House Surgeoncy, in 1950, he applied to the same hospital for a position as paid assistant surgeon. His application was rejected, and when it seemed to him that it had been rejected because he was a Brahmin, and the son of a notable physician, who thus should not need a job with a government hospital, he was persuaded that his future as a surgeon in India would be very tenuous, and he applied for an orthopaedic residency position to the Hospital for Bone and Joint Diseases in New York City. He was accepted and sailed for the United States aboard a cargo ship in 1951. He trained at the Hospital for Bone and Joint Diseases from 1951 to 1952, with the Orthopaedic Department at Iowa State University from 1952 to 1955, and at Harborview Medical Center in Seattle, Washington from 1955 to 1956. He held a position as a Research Fellow with the University of British Columbia from 1956 to 1958, and as Clinical Instructor in Orthopaedic Surgery with the University of Rochester from 1958 to 1959. At that point, intending to remain a clinician, and persuaded that the academic world posed serious obstacles to this intent, in 1960 he accepted a position as Orthopaedic Surgeon with the Group Health Cooperative of Puget Sound.

Doctor Ramamurti was a peculiarly sensitive man. Like every one of us, he brought both pleasure and pain to those he encountered, but when faced with praise on the one hand, and bitter criticism on the other, he would sometimes remark upon the seeming irony to his friends, "Now look at this—who is the real Ramamurti?" He was also a highly visible man. He rarely entered a group without leaving a distinct impression upon it of his presence and his nature. At his annoying worst, he could seem haughtily autocratic and insensitive. At his charming best, he established an immediate generous attachment. It seemed to some of us that he never felt things by halves: He was either very angry, or very glad, or very sad. He had his own criteria of a good person, and if one did not meet those criteria, he could be very aloof until contrary evidence encouraged him. But if someone did meet those criteria, his affection was constant and would be shaded only when that someone might on occasion seem to reject him. On several occasions, when certain of us saw him receive news that a friend or respected acquaintance had been misfortunate, that sometimes haughty man became instantly and very touchingly grieved.

He is remembered at Group Health as a superb surgeon and teacher, a zealous chief of his department, a loyal support to Family Practice, and a strong advocate of a Physical Therapy Department that sought not to carry people but to teach people how to restore themselves. He is remembered by his family and friends as a dear man and generous comrade.

Richard Vernon Tinker, M.D.

Introduction

Primary care is given by any clinician, however specialized, when acting in a professional relationship requiring that he or she be the physician of first call. The orthopaedist is the first to be called when his or her postoperative patient develops fever. On the other hand, the *primary care clinician* is defined today as a generalist, to whom people first come when intending to bring their problems to medical clinicians. Family practitioners, general practitioners, and some pediatricians and internists are specialists in the general and provide primary care in the contemporary sense of the term. They are extensively trained while their colleagues in the limited specialties are intensively trained.

In large, prepaid, closed-panel health care plans, like the Group Health Plans, and the Kaiser-Permanente Plans, the general and the limited specialties may become peculiarly sensitive to the divisions of clinical responsibility. The lines between primary and secondary care sharpen as specialty sections compete for the health care dollar, and as, with the addition of suburban and rural clinics, the general specialty sections outgrow the limited specialty sections. It is rare in such groups for any specialty section to be overstaffed, and they all learn to be very clear about just what riddles and solutions are best addressed by clinicians of their own particular skills and energy resources. They learn this clarity with the subscribers, whose ever-present health care needs and responses provide the facts that discipline the rhetoric of the sections.

As an orthopaedist in such a group for 16 years, as Chief of his Section for 6 years, and as one who loved to teach, Doctor Ramamurti developed a personally clear vision of the ideal line between the general specialties and orthopaedics. His vision yields to the generalist territory which many clinicians, orthopaedists and generalists alike, would assign to the orthopaedist alone. Characteristic of his method, he almost always presented his position in the particular—rarely, and then only very absentmindedly, in the abstract.

For good or bad, the completion of his text was given to an editor who is quite the opposite. As Doctor Ramamurti gave no indication as to what the introduction to his text should accomplish, it falls to this editor to use his own devices, as abstract and uncharacteristic of the author as they are. This editor intends for the introduction to accomplish three things, each speaking in its own way in defense of Doctor Ramamurti's vision of the ortho-

paedic territory of the generalist:

1. The importance of orthopaedics in primary care.

2. The character of orthopaedics in primary care.

3. An overview of the organization and character of the text.

The Importance of Orthopaedics in Primary Care

Matters of *incidence, quality, humanity, and economy* all prevail upon generalists to develop an orthopaedic expertise comparable to their medical and pediatric expertise.

Incidence. Surveys of family practice and general practice offices in groups like our own and in fee-for-service practice, indicate that about 25% of primary care work responds to complaints referable to the musculoskeletal system. Within this 25%, 10–15% of the work responds to orthopaedic injuries. Surveys of hospital emergency services indicate that about

20% of their work responds to orthopaedic injuries.

Quality. When treatment can be effected promptly, the outcome, particularly of injuries, is often more favorable.

Humanity. When treatment can be effected promptly, the afflicted are spared the pain, boredom, and inconvenience of waiting or traveling elsewhere for a therapist.

Economy. When definitively treated on the spot, patients are charged only one fee, not two, and are spared the additional costs of travel, room and board, and operating room fees.

The Character of Orthopaedics in Primary Care

The practice of orthopaedics by generalists differs in four respects from the practice of orthopaedics by orthopaedists:

1. A Reductionist Approach. Analysis of the multitudinous particular for particular purposes is facilitated when the multitude can be reduced to some common denominator. The orthopaedist becomes quite familiar with many particulars which the generalist encounters rarely. To avoid naive oversight, the generalist more than the orthopaedist must learn—and consciously analyze in terms of—a number, but a memorable number, of common denominators.

2. A Triage Approach. While every clinician must at times make sorting decisions, those who make first contact with the majority of people who bring their problems to clinicians continuously make sorting decisions: What are the problems and how do they relate to one another?

What are the clinical processes that speak to the problems? Which of these processes can a sorting physician carry out, and which must be carried out by a clinician more intensively skilled? How soon must the processes be carried out?

3. An Outpatient Approach. Outpatient treatment, when suitable, is quicker and cheaper, and sometimes safer, than is hospital operating room treatment. While there are problems that *must* be treated in a hospital operating room, and while many orthopaedists treat all other problems in the outpatient setting, some orthopaedists whose clinics are architecturally tied to hospitals find it expedient or architecturally necessary to do more of their work in the hospital operating rooms than is technically necessary. Fortunately, treatment appropriate to the outpatient setting can be learned well with less formal training than necessary for the technically complex procedures appropriate to the hospital operating room. These treatments can—and in our opinion should—be learned and applied by generalists.

4. An Incorporative Approach. A generalist learns much about the peculiarities of his or her patients and their families. Such knowledge will influence the interpretation of complaints and findings, and the choice of therapeutic responses. A person presenting a problem to a generalist may often present several other problems at the same time. The generalist, in other words, must often consider more disparate variables when assessing a clinical problem than must a secondary or tertiary care orthopaedist.

An Overview of the Organization and Character of the Text

As the majority of orthopaedic problems present as regional problems, the bulk of the text has been developed in regional chapters, 1 through 14. Chapters 7, 8, and 14 are summaries of regional information that are intended to provide an overview useful to problem assessment, and Chapter 15 collates the pediatric problems referred to in the regional text and suggests some common denominators unique to children's musculoskeletal problems. Chapters 16 through 20 deal with matters which are generally applicable to all regions. Chapter 16, dealing with outpatient anesthesia, was written by Dr. Pat Bennett, Anesthesiologist at Group Health Cooperative of Puget Sound. Doctor Ramamurti and Doctor Bennett had developed considerable respect and regard for one another over the years of their association. When he conceived the text, Doctor Ramamurti had asked Doctor Bennett to prepare the anesthesia chapter.

Each regional chapter begins with a review of essential anatomy and proceeds with a discussion of the problems of that region. Some chapters discuss injuries before the non-traumatic pain syndromes, others do the opposite. The variation reflects the editor's sense of the didactic problem—which category seemed to flow more naturally from which in a particular regional discussion.

A reading list has been appended at the end of the text. Selections were chosen to add detail beyond the scope of the text, to provide some historic perspective, to provide a different perspective on a problem than that presented in the text, or an important viewpoint at variance with the text.

The analytic and treatment methods presented in this text are not always standard, but they are, in our view, safe, effective, and entirely appropriate to the outpatient setting. Most of the material represents Doctor Ramamurti's teaching, and written intention for this text. Some of it represents the editor's additions or the suggestions of the editor's critics, Drs. Robert McGill and Robert Sherry.

Richard Vernon Tinker, M.D.

Acknowledgments

The editor wishes to point out with gratitude the help of the following individuals and groups: Carol Ramamurti for her loyalty to her husband's dream and her trust in the editor's efforts.

Robert McGill, M.D., orthopaedist with Group Health Cooperative of Puget Sound, for his detailed review of the editor's work, and his substantial clarifications, corrections, and additions to the technical detail. Doctor McGill had worked closely with Doctor Ramamurti and knew his work as an orthopaedist would know it.

Robert Sherry, M.D., family physician with Group Health Cooperative of Puget Sound, for his detailed review of the editor's work, his memory of Doctor Ramamurti's teaching, and his own insights into the outpatient problem. His suggestions often clarified Doctor Ramamurti's emphasis when the editor's interpretations of the author's first draft were less incisive than the original teaching.

Marjorie Priest, R.P.T., for her essential assistance in preparation of the material concerning scoliosis in Chapter 9. Miss Priest had worked closely with Doctor Ramamurti for more than ten years, and shared his optimistic view of the nonsurgical treatment of idiopathic scoliosis of children and adolescents.

Doug Hanson, the artist, for his superb line drawings and his visual interpretation of verbal concepts, and for his commitment to the text even when it delayed his acceptance of more permanent work.

Trudy Schaefer for her preparation of the manuscript. She had worked for Doctor Ramamurti on earlier projects and had transcribed his original draft of this text. In deference to her regard for Doctor Ramamurti and her personal involvement in the project, she continued her work for an unusually modest fee.

Doctors Robert Monroe and Michael Wanderer of the Family Practice Faculty, for their assumption of a greater burden of teaching and planning during the editor's preoccupation with Doctor Ramamurti's text.

Sara Finnegan, Vice President and Editor-in-Chief of The Williams & Wilkins Company, for her loyalty to Doctor Ramamurti's conception, her patience with delays, and her encouragement to the editor.

The Physical Therapy Department of Group Health Cooperative for use of their materials, prepared for patient instruction, and for their loyal and sober support over the years of the orthopaedic work of the Group Health Family Practice Section.

The Medical Staff of Group Health Cooperative for its endorsement and its financial support of the editor's efforts.

Richard Vernon Tinker, M.D.

Contents

CHAPTER 1
The Wry Neck

Wry neck results when the soft tissues of the neck are painfully damaged. The greater forces that damage soft tissue may damage bone as well, but fractures will be dealt with in a later chapter devoted to fractures at all spine levels. This chapter focuses entirely upon the much more common soft tissue injuries.

Essential Anatomy

To understand the course and treatment of the wry neck, the practitioner must know a few things about the functional units of the spine, and the soft tissues which control and stabilize them.

The Functional Units of the Cervical Spine (See Figure 1–1)

The occiput and the first cervical vertebra, or any two adjacent vertebrae and their articulations with one another, constitute a functional unit of the spine. The cervical spine represents eight functional units, five of which are very much alike, and three of which (the first, second, and last) are unique.

The first functional unit is the articulation between the occiput and the first cervical vertebra (the atlanto-occipital joint). (See Figure 1–2.) This unit is controlled primarily by short deep muscles anteriorly and posteriorly that extend only the width of that segment. Its movement allows for nodding, for about one-third of full flexion and extension of the head and neck, and for about 50% of lateral bending of the head and neck.

The second functional unit is the articulation between the first and second cervical vertebrae (the atlanto-axial joint). (See Figure 1–3.) It too is controlled primarily by short deep muscles anteriorly and posteriorly that extend across only the second unit and the first two units. The movement of the second unit allows for 50% of the rotational range of motion of the head and neck. Severe forces may dislocate the atlanto-axial joint only by fracturing the axial odontoid. Almost invariably, the ligaments retaining the odontoid against the anterior arch of the atlas are collectively stronger than the odontoid. However, the ligaments of a child of preschool or early school age may soften and stretch during an episode of acute pharyngotonsillitis, allowing for "spontaneous" subluxation of the atlanto-axial joint.

1

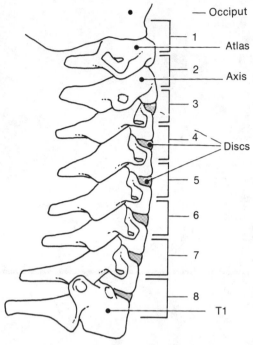

Fig. 1–1. The eight functional units.

Weight is borne across each of these first two units of the spine upon two broad surfaces, the facets.

The next five functional units are the articulations between the 2nd through the 7th cervical vertebrae. (See Figure 1–4.) These units are controlled by long and short deep muscles anteriorly and posteriorly, as well as by superficial sternomastoid and trapezius, and by the middle depth scalenus muscles. Their movement allows for about two-thirds of full flexion and extension, about 50% of rotation, and about 50% of lateral bending. In contrast to the first two units, these five units bear weight upon three broad surfaces, the two facets and the vertebral bodies. The facet articulations are synovial joints. The body articulations are fibrocartilagenous joints (the intervertebral discs). The posterolateral margins of the bodies project slightly beyond the disc to form bony pseudarthroses across each functional unit. These pseudarthroses are variably named. We

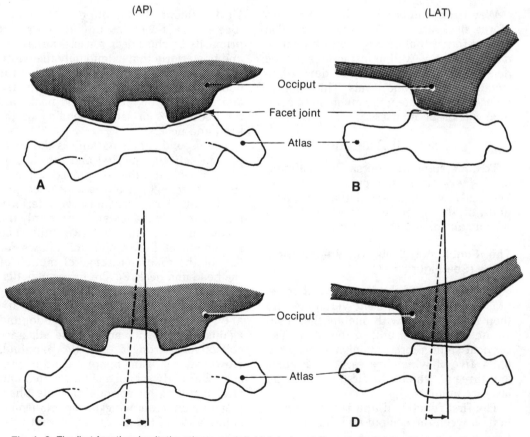

Fig. 1–2. The first functional unit: the atlanto-occipital joint. *A* and *B*, neutral. *C*, lateral bending- *D*, nodding.

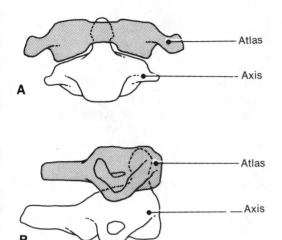

A

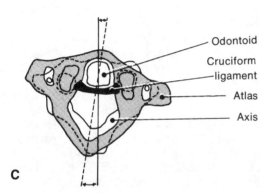

C

Fig. 1–3. The second functional unit: the atlanto-axial joint. *A*, anteroposterior, neutral. *B*, lateral. *C*, superior, rotated.

prefer the name uncovertebral joint, as it implies that they are not true joints. Whether true joints or not, because their opposed surfaces move upon one another, they are vulnerable to wear and tear, and may consequently generate spurs. Between the facet and the uncovertebral projections are grooves which together form the intervertebral or neural foramina. The nerve roots III through VII pass through these grooves and are thus vulnerable to sudden crushing injury during subluxation of any of the units and are vulnerable to the persistent crowding injury of postero-lateral herniation of disc material, or the persistent crowding injury of bony spurs from the uncovertebral and facet joints and/or swollen capsular and synovial membranes of the facet joints. The movements of the cervical spine allow for the severest injuries and greatest wear and tear across the units between C_4 and C_7.

Note that the nerve roots passing through the intervertebral foramina of those units are respectively the 5th, 6th, and 7th.

The last unit is the articulation between C_7 and T_1. (See Figure 1–5.) The C_7 vertebra is unique in two respects:

1. Its upward-directed facets are cervical-like, and its downward directed facets thoracic-like.

2. The body of each lower cervical vertebra from C_3 to C_7 is slightly larger than its superior neighbor. Hence, the body of C_7 is nearly of thoracic dimension.

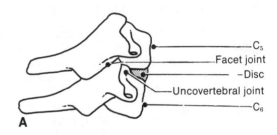

A

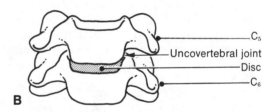

B

Fig. 1–4. The five similiar functional units: articulations between the 2nd and 7th cervical vertebrae.

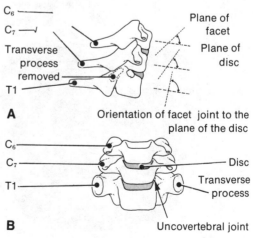

Fig. 1–5. The unique structure of the 7th cervical vertebra.

These unique characteristics allow the last functional unit of the cervical spine to be nearly characteristic of a thoracic unit, in that the vertebral bodies of C_7 and T_1 are larger and bear the bulk of the weight across the unit, and in that the articulations of these facets are no longer in the same plane as the intervertebral disc, but are nearly at right angles to it. These near-perpendicular articular surfaces allow the unit very limited movement in flexion, extension, and rotation. Severe injury or wear and tear across this unit is unusual.

The Soft Tissues of the Cervical Spine

The soft tissues of the cervical spine include the deep fascia, many layers of muscle, the thick ligaments, the synovia of the facet joints, and the intervertebral disc.

Deep Fascia. (Figure 1–6.) The deep fascia consists of three layers of dense connective tissue which separate the neck into compartments:

1. A *superficial layer* which lies beneath the platysma and surrounds all the deeper structures of the neck. It splits to invest the sternomastoid and the strap muscles anteriorly, and the trapezius posteriorly.

2. A *prevertebral layer* which surrounds the cervical sp1ne and the deep muscles that cling to the spine anteriorly and posteriorly.

3. A *pretracheal layer* which surrounds the anterior viscera (the trachea, esophagus, thyroid, and parathyroid).

4. All three layers fuse to form the *carotid sheath* which surrounds the carotid artery, the internal jugular vein, and the vagus nerve.

Muscles. (See Figure 1–7.) The muscles of the neck accessible to physical examination anteriorly are the accessory muscles of the pharynx and larynx, which in aggregate are often called the strap muscles, and the sternocleidomastoid muscle; the muscles accessible posteriorly and laterally are the trapezius and parts of the splenius capitus and cervicis, the levator scapulae, and the scalene muscles. The diagnosis of muscular injury depends upon the discovery of tenderness in these muscles. Deeper muscles that surround and lie upon the cervical spine are surely affected in painful processes, but the effect upon them of these processes cannot be uniquely demonstrated by physical examination.

Ligaments. (see Figure 1–8.) The *ligamentum nuchae* is the most superficial of ligaments. It represents a thin extension of the *supraspinatus* and *interspinatus* ligaments outward between the trapezii muscles. Indeed, while in the dorsal and lumbar spines, the supraspinatus and infrapinatus ligaments are distinct entities, in the neck they merge and lose their identities in the ligamentum nuchae. With the neck in full flexion, the ligamentum nuchae can be palpated distinctly as it extends from the spine of the 7th cervical vertebra to the prominence of occiput.

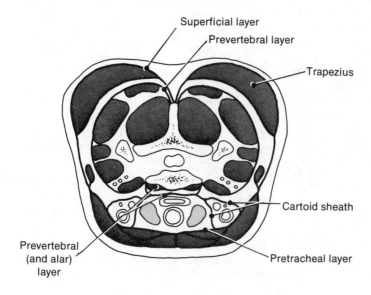

Superficial layer
Prevertebral layer
Trapezius
Cartoid sheath
Prevertebral (and alar) layer
Pretracheal layer

Fig. 1–6. The deep fascia of the neck.

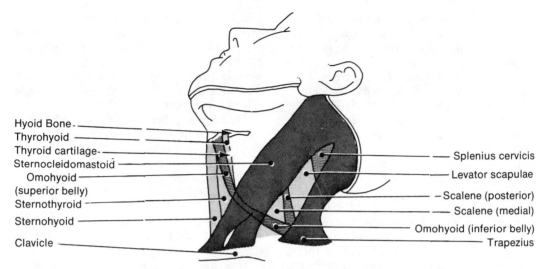

Hyoid Bone
Thyrohyoid
Thyroid cartilage
Sternocleidomastoid
Omohyoid
(superior belly)
Sternothyroid
Sternohyoid
Clavicle

Splenius cervicis
Levator scapulae
Scalene (posterior)
Scalene (medial)
Omohyoid (inferior belly)
Trapezius

Fig. 1–7. The muscles accessible to physical examination.

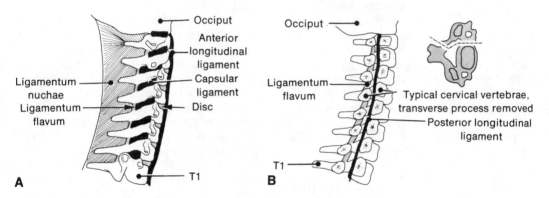

Occiput
Anterior longitudinal ligament
Capsular ligament
Disc
Ligamentum nuchae
Ligamentum flavum
T1
A

Occiput
Ligamentum flavum
Typical cervical vertebrae, transverse process removed
Posterior longitudinal ligament
T1
B

Fig. 1–8. The ligaments of the neck.

This is the only ligament that can be distinguished as such by palpation.

The *capsular ligaments* of the facet joints surround each facet joint, extending between the margins of the two articular surfaces. Palpation through the scalene and splenius muscles detects the facet column of the lateral lamina. The joints as such cannot be distinguished by palpation and, of course, tenderness of the ligaments cannot be distinguished from tenderness of the overlying muscles.

The *posterior longitudinal ligament* passes the length of the spinal column lying against the posterior walls of the vertebral bodies and discs.

The *anterior longitudinal ligament* passes the length of the spinal column lying against the anterior walls of the vertebral bodies and discs.

The *ligamenta flava* are a series of short ligaments which pass between the lamina of the posterior arches of each functional unit for the length of the spine.

Various texts assert that all these ligaments are pain sensitive except the interspinous ligaments and the ligamenta flava. However, some of our experiences have caused us to suspect that those ligaments are also pain sensitive.

The Synovia of the Facet Joints. (See Figure 1-8.) A synovial membrane lies beneath the capsular ligaments and invests and lubricates the articulations of the facets. It may be stretched along with the capsule when the facet joints are subluxed, and it has been postulated that it may be pinched between facet surfaces when they move upon one another in slight misalignment, and as may be true of all synovial joints, local degenerative and various "systemic" events can provoke an inflammation within the synovium. All these processes result in a painful synovitis.

Intervertebral Disc. (See Figure 1–8.) The disc consists of two parts, a springy ring of interwoven fibrocartilagenous bands called the *annulus,* and an hydroelastic gelatinous inner core called the nucleus pulposus. Young discs are thick, malleable, and elastic. Old discs are thin, rigid, and brittle. Greater forces are required to injure young discs than old. When a disc is injured, part of it may be so displaced as to apply force to either the anterior or posterior longitudinal ligaments sufficient to strain or rupture them. Disc material dislocated against the posterior longitudinal ligament may also protrude so far as to injure the neighboring nerve root, producing radicular pain and dysfunction. Of course, the forces that injure discs inevitably injure the anterior and/or posterior longitudinal ligaments as well. Disc material contains no pain-sensitive neuron terminals, hence the pain directly attributable to a disc injury is the pain of an associated injury to the anterior or posterior longitudinal ligament, and/or the pain of an injured nerve root.

Sudden Injury to the Cervical Spine

The damage resulting from sudden forces may be limited to the deep fascia, the ligamentum nuchae, and the muscles surrounding the cervical spine; or the injury may extend to the anterior and posterior longitudinal ligaments, the capsular ligaments and synovial lining of the facet joints, and to the intervertebral discs. Also, depending upon the severity of the trauma, ligaments may be strained, partially torn, or completely torn, discs may be ruptured, vertebrae may be fractured, and the joints may be subluxed or dislocated. Severity of trauma will depend upon the intensity of the injuring force, and the degree of protective muscle tone at the moment of its application. The greater the protective muscle tone, the lesser the injury to the ligaments, synovia, and intervertebral disc. Most cervical sprains represent hyperflexion or hyperextension injuries sustained in auto accidents. Reflex muscle contraction

and elastic rebound forces are sometimes great enough to produce a lesser opposing injury as well. (That is, a lesser rebound hyperextension injury is often associated with a primary hyperflexion injury and vice versa.) We categorize the soft tissue injuries as follows.

Mild Sprain. We define the mild sprain as a stretch injury to muscles, deep fascia, and the ligamentum nuchae. (The standard nomenclature designates a stretch injury to muscle alone, the *cervical strain.*)

Characteristic clinical features of the mild sprain are the following:

1. Pain is usually confined to the neck and is not referred either to the occiput or the upper extremities.

2. Range of movement of the neck is usually normal, though it may be somewhat painful.

3. Superficial muscles are tender, and their tone may be somewhat increased.

Treatment of the Mild Sprain.

1. The patient should rest in a position of comfort for 1–2 days. A position of comfort will be found somewhere within the arc between slight flexion and slight extension. After 2 days, bleeding and capillary oozing will have ceased, and after 3 days, pain will usually be distinctly less.

2. Ice application should be applied for 15 minutes four times daily for the first 2 days. Some people will find the ice comforting. These people should be encouraged to use it more than four times daily if they wish. After the first 2 days, heat may be used if the patient finds it to be more comforting than ice.

3. Analgesics are prescribed if muscle tone is distinctly increased, or if the patient expresses definite distress over the pain or subsequently reports that pain is keeping him awake at night. In our hands, pain not relieved by minor analgesics (aspirin 600 mg., acetaminophen 600 mg., or propoxyphene 100 mg.), and a minor tranquilizer (Valium or Librium 5–10 mg.), has rarely yielded to the addition of a narcotic. Continuous distress over pain has at this point usually indicated a misunderstanding between ourselves and the patient. Whether we have done so initially or not, we make a determined effort at this time to clarify the patient's expectations of the injury, of ourselves, and of any third party. We try

to help the patient acknowledge resentment, anxiety, or depression, and separate these from the pain, and we try to bring their expectations of the injury and of treatment into closer congruence with the tissue pathology and the biology of healing.

4. If the patients' reaction to the injury causes them to be inactive for more than 3 days, we advise the addition of range of motion and isometric exercises to prevent stiffening and weakening.

Severe Sprain. We define severe sprain as injury not only to the muscles, deep fascia, and ligamentum nuchae, but to the deep longitudinal ligaments, the capsular ligaments, and the synovia of the facet joints as well. (Standard nomenclature designates this injury the *cervical sprain.*) Greater force is required to tear the anterior and posterior longitudinal ligaments than to tear the capsular ligaments, and all ligaments are more vulnerable if the spine is at all rotated at the time of injury. Signs of severe sprain usually imply a momentary subluxation of certain functional units at the time of injury. Nerve roots may be contused during the subluxation. They too are more vulnerable if the spine is at all rotated at the time of injury. Clinical characteristics of the severe sprain are the following:

1. Pain is fairly intense at the moment of injury, momentarily subsides somewhat, only to increase with time.

2. Often the pain is felt initially in the back of the neck and sooner or later is referred upward to the occiput, downward to the interscapular region, and outward to both shoulders and upper extremities. Occasionally, extremity pain will show a radicular distribution in one arm or the other.

3. Movement of the cervical spine is painful and limited in all directions.

4. Neurological examination of the upper extremities is usually quite normal, even in the face of radicular pain and dysesthesia.

5. Symptoms which have been attributed to injury of the cervical sympathetic chain and the brain stem will occur perhaps half the time. These are subjective vertigo, blurred vision, tinnitus, periods of faintness, and palpitations.

6. As long as recovery is not delayed by psychologic complications, a usual sense of well-being is often restored after 2 months. Occasionally, symptoms may persist for the better part of a year. Radicular symptoms are more likely to occur and persist in the face of degenerative changes of facet, uncovertebral, and disc joints.

7. Evaluation of all severe cervical sprains should include cervical spine x-rays. Anteroposterior, lateral, oblique, and open-mouth views must be obtained. These views are inspected for vertebral alignment, for fracture, for previous degenerative change, and for soft tissue swelling between the spine and the esophagus. Such soft tissue swelling would suggest fracture or an injury to an intervertebral disc and the anterior longitudinal ligament. When history suggests the trauma to have been severe, if the routine views show normal alignment of the vertebrae, views of the spine are taken with the spine laterally bent and with the spine in extension. If any functional units are unstable, these views will reveal it. Usually, x-rays of a cervical sprain, without fracture or persistent dislocation or subluxation, are normal except for a straightening of the cervical spine which some attribute to reactive increase in muscle tone, and others to the artifact of positioning for the x-ray.

Treatment of the Severe Sprain.

1. The neck should be immobilized as necessary for comfort. Usually, a soft collar is required. The position of immobilization should be determined by trial and error and will lie somewhere within the arc between slight flexion and slight extension. (See Figure 1–9.) The duration of immobilization will depend upon the patient's distress when not immobilized, but should not exceed 4 weeks. In our opinion, early movement brings about a better result than prolonged immobilization.

2. The use of ice and heat is prescribed as for minor sprains.

3. Analgesics are prescribed as for minor sprains.

4. Active range of motion and isometric exercises must begin after 1-week immobilization. (See Figure 1–10.) These exercises are performed at first in the collar, and when a diminution of pain allows, without the collar. However, the unstable

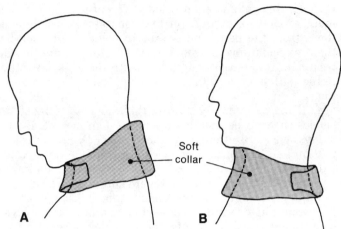

Soft collar

Fig. 1–9. Applications of the soft collar. *A*, flexion. *B*, extension.

A   **B**

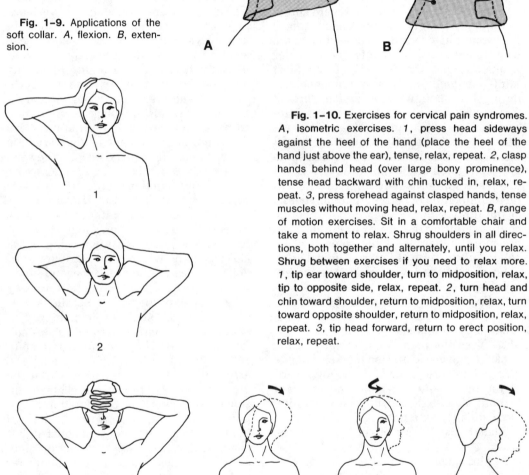

Fig. 1–10. Exercises for cervical pain syndromes. *A*, isometric exercises. *1*, press head sideways against the heel of the hand (place the heel of the hand just above the ear), tense, relax, repeat. *2*, clasp hands behind head (over large bony prominence), tense head backward with chin tucked in, relax, repeat. *3*, press forehead against clasped hands, tense muscles without moving head, relax, repeat. *B*, range of motion exercises. Sit in a comfortable chair and take a moment to relax. Shrug shoulders in all directions, both together and alternately, until you relax. Shrug between exercises if you need to relax more. *1*, tip ear toward shoulder, turn to midposition, relax, tip to opposite side, relax, repeat. *2*, turn head and chin toward shoulder, return to midposition, relax, turn toward opposite shoulder, return to midposition, relax, repeat. *3*, tip head forward, return to erect position, relax, repeat.

A   3   **B**   1   2   3

injury should be exercised within the collar for the full 4 weeks before beginning exercises without the collar. The force of the isometrics should be limited to that which barely produces pain, and the extent of range of motion without the collar should be limited to that which barely produces pain. With the collar, the extent of range of motion is, of course, limited by the collar. As long as pain does not worsen, the exercises should be performed to the point of fatigue four times daily. Should pain worsen, the duration but not the frequency of exercise should be decreased.

We strongly advise the involvement of a physical therapist after the 1st week of immobilization whenever possible.

5. Manipulative treatments, including traction, are contraindicated in the acute stage. Whereas traction has been advised for initial immobilization of all soft tissue injury, we use it only for those that have presented with a persistent, subluxed, or frankly dislocated relationship. Even those injuries which prove on x-ray to be unstable on lateral flexion or extension are in our opinion adequately treated by soft cervical collar as long as the alignment at rest is normal. The unstable severe sprain will require collar immobilization for 4 weeks.

If neck pain and stiffness persist after 6–8 weeks, steady or intermittent cervical traction may then prove beneficial. The proper direction of traction straightens the cervical spine and slightly flexes the atlanto-occipital joint. Two ways of achieving this direction of traction are diagrammed in Figure 1–11. It is often safe to begin with a traction force equal to the weight of the patient's head (10 pounds in average adults). The occasional patient is afraid of traction and tenses the neck muscles during it. These individuals will not benefit unless they can be taught to trust the traction. Beginning with a traction force half the weight of the head, and taking time to explain and re-explain, will often guide them securely into it. Weight may be increased up to three times the weight of the head as pain allows, and benefits direct.

Radicular pain is usually benefited by steady traction. One may theorize that with weight off the discs, they imbibe fluid, so that when traction is removed, the intervertebral space remains wider, sometimes for a period of hours. If the persistence of radicular symptoms is reflecting a swelling of the nerve root as well as the surrounding structures, sufficiently frequent traction, by decreasing the compression of the nerve, may allow the nerve to heal and its swelling thus to subside. Eventually, the nerve could thus

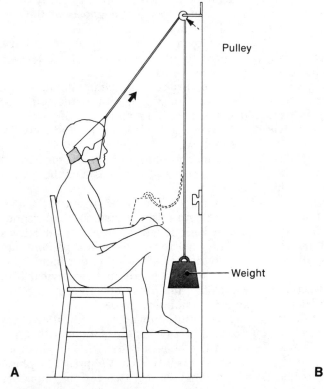

Pulley

Weight

A

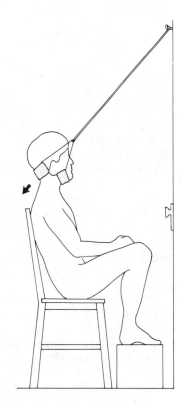

B

Fig. 1–11. *A*, cervical traction by counterweight. *B*, cervical traction by body weight.

again become small enough to pass uncompressed through the still-narrowed intervertebral foramen. *Ligamentous pain is often more likely to yield to intermittent traction,* which one may theorize will "pump" tissue fluid out of the congested ligaments, restoring to them a compliance that will allow a degree of active motion that can stave off the recurrence of congestion. Again we advise that these treatments be guided by a physical therapist whenever possible.

6. The symptoms that have been attributed to cervical sympathetic chain injury and brain stem contusion cannot be treated as such. We advise our patients that they will pass, usually as the neck improves, occasionally some time after full neck recovery. Whether resentment, conversion, or depression tend to augment or fix these symptoms cannot be stated with any certainty. Whenever these psychologic phenomena appear, they should, of course, be treated in their own right, regardless of other symptoms. The right psychiatrist's help can be beneficial, if the referral is made tactfully.

Injury to the Cervical Disc

Cervical disc injuries and degenerative changes usually occur between units C_5-C_6 and C_6-C_7, as these are the units of greatest movement. When disc protrusion occurs as a result of trauma, radicular pain persists, unresponsive to the conservative treatments described above.

Characteristic clinical features of disc protrusion are as follows:

1. Pain is felt not only in the back of the neck, the interscapular region, and the outer aspects of the shoulders, but also along the lateral aspect of one arm, the radial aspect of that forearm, and into the thumb, index, or middle fingers of that hand.

2. When the C_5-C_6 disc is involved, the biceps jerk may be diminished, and paresthesias will be referred to the thumb and index finger. When the C_6-C_7 disc is involved, the triceps jerk may be diminished, and paresthesias will be referred to the middle finger. The paresthetic fingers may be hypoesthetic to sensory examination as well.

Because inexperienced physicians confuse cervical disc syndrome with thoracic outlet syndrome, let it be parenthetically stressed that pain of the cervical disc syndrome radiates to the lateral aspect of the arm, the radial aspect of the forearm, and into the thumb, index, and middle fingers. On the other hand, the pain of nerve root or brachial trunk compression within the thoracic outlet, which usually involves the C_8 and T_1 nerve roots, usually refers along the inner aspect of the arm, the ulnar aspect of the forearm, and into the fifth finger.

3. Movement of the neck, particularly extension of the cervical spine, or straining, as during coughing and sneezing, will often accentuate the pain and cause paresthesias.

4. X-rays may show narrowing between C_5-C_6, and C_6-C_7, or actual arthritic changes with osteophytic lipping and encroachment upon the intervertebral foramina at those levels. X-rays may also be normal or show osteophytic encroachment on intervertebral foramina, other than the ones which fit the symptoms. X-ray is the least useful tool for diagnosis of the cervical disc injury.

Treatment of the Cervical Disc Injury. Many patients respond to the following conservative treatment:

1. The neck should be immobilized in a position of comfort with a soft collar, as described for the major cervical sprain.

2. When muscle tone is reactively increased, we advise that heat or ice be applied in an attempt to relax the muscles. If either is successful, we instruct the patient to continue it.

3. Analgesics may be prescribed as for cervical sprains. Occasionally, narcotics are of benefit when the minor analgesics do not give relief and when patients are greatly distressed. Why in our hands narcotics are of benefit in the cervical disc syndrome, and not of benefit after cervical sprains is not clear to us.

4. Anti-inflammatory medications occasionally may benefit. One can theorize that they benefit when the neighboring facet joint is inflamed. We prescribe phenylbutazone 100 mg. two to four times per day, or dexamethasone 0.04 mg./kg./day, at which time, whether or not benefit has

accrued, we discontinue these drugs, remembering to taper the Dexamethasone over the 2nd week. Prednisolone 0.3 mg./kg./day may be used in lieu of dexamethasone.

5. If isometric exercises do not increase radicular pain, they should be performed to fatigue four times per day.

6. Steady traction should be tried for 15 minutes by the methods described in the previous section. Weights of 10–30 pounds (one to three times the head weight) are used, and—if comforting—the treatment is repeated as soon after the reappearance of pain as possible, or at least four times daily.

7. If symptoms persist on conservative treatment longer than the patient will endure, or longer than 3 months, or if radicular muscle weakness appears, the patient should be referred to an orthopaedist or neurosurgeon for further evaluation and possible surgical treatment.

Wry Neck without Recognized Injury

The onset of the painful stiff neck which develops without a recognized injury may be sudden or gradual. *Sudden onsets* seem usually to occur while the neck is in motion, or while the individual is making an intense muscular effort. The pain is severe, usually resulting in a marked reactive increase in neck muscle tone, and a severe constraint on neck motion. Often the neck is held by pain within a few degrees of a position of slight rotation and lateral bending. *Gradual onsets* usually begin as pain noted just before the limit of motion in one direction or another, which progresses over a few hours to become variably intense and to encroach more and more upon the range of motion. Ultimately, the reactive increase in muscle tone may be as great and the range of motion as restricted as they are in the syndrome of sudden onset.

The Basic Syndromes

We have found it clinically useful to regard the syndromes of the wry neck without recognized injury to be three: the facet syndrome, the cervical disc syndrome, and acute cervical myalgia. The

clinical features of each of the three are quite distinct from one another.

The Facet Syndrome. 1. Onset may be sudden or gradual, and pain will be felt in one posterior triangle or the other, and may be referred into the interscapular region of the same side, and into the occiput of the same side.

2. In time, the shoulder and arm may begin to ache, but the distribution of pain is not radicular.

3. Range of motion in extension and in one direction of rotation and lateral bending is usually severely constrained by pain. Range of motion in other directions is variably constrained.

4. Tenderness of one or several segments of one facet column is elicited by modest pressure through the splenius and scalene muscles where they overlie the facet column laterally. Similar tenderness is usually not elicited on the other side. The tender side is usually the side toward which the head and neck cannot turn without intolerable pain.

5. Manual traction with the patient supine and the neck in slight flexion will often decrease the pain and allow a modest increase in range of motion, as long as the traction is applied. (See Figure 1–12.)

6. With the patient in the same supine position, and the head and neck slightly flexed, an abrupt forward thrust on the spines of the involved unit and/or an abrupt lateral thrust on the facets of the

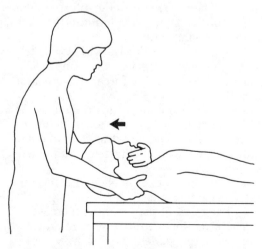

Fig. 1–12. Manual traction: slowly augment traction, hold for several seconds, release and repeat several times.

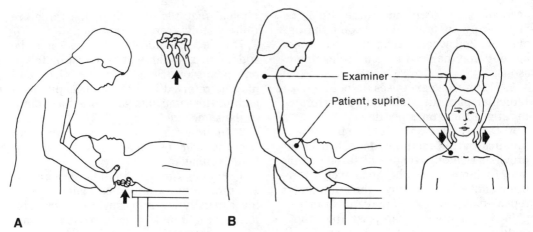

Fig. 1–13. *A,* forward thrusts. Firm vertical thrusts with index and 3rd fingers at successive spinous levels. *B,* lateral thrusts. Firm lateral thrusts with each thumb at successive facet levels.

involved unit will sharply intensify the pain. (See Figure 1–13.)

7. Anteroposterior, lateral, and oblique x-ray views of the cervical spine may show interspace narrowing and joint margin spurring. These degenerative changes are not always evident, nor does the location of the severest x-ray change always correlate with the location of the pain process suggested by symptoms and physical signs. We rarely find x-rays to make a difference, and we tend to order x-rays only when the question of vertebral bone pain remains.

The Disc Syndrome. 1. Onset may be sudden or gradual, and pain will be felt in one posterior cervical triangle or the other, and may be referred into the interscapular region of the same side, and into the occiput of the same side.

2. Pain and paresthesias will also be felt along the outer aspect of the arm, and in the radial aspect of the forearm, hand, and first three fingers.

3. Range of motion is constrained, as for the facet syndrome, but the pain that constrains movement includes the radicular arm pain as well as the neck and interscapular pain.

4. Tenderness can be elicited as it is in the facet syndrome.

5. The relief of pain and the increase in range of motion afforded by *manual* traction with the patient supine may be as great as for the facet syndrome, but its immediate effect on radicular pain dimin-

ishes the longer the radicular symptoms persist.

6. An abrupt forward thrust on cervical spines intensifies neck and interscapular pain as it does in the facet syndrome. It usually does not affect the radicular symptoms.

7. The biceps deep tendon reflex may be obtunded, and paresthesias and hypoesthesias may be localized in the thumb and index finger when the C_5–C_6 disc has herniated, and the triceps deep tendon reflex may be obtunded, and paresthesias and hypoesthesias be localized in the index and middle fingers when the C_6–C_7 disc has herniated.

8. Anteroposterior, lateral, and oblique x-ray views may or may not show narrowing of the implicated joint space. We rarely find x-rays to make a difference and tend to order them only when surgical decompression is planned, or unusual features cause us to suspect bone pathology.

Acute Cervical Myalgia. 1. Onset is gradual, and pain is felt in one or the other posterior cervical triangles.

2. Occasionally, pain may refer into the ipsilateral shoulder, interscapular region, and occiput.

3. Range of motion is usually less restricted by myalgia than by the facet and disc syndrome. Greatest restriction is usually in those directions that stretch the affected muscle.

4. A tender focus can often be discovered by careful palpation of the trapezius,

splenius capitis, and levator scapulae on the painful side. If deep cervical myalgia exists, we cannot diagnose it. Perhaps some individuals whose neck findings do not exactly match with our categories are suffering a deep cervical myalgia.

5. Traction and forward thrusts on the vertebral spine have no effect on the pain or the range of motion.

6. X-rays are not indicated when the syndrome is characteristic of acute cervical myalgia alone.

Treatment of the Syndrome

The facet syndrome of sudden onset will occasionally yield dramatically to gentle manipulation. A modification of one of the diagnostic maneuvers used to distinguish the cause of a wry neck constitute this occasionally curative manipulation. (See Facet Syndrome paragraph 5 above.) With the patient supine, we smoothly apply firm traction with the head and neck in slight flexion. We apply and release this traction slowly and smoothly for 1–2 minutes, then, during continuous traction, we gently attempt rotational and lateral bending movements. During these efforts, the patient must relax. Gentle reassuring instructions and slow movements attempted repeatedly to the point of initial pain only will usually, in time, encourage relaxation, and occasionally will yield a dramatic increase in range of motion, which will persist after the manipulation ends. There are few successes which leave a physician feeling more useful to his patient, but the resultant self-esteem will be tempered by the recognition that no one can prove to general satisfaction what these beneficent effects represent: whether the relocation of a subluxation, a mobilization of tissue fluid from congested deep ligaments or synovia, a restoration of blood flow through ischemic deep ligaments or synovia, or some event as yet unimagined.

The facet syndrome of gradual onset and the syndrome of sudden onset which has not been lastingly relieved by manipulation are treated as is the severe neck sprain, except that traction is recommended when it affords temporary relief during the diagnostic manipulation.

The disc syndrome is treated as is the traumatic disc syndrome. See the previous discussion in this chapter on pages 7 through 11. Recently, very large doses of corticosteroids (equivalent to 0.15 mg. of dexamethasone/kg. of body weight/day) have been advocated in orthopaedic literature. We have as yet not had sufficient experience with that regimen to comment.

Acute cervical myalgia is treated as the mild cervical sprain, except that the exercise regimen emphasizes the movements which stretch the tender muscle.

The Atlanto-Axial Subluxation

A preschool or early school child with a wry neck must be suspected of this uncommon disorder. Unless an obvious cervical myalgia can be demonstrated in a child with only modest reduction in range of motion, standard cervical x-rays must be obtained to allow a two-dimensional inspection of the atlanto-axial joints. The child in great distress, whose neck is quite immobile, will occasionally be shown to have suffered a subluxation of that joint. Such a subluxation is most likely to occur after an upper respiratory tract infection, particularly after an acute pharyngotonsillitis.

The child presents as one with a facet syndrome, except the tenderness will be greatest in the upper third of the spine. We send all these children for x-ray before we examine them. Among those whose x-rays demonstrate an atlanto-axial subluxation are a few who will be "cured" by manual traction during the initial evaluation. Those who are should be protected from a recurrence by immobilization in a soft collar for at least 1 week and until full range of motion is painless. Those who are not should be treated in bed with steady head weight, horizontal traction, released only during meals. Such treatment is easiest to effect in a hospital. If neck x-rays do not demonstrate an atlanto-occipital subluxation, the children are treated as is anyone with a facet syndrome.

CHAPTER 2
The Thoracic Outlet Syndrome

Essential Anatomy

The brachial plexus is formed by the low cervical nerve roots (5th through 8th) and the first thoracic nerve root. Upon their exit from the intervertebral foramina, the neurons of the plexus begin a long and hazardous journey to the periphery—hazardous in that there are several points along their pathway at which they are vulnerable to compressive injuries. As the plexus descends from above, it courses laterally over the first rib, in the triangle formed by the first rib and and anterior and medial scalene muscles. It is at this point that the subclavian artery and vein rise from below and join the brachial plexus in its journey toward the axilla. As these neurovascular structures pass beyond the scalene triangle, they enter a rigid narrow space formed by the clavicle anterosuperiorly, and the first rib posteroinferiorly. Continuing toward the axilla, the neurovascular structures pass below the beak-like coracoid process. The insertion of the pectoralis minor to the tip of this process creates a narrow space between the muscle, the process, and the rib cage, through which the neurovascular

structures pass. Thus, in their journey from the region of the base of the neck to the axilla, they are subject to compression at three points: (See Figure 2-1.)

1. Supraclavicular—above the level of the clavicle, in the triangle formed by the first rib and the anterior and medial scalene muscles.

2. Costoclavicular—in the space between the clavicle and the first rib.

3. Infraclavicular—beneath the coracoid process, where they pass deep to the pectoralis minor's insertion to the coracoid process.

The Character of Neurovascular Symptoms

Compression of neural structures alone produces a characteristic pattern of symptoms. These are:

1. Paresthesias and dysesthesias (numbness, tingling, burning pain, spontaneously or in response to light touch),

2. along the distribution of the compressed neural structures,

3. without the edema or color change that would herald a vascular compression.

Vascular compression alone causes a

different characteristic pattern of symptoms:

1. Pain which is diffuse along the extremity and which does not have a nerve root distribution, and may be in the form of an ache or of a burning or pulsing pain, which is particularly felt in the fingertips.

2. Parts peripheral to the compression may become swollen,

3. and they may become cyanotic or pallid.

4. Peripheral artery pulsations may not be palpable.

Though the syndromes of neural and vascular compression are thus distinct from one another, the compression syndromes that are caused from pressures in the thoracic outlet are variable combinations of the two.

The Syndromes

Supraclavicular Compression

Characteristic features of supraclavicular compression are presumed to result from the effects of pressure upon neurons of the lower roots of the brachial plexus in one of four structural circumstances: (a) in passage over a protruding cervical rib, which is a rib-like enlargement from a transverse process of the 7th cervical vertebra; (b) in passage over a fibrous band, which extends from the transverse process of C_7 to the first rib; (c) in passage over the first rib through a narrowed scalene triangle (the scalenus anticus syndrome); (d) in passage over the first rib when traction upon the plexus and artery is augmented by an exaggerated shoulder droop.

While, for many years, reactive spasm of the scalenus anticus muscle has been considered to be a contributing factor, its etiologic reality has not been proven; and while symptoms often occur when a cervical rib or a fibrous band encroaches on the supraclavicular space, symptoms may also be present without such encroachment. Indeed, merely an excessive drooping of the shoulder, with the consequent traction upon the plexus and artery over the first rib, may be the sole cause of compression. An excessive drooping of the shoulder is seen as a developmental variant perhaps more often in young women than in young men, and is seen with the muscular wasting and lethargy of an unconditioned middle age or a catabolic illness. (While the syndrome of supraclavicular compression is usually more neural than vascular, there may be some compression of the subclavian artery. Again, this vascular compression is more common in those with the greater shoulder droop.)

The characteristic clinical features are:

1. Pain, paresthesias, and dysesthesias

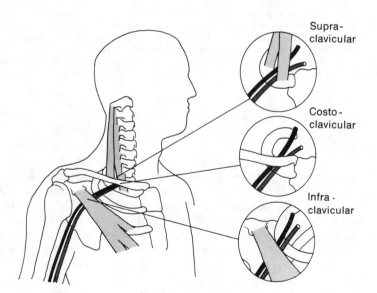

Fig. 2–1. Point of neurovascular compression in the thoracic outlet.

Supra-clavicular

Costo-clavicular

Infra-clavicular

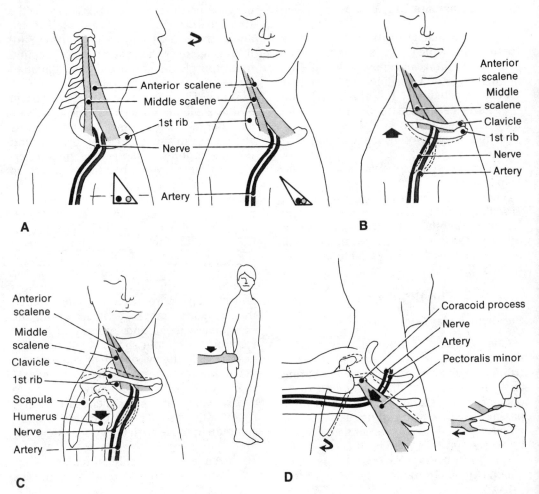

Fig. 2-2. Mechanisms of the Adson maneuvers. *A*, rotation of the head and neck toward the affected side compresses the neurovascular structures between the anterior and middle scalene muscles. *B*, a full inspiration elevates the first rib which thus stretches out the neurovascular structures and also further narrows their passage between the first rib and the middle and anterior scalene muscles. *C*, downward traction on the arm stretches out the neurovascular structures and also narrows their passage between the first rib and the clavicle. *D*, abduction and extension of the shoulder stretches out the neurovascular structures and retracts the scapula, thereby stretching the pectoralis minor tightly over the ribs, narrowing the neurovascular passage between the pectoralis minor and the ribs.

along the medial aspect of the arm, ulnar aspect of the forearm and hand, and into the little finger.

2. The Adson maneuvers may be positive. There are three Adson maneuvers: (See Figure 2-2, *A–D*.)

a. With the patient's chin rotated toward the affected side and elevated to hyperextend the neck, the patient is instructed to take a deep breath.

b. With the patient's chin rotated toward the affected side and elevated to hyperextend the neck, the examiner ap-

plies traction downward on the affected extremity.

c. With the patient's chin rotated toward the opposite side, and the affected shoulder abducted to 90°, the examiner extends the shoulder maximally.

The test maneuvers are diagnostic of the supraclavicular compression syndrome when any of the three provoke the typical pain and paresthesias of neural compression. The third maneuver may provoke the diagnostic symptoms in those suffering the hyperabduction syndrome as well (see be-

low). While these maneuvers may also obliterate the radial pulse, that finding is not
diagnostic as they will obliterate the pulse
in a good percentage of normal individuals.

Costoclavicular Compression

Characteristic features of costoclavicular compression result from compression
of the neurovascular structures as they
pass between the clavicle and the first rib.
This space may be narrowed by drooping
of the shoulder or by an abnormal config-
uration or elevation of the first rib. The
costoclavicular space is especially narrowed if the shoulders are forcibly pulled
downward and backward for prolonged
periods of time, as by a heavy pack, or the
postural intention of a soldier on parade.
Indeed, the onset of the syndrome may
very often be correlated with a prolonged
period of heavy backpacking, or heavy
weight lifting.

Unlike supraclavicular compression,
costoclavicular compression characteristically produces vascular symptoms before
neural symptoms. Patients with this disorder will usually complain of painful pulsations in the fingers, and their extremity
will appear pale or cyanotic. If neural
symptoms are present, patients will also
complain of pain, paresthesias, and dysesthesias along the medial aspect of the arm,
the ulnar aspect of the forearm, and the
little finger. These neural symptoms can
be increased by downward and backward
traction on the arm. (See Figure 2–2C.)

Infraclavicular Compression: (The Hyperabduction Syndrome)

Characteristic features of the hyperabduction syndrome result from compression of the neurovascular structures as
they pass between the pectoralis minor
and the rib cage, and from their sharp
angulation beneath the coracoid during
full hyperabduction and extension of the
shoulder. The syndrome usually emerges
in those who work for prolonged periods
with their arms stretched overhead, or
sleep in positions which hyperabduct one
or both shoulders. Presumably, these maneuvers apply the greatest stretch and
compression upon the medial cord of the
brachial plexus (constituted by neurons
from the lower roots), as paresthesias, dysesthesias, and neural pain tend once again
to be referred through the medial aspect of
the arm, the ulnar aspect of the forearm
and hand, into the little finger. Like supraclavicular compression, and unlike costoclavicular compression, infraclavicular
compression characteristically produces
neural symptoms before vascular. When
hyperabduction sufficiently compresses
the axillary artery as well as the plexus,
the patient will also complain of a generalized aching in the arm, and of burning
and painful pulsations in the fingers. The
examiner may gain further confidence in
the diagnosis when upon hyperabducting
and extending the shoulder, paresthesias
characteristic of neural compression result. (See Figure 2–2D.)

The Distinction of Thoracic Outlet from Other Shoulder-Arm Pain Syndromes

While we try to delineate the area of
compression between the base of the neck
and the axilla, whether supraclavicular,
costoclavicular, or infraclavicular, the essential clinical picture of the thoracic outlet syndrome is about the same: pain extending down the medial aspect of the arm
and forearm to the little finger, paresthesias and dysesthesias in the same region,
constant ache of the entire arm, burning
painful pulsations of the fingers, and pallor
or cyanosis. This syndrome when augmented by the manipulations described
above is quite distinct from the other
causes of shoulder-arm pain. No other syndromes produce neuritic pain of ulnar distribution, and only two other conditions
produce neuritic pain extending the length
of the arm: a rare form of brachial neuritis
which occasionally may be associated
with a clumping of vesicles suggestive of
herpes zoster, and the more common cervical disc syndrome.

As the novice may often confuse a cervical disc for a thoracic outlet syndrome
and vice versa, it must be particularly
stressed that the thoracic outlet syndrome
contrasts very distinctly from the syndrome caused by compression of nerve
roots due to cervical disc herniation. The

cervical disc syndrome usually involves the 5th, 6th, and 7th cervical nerve roots, and these nerve roots produce symptoms along the lateral aspect of the arm, the radiodorsal aspect of the forearm, into the thumb and index finger.

Causalgia and occlusions of the axillary and brachial artery and veins may be distinguished from vascular compression in the thoracic outlet by the persistence of their symptoms and signs regardless of posture and by the absence of brachial neuritic symptoms.

Treatment

Conservative management of the supraclavicular and costoclavicular variants of the thoracic outlet syndrome is identical. Specific exercises are prescribed to strengthen the muscles of the shoulder girdle, and prevent the sagging or droop of the shoulder which is supposed to bring on these symptoms. (See below.) If the symptoms have been brought on by backpacking or heavy carrying, or any other activity that produces downward traction on the shoulder, these activities should be modified to avoid such traction.

Individuals who suffer the hyperabduction syndrome, should be instructed to avoid positions of hyperabduction during sleep, and to minimize or avoid the position during work.

When the patient complies with treatment, improvement often follows within 1–2 months. When compliance does not yield benefit after such an interval, the patient may desire orthopaedic referral. The only absolute indication for orthopaedic referral is progressive weakness in the ulnar distribution.

Shoulder-Girdle Exercises for Thoracic Outlet Syndrome

The following exercise instructions are given to patients with the thoracic outlet syndrome by the Group Health Cooperative of Puget Sound Physical Therapy Department.

At the beginning, each exercise is done 10 times in succession twice a day. As the shoulders and neck gain strength, the number of times each exercise is done consecutively can be increased.

Exercises.

1. Stand erect with the arms at the sides holding in each hand a 2-pound weight (sandbags or bottles, jars or sacks filled with sand). (a) Shrug the shoulders forward and upward. (b) Relax. (c) Shrug the shoulders backward and upward. (d) Relax. (e) Shrug the shoulders upward. (f) Relax and repeat.

2. Stand erect with the arms out straight from the sides at shoulder level; hold a 2-pound weight in either hand (palms should be down). (a) Raise the arms sideways and up until the backs of the hands meet above the head (keep elbows straight). (b) Relax and repeat.

Note. As strength improves and exercises 1 and 2 become easier, then the weights should be made heavier, increasing to 5–10 pounds.

3. Stand facing a corner of the room with one hand on each wall, arms at shoulder level, palms forward, elbows bent, and abdominal muscles contracted. (a) Slowly let the upper part of the trunk lean forward and press the chest into the corner. Inhale as the body leans forward. (b) Return to the original position by pushing out with the hands. Exhale with this movement.

4. Stand erect with the arms at the sides. (a) Bend the neck to the left, attempting to touch the left ear to the left shoulder without shrugging the shoulder. (b) Bend the neck to the right, attempting to touch the right ear to the right shoulder without shrugging the shoulder. (c) Relax and repeat.

5. Lie face down with the hands clasped behind the back. (a) Raise the head and chest from the floor as high as possible while pulling the shoulders backward and the chin in. Hold this position for a count of three. Inhale as the chest is raised. (b) Exhale and lower the arms to the sides. (c) Repeat.

6. Lie down on the back with arms at the sides with a rolled towel or a small pillow under the upper part of the back between the shoulder blades and no pillow under the head. (a) Inhale slowly and raise the arms upward and backward overhead. (b) Exhale and lower the arms to the sides. (c) Repeat 5–20 times.

CHAPTER 3
The Shoulder

Essential Anatomy

The shoulder may be studied as a complex of four joints:

1. The scapulothoracic joint.
2. The glenohumeral joint, which is the joint usually referred to by the term "the shoulder joint," or "socket."
3. The acromioclavicular joint.
4. The sternoclavicular joint.

The Scapulothoracic Joint

The scapula is fixed to the thoracic rib cage by muscular attachments and a bony strut, the clavicle. The deep muscular attachments posteriorly spring from the cervical and thoracic spines, and insert upon the medial border and inferior angle of the scapula. These are: the levator scapulae, the rhomboides minor, and rhomboides major, inserting onto the upper, middle, and inferior thirds respectively of the posterior surface of the medial margin of the scapula. A larger muscle, the serratus anterior, is attached anteriorly to the upper eight to nine ribs and circles around the thorax posteriorly to be attached to the anterior surface of the medial margin and inferior angle of the scapula. The greatest bulk of the serratus anterior attaches to the inferior angle. Superficial to these muscles posteriorly, the triangular trapezius muscle arises from the spinous processes of the cervical and thoracic spine, to insert into the spine and acromion of the scapula. The latissimus dorsi, arising from the lower half of the vertebral spine and iliac crest, and inserting on the anterior aspect of the upper third of the humerus, while it bridges the scapula without regular attachment to it, nonetheless exerts strong control over the scapula.

Anteriorly, the scapula is controlled by the pectoralis major—though it also bridges the scapula—and the pectoralis minor, which inserts upon the coracoid process of the scapula.

These muscles control the stability and effect the six movements of the scapula. The movements and their prime controllers are the following (see figure 3–1):

Elevation. Trapezius, levator scapulae, rhomboidei major and minor.

Depression. Latissimus dorsi, pectoralis major.

Upward rotation. Serratus anterior, trapezius.

Downward rotation. Levator scapulae, rhomboidei major and minor, pectoralis minor.

Protraction. Serratus anterior, pectoralis minor, pectoralis major.

Retraction. Trapezius, rhomboidei major and minor.

The bony anchor of the scapula to the thoracic cage is the clavicle, which articulates laterally with the acromion at the acromioclavicular joint, and medially with the sternum at the sternoclavicular joint.

The clavicle is shaped like half a bow, convex to the front medially, and concave to the front laterally.

The Glenohumeral Joint

The glenohumeral joint is a very mobile joint and, unlike the acetabulum or socket of the hip joint which is quite deep and

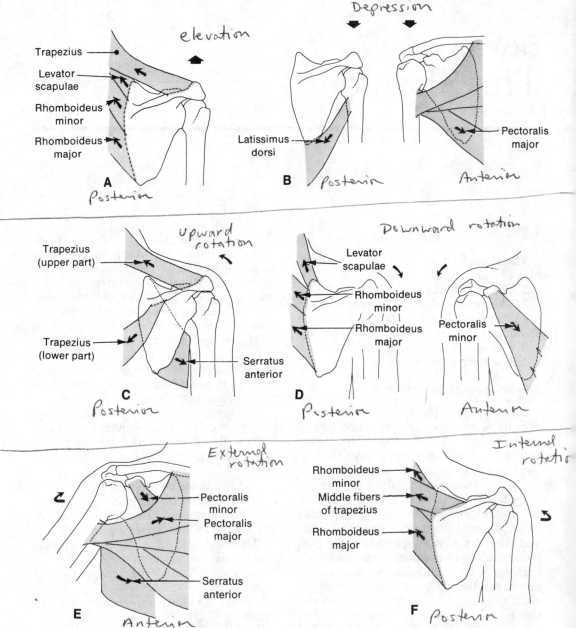

Fig. 3–1. The motions of the shoulder girdle. *A*, elevation, posterior view. *B*, depression. *Left*, posterior view. *Right*, anterior view. *C*, upward rotation, posterior view. *D*, downward rotation. *Left*, posterior view. *Right*, anterior view. *E*, protraction, anterior view. *F*, retraction, posterior view.

cup-shaped, the socket of the shoulder joint is more or less flat with a mildly concave surface. This surface articulates with the spherical head of the humerus. The glenohumeral joint depends considerably on the strength and integrity of the ligaments and surrounding muscles for its stability. Surrounding the capsule of the shoulder joint are four important tendons: the supraspinatus along the superior aspect of the capsule of the shoulder joint, the infraspinatus and teres minor along the posterior aspect of the capsule of the shoulder joint, and the subscapularis along the anterior aspect of the capsule of the shoulder joint. (See Figure 3–2.) The supraspinatus muscle arises from the supraspin-

ous fossa of the scapula, and passes underneath the acromion along the superior aspect of the capsule of the shoulder joint, to be inserted into the superior facet of the greater tubercle of the humerus, which is located just lateral and distal to the spherical head of the humerus. The infraspinatus arises from the infraspinous fossa and passes along the posterior aspect of the capsule of the shoulder joint, and is inserted into the middle facet of the greater tubercle of the humerus. The teres minor arises from the lateral margin of the scapula, and is inserted into the inferior facet of the greater tubercle of the humerus. The subscapularis arises anteriorly from the subscapular fossa of the scapula and

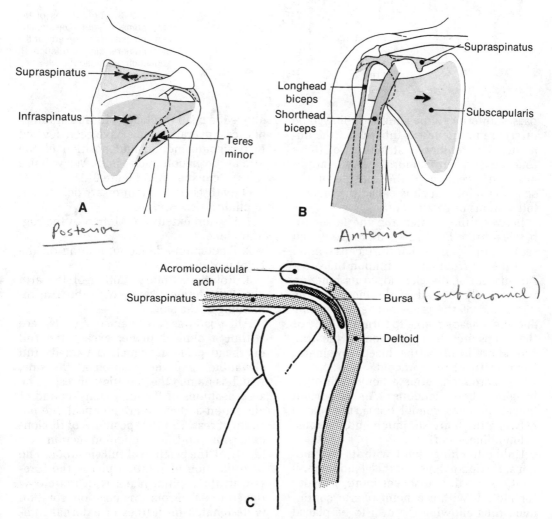

Fig. 3–2. *A* and *B*, the myotendinous cuff. *A*, posterior view; *B*, anterior view. *C*, the subacromial bursa.

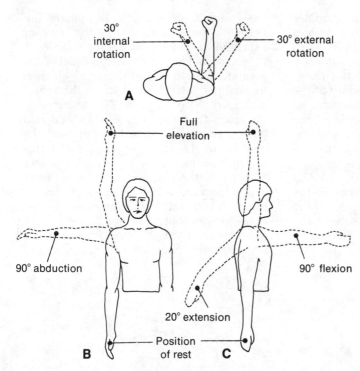

Fig. 3–3. The motions of the glenohumeral joint. Designating motion positions of the arm at the glenohumeral joint. *A*, rotation. *B*, abduction/adduction. *C*, flexion/extension.

passes anterior to the shoulder joint, to be inserted into the lesser tubercle of the humerus. The tendinous structures of these four muscles form a more or less continuous reinforcement to the capsule of the shoulder joint, which is called the musculotendinous or rotator cuff.

Between the greater and the lesser tubercles of the humerus is a groove which receives the long head of the biceps tendon as it passes from its origin upon the superior margin of the glenoid, to its junction with the short head of the biceps at the distal end of the groove. There, the long and short heads merge to form the belly of the biceps muscle on the front of the arm. The short head of the biceps originates from the tip of the coracoid.

The acromion forms a bony arch overhanging these tendons. An important bursa, the subacromial bursa, is situated between the bony acromion and the musculotendinous cuff.

Unlike the hinge joint with its two motions, flexion-extension, the glenohumeral joint, as a ball-and-socket joint, provides for motion within a hemispheric continuum, thus allowing the arm to be placed above the head through an infinite number of arcs. Several systems have been devised to designate motion and position of the arm at the glenohumeral joint. We will use the system shown in Figure 3–3.

Only three arcs of motion are designated in clinical description:

1. Flexion-extension. Motion in the sagittal plane.

2. Abduction-adduction. Motion on the frontal plane.

3. Rotation. Rotary motion of the arm about the humeral axis, with the arm remaining at the side.

All positions are named by degrees within a clinical plane, except the full overhead position, which is named "full elevation," and the position at the side, which is named the "position of rest." The zero positions of flexion-extension and of abduction-adduction are identical, the position of rest. The 180° positions of flexion-extension and abduction-adduction are identical, the position of full elevation. The zero position of rotation places the forearm in the sagittal plane with the elbow flexed to 90°. From this position, rotation is designated in degrees of external rotation as the forearm is directed away from the body and in degrees of internal rotation as the forearm is directed across the body.

The term *hyperabduction* refers to abduction beyond 90°.

The Acromioclavicular Joint (See Figure 3–4)

The lateral end of the clavicle articulates with the medial articular facet of the acromion to form the acromioclavicular joint. The capsule of the acromioclavicular joint is reinforced by a superior and inferior acromioclavicular ligament. The superior acromioclavicular ligament is stronger than the inferior acromioclavicular ligament. A fibrocartilagenous disc is contained within the acromioclavicular joint. Perhaps the ligament most important to the stability of the acromioclavicular joint is the coracoclavicular ligament, which consists of two tough fasciculae which stretch between the coracoid process and the undersurface of the clavicle.

The Sternoclavicular Joint (See Figure 3–5)

The medial end of the clavicle articulates with the sternum to form the sternoclavicular joint. There are quite a few similarities between the sternoclavicular joint and the acromioclavicular joint. A capsular ligament surrounds the joint between the articular surface on the medial end of the clavicle, and the articular surface on the manubrium sterni. This capsule is rein-

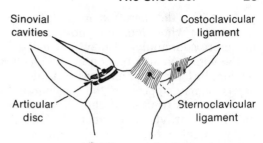

Fig. 3–5. The sternoclavicular joint: its synovial cavities, disc, and ligaments.

forced by anterior and posterior sternoclavicular ligaments. An intra-articular fibrocartilagenous disc lies within this joint, similar to the intra-articular fibrocartilagenous disc in the acromioclavicular joint. The upper margin of this disc is attached to the superior and posterior aspect of the clavicle, and its lower margin is attached to the margin of the first rib at its junction with the sternum. It divides the sternoclavicular joint into two compartments. As in the acromioclavicular joint, there is a strong extra-articular ligament, the costoclavicular ligament, which stretches from the medial end of the clavicle to the first rib and is responsible for the stability of the sternoclavicular joint. The importance of this ligament to the sternoclavicular joint is similar to that of the coracoclavicular ligament to the acromioclavicular joint.

Degenerative and Traumatic Disorders of the Shoulder

The disorders of the shoulder affect the musculotendinous structures, the bony structures, and the acromioclavicular, sternoclavicular, and glenohumeral joints and their ligaments.

Musculotendinous (Rotator) Cuff Pain Syndrome

With advancing age, degenerative changes are known to occur in the musculotendinous cuff. There is constant friction between the musculotendinous cuff and the undersurface of the acromion, particularly during abduction movements. People who have to use their arms overhead are particularly prone to such degen-

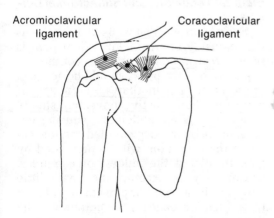

Fig. 3–4. Ligaments of the acromioclavicular joint.

eration. The degeneration may diffusely involve the whole musculotendinous cuff, or—more commonly—it may be localized in the supraspinatus tendon or the biceps tendon. Inflammatory changes and calcific deposits may appear in the degenerated tendons. This process of chronic attrition may lead to fraying and eventually to partial or complete tearing of the tendons.

Supraspinatus Tendinitis. The patient is usually middle-aged, with subacute or chronic symptoms of pain in the shoulder. The history usually suggests a course of periodic remissions and exacerbations, and a history of trauma, usually relatively minor, may be elicited. Characteristic clinical features are the following:

1. Pain usually centers in the shoulder, but may be referred to the insertion of the deltoid on the outer aspect of the arm. The more intense or prolonged the pain, the more likely is the entire arm to ache and develop paresthesias.

2. Tenderness may be elicited on the top of the shoulder just distal to the acromion, in the sector of the supraspinatus tendon.

3. Abduction movements up to 80° may be possible with minimal pain, but further abduction between 80° and 120° is painfully inhibited.

4. In advanced cases, abduction may be impossible beyond 45°.

5. X-rays of the shoulder may show sclerosis or cystic changes in the greater tubercle, erosion of the undersurface of the acromion, calcific deposits along the course of the supraspinatus tendon, or a perfectly normal shoulder.

Bicipital Tendinitis. Bicipital tendinitis emerges from a similar process of degeneration along the anterior aspect of the musculotendinous cuff and the adjacent long head of the biceps tendon.

Characteristic clinical features are the following:

1. Pain is felt in the anterior aspect of the shoulder and may be referred along the front of the arm. The more intense or prolonged the pain, the more likely is the entire arm to ache and develop paresthesias.

2. Tenderness may be elicited over the long head of the biceps and the bicipital groove, and the thickened biceps tendon may be rolled underneath the examining finger—a maneuver which provokes severe pain.

3. Flexion will be quite painful with the elbow extended and the forearm supinated and less painful with the elbow flexed and the forearm pronated.

4. Rotational movements are restricted by pain.

5. With the forearm in supination, flexion of the elbow against resistance causes pain in the anterior aspect of the shoulder.

6. X-rays of the shoulder may show calcific deposits along the course of the bicipital tendon, or nothing abnormal at all.

Subacromial Bursitis. Perhaps the most acute and intensely painful degenerative disorder of the shoulder is an inflammation of the subacromial bursa. In our experience it is the least common of the musculotendinous cuff disorders. This usually accompanies other degenerative changes in the shoulder, and the patient often admits to repeated or long-standing symptoms of tendinitis of the shoulder.

Characteristic clinical features are the following:

1. The onset is acute.

2. Pain in the shoulder is severe.

3. Any movement of the shoulder increases the pain.

4. The shoulder is diffusely tender.

5. Redness and edema of the skin and swelling of the shoulder are often distinct.

6. The body temperature may be elevated, and the erythrocyte sedimentation rate increased.

Treatment of Supraspinatus Tendinitis, Bicipital Tendinitis, and Subacromial Bursitis.

Exercise. (See Figure 3–6.) Exercise is the mainstay of treatment. When pain is severe, rest in a sling and the continuous application of ice packs should be advised, but as early as pain allows, in a matter of days if not hours, active movement should be started. While abduction, causing impingement of the degenerated tendon beneath the acromion, will be prevented by pain in all but the mildest of examples, flexion may be accomplished with little pain as it avoids impingement of the frayed tendon beneath the acromion. The "gravity assisted" pendulum exercise is

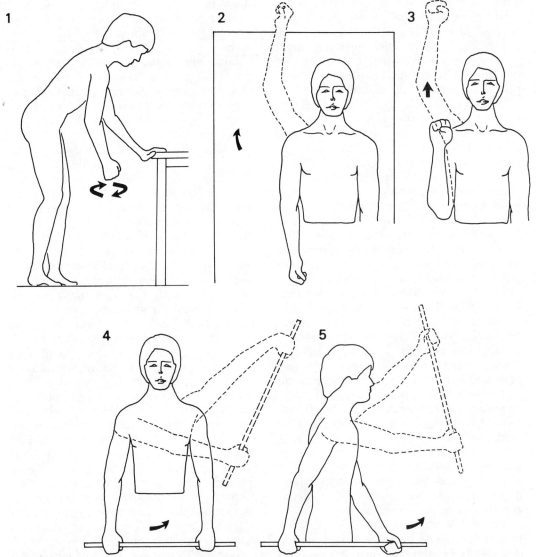

Fig. 3–6. Exercises for rehabilitation of the shoulder. *1*, gravity-assisted pendulum exercise. *2*, hyperabduction, patient supine. *3*, hyperabduction, patient standing. *4*, hyperabduction with rod assistance. *5*, hyperflextion with rod assistance.

the easiest form of active movement and can usually be performed very early in the course of the disorders. As pain allows, the exercise program should progress as follows: The arc of the pendulum swing should increase until the arm is nearly horizontal; then, standing flexion to full elevation, if necessary with the gentle assistance of a pulley or a rod; then, supine and finally standing abduction to full elevation should be attempted. With the elbow flexed, as it is when vertically pressing a weight, the moment-arm resisting flexion or abduction is less and the strain on the musculotendinous cuff is proportionally less. We advise that the unassisted standing exercise be performed with the arm in this attitude.

Therapeutic exercise always runs the course between the Scylla of overzealous efforts to restore motion and the Charybdis of overgentle protection from pain. Either error can result in a frozen shoulder. The tactful physical therapist is most capable of guiding the patient through the safe course. When pain is severely immobilizing, or when less painful examples do not improve after 2 weeks encouragement to abide by the therapeutic regimen, we recommend that a tactful physical therapist be employed, if available.

Drugs. Anti-inflammatory medication may be used and the regimen chosen depends upon the preference of the practitioner. We like to begin with aspirin or sodium salicylate 10-15 grains four times daily. Tinnitus-inducing doses are not necessary, and we advise a decrease in dose when patients complain of tinnitus. When aspirin has failed to give benefit after 1 to 2 weeks' trial, we may employ phenylbutazone 100 mg. two or three times daily for 2-3 weeks, or indomethacin 25 mg. two or three times daily for 2-3 weeks. When aspirin is contraindicated, we do not substitute phenylbutazone or indomethacin. Prednisolone 0.3 mg./kg./day or dexamethasone 0.04 mg./kg./day for 1 week is usually safe and can be quite helpful in the acute stage. We sometimes use it when pain and immobility are very severe and when the other drugs are contraindicated. The dangers of these drugs are briefly reviewed in Chapter 19 on Arthritis. The reader is also referred to Robert L. Roe, "The Anti-Inflammatory Agents Used in Rheumatic Disorders," *Primary Care*, Vol. 2, No. 2, June 1975, pp. 259-273. Many physicians use higher doses of these drugs and for longer duration than we.

Physical Modalities. When pain is severe, when signs of acute inflammation are visible, and following corticosteroid injections, cold applications should be prescribed. Heat application may be prescribed after the initial severity of pain lessens, and any physical signs of inflammation have disappeared. Heat application may be of any kind, but moist heat or heat after application of a liniment has seemed to us to be more comforting. Some individuals discover that heat increases their pain, and for these, we recommend that ice be continued. Some individuals discover that liniment alone is comforting. If physical therapy facilities are available, ultrasound or the use of diathermy may be helpful, although we believe that in most cases they are not superior to the application of moist heat or ice. Heat or cold should be applied for 15-20 minutes four to six times daily.   *Lidocaine also*

Local Injections. Any corticosteroid prepared for intra-articular use may be injected into the tender area. Rapid relief of symptoms often follows. With the patient sitting, we identify the tender area and inject 1 cc. of corticosteroid directly into that area. We habitually use Depo-Medrol 40 mg. or 80 mg./cc. or Kenalog 10 mg. or 20 mg./cc., but any intra-articular corticosteroid is acceptable. Some physicians suspect that calcium deposits in degenerated tendons perpetuate the painful process and that injection into these deposits facilitates diffusion of the calcium out of the tendon and thereby yields more lasting remission. Repeated injections should be avoided, as, with time, they have deleterious effects on the structures receiving the injection. It has been our practice to restrict injections of corticosteroids to trimonthly intervals, so that a patient does not get more than four local injections of corticosteroids a year. We prefer local corticosteroids to systemic corticosteroids, phenylbutazone, and indomethacin, and we employ the injection rather than the oral drugs in every case unless the patient refuses, or the quarterly or yearly limit would be exceeded, or the pain at rest is intense. When pain at rest is intense, we employ all the other treatment modes first, and sometimes follow with an injection at a later, more comfortable but tenacious stage of convalescence.

Surgical Treatment. The various painful syndromes of the myotendinous cuff may be disablingly recurrent or persistent. For some individuals who are subject to frequent recurrences, therapeutic exercises must be continued indefinitely, and when 2-3 months of compliance with therapy have failed to yield a remission from a particular episode, the patient may have to be referred to a surgeon. Partial acromionectomy, excision of the acromioclavicular joint, or excision of the coraco-acromial ligament, all have their advocates, and are all intended to prevent impingement.

Tendinious (Rotator) Cuff Syndrome.

The primary care physician often serves patients with tendinous cuff pain which does not clearly fit any of the three entities described above. There are no visible signs of inflammation as one would expect with a subacromial bursitis; the supraspinatus and bicipital tendons are not uniquely tender; and the bicipital tendon is not thickened. Often, tenderness will be elicited anteriorly or posteriorly only after maximum external or internal rotation respectively. Occasionally, the entire tendinous arc, or more than one point on the tendinous arc, will be tender. As in the three more specific entities, patients who present these findings may also complain bitterly of pain and may show great reduction in their range of motion. Treatment is identical to that for the specific entities, except that the location of any corticosteroid injection will, of course, be different. We do not employ injections when tenderness is diffuse. Once again, specific exercises are the foundation of treatment.

Except in the face of visible signs of inflammation, as are characteristic of subacromial bursitis, some physicians doubt the accuracy of the inflammation thesis and wonder whether pain syndromes in the region of the tendinous cuff (or, indeed, in any musculotendinous structure) could represent a less generally recognized pain process than inflammation. They will apply the term tendinous cuff syndrome, rather than tendinitis or bursitis, to any episode of tendinous cuff pain not accompanied by visible signs of inflammation, or by a tender and thickened bicipital tendon. (See also the discussion of myofascial pain syndrome in Chapter 19.)

Musculotendinous (Rotator) Cuff Tear.
(See Figure 3–7.) While a tear of the musculotendinous cuff may occur as a primary process, secondary to major trauma in young individuals who may not have had previous symptoms referable to the shoulder, major trauma is not required for a tear of the musculotendinous cuff. A fall on the outstretched arm or repetitive ordinary strain may apply enough force to the tendinous cuff to produce a rupture of the tendinous fibers if there are pre-existing degenerative changes. The patient may describe a history of supraspinatus tendinitis

or bicipital tendinitis, or chronic shoulder pain with exacerbations or remissions over the years. Their visit may be preceded by a sudden fall which produces an increase in the severity of pain and a new weakness of abduction of the shoulder.

The characteristic clinical features are the following:

1. Pain in the shoulder and tenderness, usually over the middle third of the musculotendinous cuff (supraspinatus tendon).

2. In the case of massive tears, an inability to abduct the shoulder, and in the case of minor tears, weak and incomplete abduction accompanied by pain.

3. Palpable crepitation during passive or active abduction movements of the shoulder.

4. In massive tears, and particularly in thin patients, a palpable cleft on the superior aspect of the shoulder, just distal to the acromion.

5. Painless or tolerable passive abduction beyond the range of active abduction. This is a classic sign of musculotendinous cuff tear and may be expected when weakness is more troublesome than pain.

6. Noticeable atrophy of the supraspinatus or the infraspinatus muscles after symptoms have been present for some time.

7. A characteristically abnormal arthrogram. Arthrography of the shoulder may reveal a full thickness tear when the dye escapes from the shoulder joint superiorly into the subacromial region.

Treatment of the Musculotendinous Cuff Tear.
There is still some controversy about the treatment of rotator cuff tears.

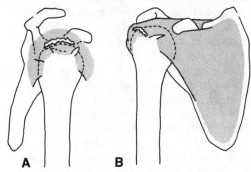

A **B**

Fig. 3–7. Myotendinous cuff tear. *A*, lateral; *B*, anterolateral.

Judgment must be exercised in selecting patients for surgical treatment. Incomplete tears in any individual who has very little restriction of abduction and only slight weakness, and full thickness partial tears in middle-aged individuals who are not athletically inclined, may respond quite satisfactorily to conservative measures of treatment. Even massive tears in the very elderly should have a trial of conservative treatment.

The conservative method of treatment is similar to the treatment discussed for the other painful musculotendinous cuff degenerations:

1. Exercise. The patient should be instructed in exercises of the shoulder. Whether or not and in what form active exercise should be employed early in convalescence is debated. It is perhaps safest to rely on passive and on gravity-assisted active exercises only, during the first 6 weeks of convalescence. During the 7th week, active supine abduction can usually begin and advance to active standing flexion. Perhaps active abduction should not be attempted at all. The services of a tactful physical therapist should be employed whenever possible.

2. Drugs. Anti-inflammatory medications can be helpful when the pain is severe, or signs of inflammation are visible.

3. Physical Modalities. Heat application to the shoulder for 15–20 minutes in the form of moist heat, four to six times daily, may help in the reparative process, but cold is usually preferable when pain is severe or signs of inflammation are visible.

4. Local Injections. Injection of Lidocaine and its analogs into this region may decrease the pain and allow the patient to carry out the exercise program diligently. When a diagnosis of tendinous cuff tear has been made, we prefer not to inject corticosteroids locally.

5. Surgical Treatment. Surgical treatment is indicated when a full thickness tear of the rotator cuff is suspected in a young adult, and when conservative measures were indicated and have been encouraged diligently without benefit for 8 weeks. Surgical treatment is varied and includes repair of the musculotendinous cuff, partial acromionectomy, and excision of the acromioclavicular joint.

Acromioclavicular Joint Pain Syndromes

The Acute Acromioclavicular Joint Pain Syndrome. Internal derangement of the acromioclavicular joint may occur in young athletes, particularly those who employ overhand actions as do baseball pitchers and tennis players. These individuals possibly suffer an injury to the fibrocartilagenous disc in the acromioclavicular joint. Characteristic clinical features are the following:

1. Pain is felt in the shoulder and may sometimes be referred down the arm.

2. Abduction beyond 90° causes pain, hence overhand actions are inhibited.

3. Fullness or swelling may be evident over the acromioclavicular joint, and tenderness is localized to the acromioclavicular joint.

4. When the patient is advised to protract the arm and shoulder forward across the body, pain is referred to the acromioclavicular joint. (See Figure 3–8.)

5. When the patient holds both upper extremities across the chest, with the right hand over the left shoulder, and the left hand over the right shoulder, and the elbow by the side of the body, if the examiner simultaneously stabilizes the clavicle and abruptly forces the elbow upward, pain will be felt in the acromioclavicular joint. (See Figure 3–8.)

6. X-rays of the acromioclavicular joint may show a widening of the joint space, some irregularity or cystic changes of the articular ends of the bone, or radiographically normal structures.

Treatment of the Acute Acromioclavicular Joint Pain Syndrome.

Exercise. If the symptoms are particularly severe, the young patient must be advised to avoid athletic activities which require overhand actions, until symptoms abate.

Physical Modalities. Heat or ice application to the acromioclavicular joint may afford some pain relief.

Drugs and Local Injections. Anti-inflammatory drugs or corticosteroid injection into the acromioclavicular joint may give dramatic relief, particularly when there is visible evidence of inflammation.

Surgical Treatment. If symptoms are persistent, the patient may require referral

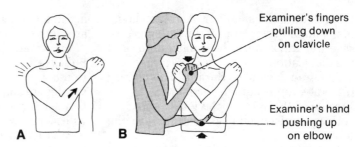

Examiner's fingers pulling down on clavicle

Examiner's hand pushing up on elbow

Fig. 3-8. Tests for acromioclavicular pain.

A

B

to an orthopaedist, but rarely will surgical treatment be necessary. Excision of the outer end of the clavicle may be the surgical treatment of choice.

Acromioclavicular Joint Arthritis. In people of older age, arthritic changes may occur in the acromioclavicular joint, and result in symptoms similar to those of the acute acromioclavicular pain syndrome.

Characteristic clinical features are the following:

1. Pain is felt in the shoulder, particularly during hyperabduction of the shoulder beyond 90°.

2. Swelling may be evident over the acromioclavicular joint, and an irregularity of the articular ends of the clavicle and acromion, suggestive of bony spurs, may be palpable.

3. Tenderness may be well localized to the acromioclavicular joint.

4. The tests for acromioclavicular joint pain mentioned above will usually elicit pain.

5. X-ray will show degenerative changes about the acromioclavicular joint.

Treatment of Acromioclavicular Joint Arthritis.

1. Exercise. Hyperabduction movements and the use of the arm overhead should be avoided.

2. Physical Modalities. Heat should be applied to the acromioclavicular joint for 20 minutes four to six times daily, until pain remits.

3. Drugs and Local Injections. Anti-inflammatory medications or injection of corticosteroid into the acromioclavicular joint may give dramatic relief, particularly when there is visible evidence of inflammation.

4. Surgical Treatment. If symptoms are persistent, the patient may require referral to an orthopaedist for consideration of surgical treatment. Excision of the outer end of the clavicle may be the surgical treatment of choice.

Fractures of the Clavicle and Injuries of Its Joints

Fractures of the clavicle can occur at the sternal or medial end of the clavicle, through the lateral or acromial end of the clavicle, and through the middle third of the clavicle at the junction of the convex medial half and the concave lateral half, where it appears as though the bone twists on itself as it changes direction. Fractures of the acromial and sternal thirds are sustained by great forces applied directly to the fracture points—forces identical to those that dislocate the acromioclavicular and sternoclavicular joints. Forces of such violence are most likely to be encountered by adolescents and young adults. The medial epiphysis at the sternal end of the clavicle appears at about the 18th year, and does not usually fuse with the shaft until about the 25th year. Hence, forces injuring the sternal third of the clavicle prior to the 25th year may produce epiphyseal separation rather than the metaphyseal fracture, which they will produce in later years. The epiphyseal separation is very likely to be mistaken for a sternoclavicular dislocation. As the mechanism of injury and the evaluation of fractures of the acromial and sternal thirds of the clavicle are very similar to those of dislocations of the associated joints, discussion of these fractures is deferred to the discussion of the injuries to the associated joints.

Injuries to the Acromial End of the Clavicle. Acromioclavicular joint injuries are usually suffered by the young and by middle-aged adults who participate in athletics. The injuries usually result from a direct fall onto the shoulder. Acromioclavicular joint injuries are of three degrees of severity: the sprain, the subluxation, and the dislocation.

Acromioclavicular Sprain. This injury probably represents a partial tear of the capsule of the acromioclavicular joint.

Characteristic clinical features are the following:

1. A young or middle-aged individual has suffered a severe trauma to the shoulder.

2. The acromioclavicular joint is tender and may be slightly swollen.

3. Attempted abduction of the shoulder beyond 60° causes pain.

4. X-rays obtained with the patient standing and holding 10-pound weights in either hand will show a normal acromioclavicular joint.

Treatment of the Acromioclavicular Sprain.

1. Exercise. Initially, the patient should have his arm splinted in a sling. Early movements should be started as soon as the pain has disappeared, but hyperabduction should be avoided for 3 weeks, and heavy lifting should be avoided for at least 6 weeks.

2. Physical Modalities. Ice packs to the acromioclavicular joint may decrease pain during the acute stage. Moist heat may give comfort during later convalescence.

Acromioclavicular Subluxation. (See Figure 3–9.) This injury represents a complete tear of the capsule of the acromioclavicular joint, particularly through the superior acromioclavicular ligament.

Characteristic clinical features are the following:

1. A young or middle-aged individual has suffered a severe trauma to the shoulder.

2. The acromioclavicular joint is markedly tender and swollen.

3. The outer end of the clavicle may protrude slightly upward.

4. Attempted abduction of the shoulder beyond 60° provokes pain.

5. X-rays obtained with the patient standing may show a normal acromioclavicular joint, while x-rays obtained with the patient holding 10-pound weights in either hand may show a widening of the acromioclavicular joint on the injured side as compared to the normal.

Treatment of the Acromioclavicular Subluxation. Acromioclavicular subluxation is treated similarly to the acromioclavicular sprain, though the shoulder may be painful for a longer period, and the convalescence will be likewise extended. Hyperabduction of the shoulder beyond 90° should not be permitted for at least 3–4 weeks, and the patient should avoid heavy lifting for at least 2 months. The functional result will be quite satisfactory, though there may be a permanent prominence of the outer end of the clavicle.

Acromioclavicular Dislocation. (See Figure 3–9.) This injury represents not only a tearing of the acromioclavicular joint ligaments, but also a tearing of the important coracoclavicular ligaments. These disruptions permit the sternomastoid to pull the clavicle upward, while the weight of the extremity pulls the shoulder downward.

Characteristic clinical features are the following:

1. A young or middle-aged individual has suffered a severe trauma to the shoulder.

2. The acromioclavicular joint is markedly tender and swollen, and may be ecchymotic.

3. The outer end of the clavicle will usually be projecting superiorly.

4. Any movement of the shoulder beyond a few degrees usually causes pain in the acromioclavicular joint, but some patients may be able to abduct the shoulder up to 60° without complaints.

5. X-rays obtained with the patient in the standing position will show the superior displacement of the clavicle, the dislocation of the acromioclavicular joint, and an increase in space between the coracoid process and the undersurface of the clavicle, as compared to the normal shoulder.

Treatment of Acromioclavicular Dislocation. There is quite a difference of opinion regarding treatment of acromioclavicular dislocation because functional results seem to vary, regardless of what is done. The surest way that a displaced clavicle can be realigned to the acromion successfully, and maintained in that position is by

Acromioclavicular ligament

Coracoclavicuar ligament

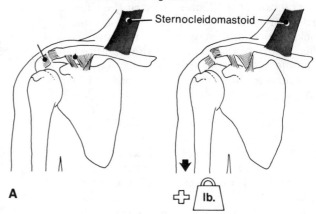

Sternocleidomastoid

A

Sternocleidomastoid

lb.

Acromioclavicular ligament

Coracoclavicular ligament

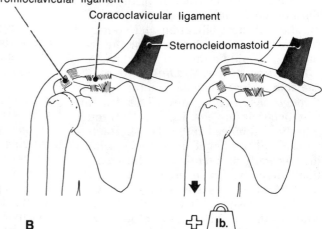

Sternocleidomastoid

Fig. 3–9. Acromioclavicular
joint injuries. *A*, acromioclavicular
subluxation. *B*, acromioclavicular
dislocation.

B

Sternocleidomastoid

lb.

internal fixation of the acromioclavicular joint with any fixation device preferred by the surgeon. On the other hand, it is our belief that functional results are just as satisfactory just as often with non-surgical methods of external bracing, or indeed with no bracing at all but merely with a sling for comfort. Occasionally anatomic healing will be achieved by external bracing.

There are different acromioclavicular braces, the purpose of which is to depress the superiorly displaced clavicle with the arm held in a sling. They may partially reduce the dislocation of the joint and facilitate healing compatible with comfortable participation in all but the most vigorous shoulder activities. The acromioclavicular brace that we use is illustrated in

Figure 3–10. Appropriate padding should be applied underneath the straps to prevent skin irritation. The brace should be tightened periodically, perhaps at weekly intervals, and the patient should be checked repeatedly for skin complications. The immobilization should be continued for a period of 6 weeks, after which the arm should be held in a sling, but removed three or four times daily for active gravity-assisted exercises of the shoulder. The sling may be discontinued after 8–9 weeks.

In our opinion, surgical treatment by open reduction and internal fixation of the acromioclavicular joint is absolutely indicated only for those concerned about the cosmetic result.

For all other patients, conservative methods of treatment should give satisfactory results as often as do surgical methods.

Fracture of the Outer Third of the Clavicle. Forces that can dislocate the acromioclavicular joint may instead fracture the outer third of the clavicle. If the fracture is complete, the outer third usually remains attached to the acromion and coracoid by the acromioclavicular and coracoclavicular ligaments, and the medial two-thirds are pulled upward by the sternomastoid. The acromioclavicular joint is often sprained and may be subluxed, but is rarely dislocated when a fracture occurs.

Treatment of Fracture of the Outer Third of the Clavicle. Treatment employs the acromioclavicular brace, as modified for reduction of the fracture of the middle third of the clavicle. (See Figure 3–13.) The duration of immobilization and course of rehabilitation are as advised for the fracture of the middle third of the clavicle.

Fractures of the Middle Third of the Clavicle. Most clavicle fractures occur through the middle third. This fracture may occur at any age, from birth through senility, and indeed is the clavicle fracture occasionally inflicted upon the newborn, inadvertently or intentionally during a difficult delivery. However, this fracture is most likely to be sustained by a growing child as a result of a fall upon the outstretched hand. When the fracture is complete, the medial or proximal fragment of the fractured clavicle is displaced upward, due to the pull of the sternomastoid muscle, and the lateral or distal fragment is displaced downward and anteriorly by the weight of the arm. (See Figure 3–11.)

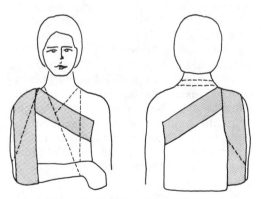

Fig. 3–10. Acromioclavicular brace.

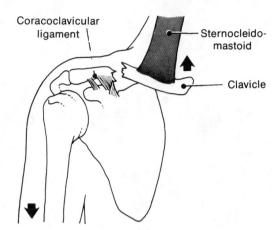

Fig. 3–11. Complete fracture of the middle third of the clavicle.

Neurovascular injury, though it may occur, is fortunately not common in fractures of the middle third of the clavicle. There is a higher incidence of vascular injury in fractures of the sternal end of the clavicle, particularly when this injury is combined with a fracture of the first rib. As a matter of fact, all the vascular injuries accompanying the fractures of the clavicle that we have seen have accompanied fractures of the sternal end of the clavicle. However, gross displacement of fractures of the middle third of the clavicle may cause neurovascular injury. Hence, those complications must always be looked for.

Pressure on the cords of the brachial plexus may cause paresthesia and dysaesthesia along cord distribution in the upper extremity, and pressure on the vascular structures will cause the usual symptoms and signs of vascular insufficiency. These are:

1. Disappearance of the radial and ulnar pulses.

2. Edema and swelling of the fingers.

3. Inadequate capillary return to allow brisk suffusion of nailbeds after blanching of nailbeds on pressure.

4. Diffuse aching over the extremity.

5. Burning pulsing pain at the tips of the fingers.

Treatment of Fractures of the Middle Third of the Clavicle. The figure-of-eight splintage, as shown in Figure 3–12, is the traditional method of treatment of frac-

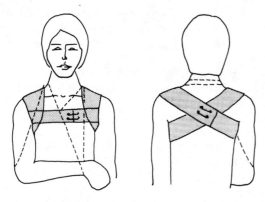

Fig. 3–12. Figure-of-eight splint for fractures of the middle third of the clavicle.

tures of the clavicle. The therapeutic intention is to pull the lateral distal fragment upward and posteriorly to align it with the medial fragment, which is displaced superiorly. A few refinements in the application of the figure-of-eight splintage may insure better reduction of the fracture. A thick pad in the axilla on the affected side may help to elevate the lateral fragment more effectively; the tendency of the loop of the figure-of-eight bandage over the shoulder to displace laterally can be prevented by tying the two shoulder loops to each other, as shown in Figure 3–12; the additional suspension of the extremity in a short sling may facilitate elevation of the outer fragment of the shoulder. A commercially obtainable clavicular brace may serve the same purpose as the figure-of-eight bandage, but should be modified as mentioned above. We personally do not believe that the figure-of-eight splintage, even with the suggested refinements, does very much to correct the displacement, and we have found that a modification of the acromioclavicular brace, diagrammed in Figure 3–13, has provided a more satisfactory correction.

However, while apposition necessary for healing is usually secured by one of these methods, accurate anatomic repositioning of the fragments is seldom obtained by either. Fortunately, it is not necessary to secure anatomic reduction in most cases, as moderately displaced and uncomplicated fractures of the clavicle generally tend to heal with full restoration

of shoulder function, and with a cosmetic deformity that is acceptable to the patient. Indeed, in children and younger adolescents, remodelling of the growing bone will often completely correct a rather marked deformity within 1–2 years. Older adolescents and adults must be apprised of the degree of deformity expected. If the patient expresses dissatisfaction with that prediction, referral to an orthopaedist for consideration of open reduction and fixation may be necessary.

When the fracture is managed conservatively by splintage, movements of the shoulder should be restricted for the first few weeks. Abduction of the shoulder up to 90° may be permitted in the young child, but hyperabduction should be prevented for at least 4 weeks. In the adolescent patient, hyperabduction may have to be prevented for about 6 weeks. The splintage may be continued beyond 6 weeks, as necessary for comfort. Generally, clinical union of these fractures occurs in about 6 weeks, though radiologic union may not be complete for 3 months.

Surgical reduction and immobilization may be required in five circumstances.

1. If there is injury to the overlying skin.

2. If the displacement of the fracture is so great that the medial end protrudes high, and there appears to be impending laceration due to the marked deformity.

3. If the fracture is complicated by neurovascular injury.

4. Only occasionally and usually in de-

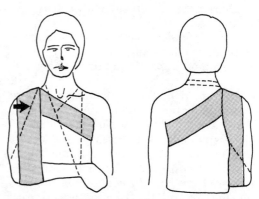

Fig. 3–13. Acromioclavicular brace, modified for middle third fractures of the clavicle. The acromioclavicular brace is modified by placing the vertical strap closer to the neck.

ference to local standards, if conservative bracing techniques do not establish apposition of the fragments.

5. If an older adolescent or adult does not accept an expected residual deformity.

Injuries to the Sternal End of the Clavicle. Charles A. Rockwood, Jr. has presented a good description and classification of injuries to the sternal end of the clavicle. (See Charles A. Rockwood, Jr., and David P. Green, eds., *Fractures*, J. E. Lippincott, Co., 1975, Vol. 1, pp. 756–787.) The following is an outline of that presentation:

Sternoclavicular Joint Injury.
Sprain of the Sternoclavicular Joint.
Subluxation of the sternoclavicular joint.
Dislocation of the sternoclavicular joint.
Anterior Dislocation.
Posterior Dislocation.
Habitual Dislocation.
Epiphyseal Separation of the Sternal End of the Clavicle.
Fracture of the Sternal End of the Clavicle.

Injuries to the sternal end of the clavicle are not common, as they result only from uncommonly directed and strong forces.

Sprains and Subluxations of the Sternoclavicular Joint. (See Figure 3–14.) The sprain represents a partial tear of the sternoclavicular ligaments, and the subluxation represents a complete tear of the sternoclavicular ligaments.

Characteristic clinical features are the following:

1. Pain, tenderness, and swelling at the sternoclavicular joint.

2. Pain on hyperabduction of the shoulder.

Treatment of Sternoclavicular Sprains and Subluxations. The treatment is essentially symptomatic. A sling or figure-of-eight splintage as necessary is used for comfort, and ice packs are applied until the initial pain and swelling have subsided. Range of motion of the shoulder is maintained, except that hyperabduction is avoided for 2–3 weeks.

Dislocations of the Sternoclavicular Joint. (See Figure 3–14.) This injury represents a tear of the costoclavicular ligament

as well as the sternoclavicular ligaments.

Characteristic clinical features as described by Charles A. Rockwood, Jr. are the following:

Anterior Dislocation.

1. Pain and tenderness at the sternoclavicular joint are severe.

2. Any movement of the shoulder causes severe pain.

3. Pain is increased when the patient is supine, and the patient prefers to be in the sitting position, holding the arm on the injured side.

4. The displaced medial end of the clavicle is quite visible.

Posterior Dislocation.

1. Pain and tenderness of the sternoclavicular joint are severe.

2. Any movement of the shoulder causes severe pain.

3. Pain is increased when the patient is supine, and the patient prefers to be in the sitting position, holding the arm on the injured side.

4. The usual prominent medial end of the clavicle is not visible or palpable due to its displacement posteriorly.

5. Posterior dislocation of the sternoclavicular joint may cause pressure on the great vessels or on the trachea, or on the esophagus, and the dislocation itself or associated injuries to the chest wall may also result in a pneumothorax. These complications will be manifested by:

a. Venous congestion in the neck.

b. Evidence of partial or complete airway obstruction.

c. Difficulty in swallowing.

d. If a pneumothorax is extensive, the patient may complain of air hunger, and breathing will be rapid, and breath sounds will be diminished over the area of the pneumothorax. A tension pneumothorax will be suggested by the usual signs of vascular collapse.

An x-ray may be necessary to confirm the diagnosis of a sternoclavicular dislocation. Since the usual roentgenograms of the sternoclavicular joint are difficult to interpret, the technique suggested by Charles A. Rockwood, Jr., may be more diagnostic. The patient is placed supine on the table. The x-ray tube is tilted at a 45° angle from the vertical, and is centered directly at the manubrium. A cassette is

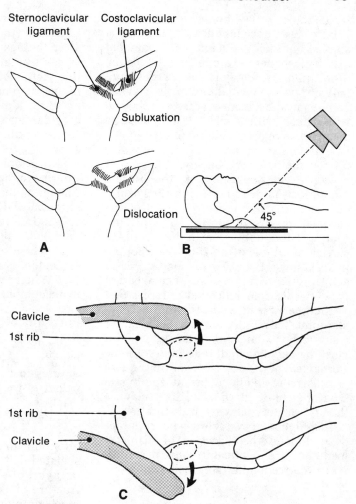

Fig. 3–14. Injuries to the sternoclavicular joint. *A*: *Top*, subluxation. *Bottom*, dislocation. *B*, x-ray orientation, patient supine. *C*, *Top*, superior view of posterior dislocation. *Bottom*, superior view of anterior dislocation.

placed behind both shoulders and the neck. (See Figure 3–14.) When such x-rays are obtained, the anterior dislocation would show the sternal end of the clavicle riding higher than the interclavicular line, and a posterior dislocation of the sternoclavicular joint would show the clavicle lying below the interclavicular line. (See Figure 3–14.)

Treatment of Sternoclavicular Dislocations. (See Figure 3–15.) Anterior Dislocation. The sedation protocol described later in this chapter for reduction of shoulder dislocation is often adequate, but anesthesia may be required. The patient is placed at the edge of the table with a sandbag underneath the scapula. The injured arm is abducted to 90°, and extended to the point of resistance (about 15°). Traction is applied in this abducted and extended axis. While traction is being applied to the abducted arm, the medial end of the clavicle is pushed backward to relocate it into the sternoclavicular joint. Reduction will be easy, but it may be unstable. A figure-of-eight splintage should be applied as external fixation for a period of 3–5 weeks. Whether anatomic healing is achieved or not, satisfactory painless function usually results, and seemingly no more often in cases that heal anatomically than in those that do not.

Posterior Dislocation. When pressure on the great vessels or trachea is posing a threat to life, reduction of the dislocation will be an emergent concern. Unless the patient is in extremis, anesthesia or sedation should be used. The patient is placed at the edge of the table with a sandbag underneath the scapula. The injured arm is abducted to 90°, and extended to the point of resistance (about 15°). Traction is applied in this abducted and extended axis. This maneuver alone may reduce the dislocation, but it may be necessary to pull outward on the medial end of the clavicle at the same time. In most cases, the clavicle will reduce with a click. If reduction is obtained, a figure-of-eight splintage must be maintained for 3–5 weeks. *In extremis, a strong half-Nelson can save a life.*

Epiphyseal Separation of the Sternal End of the Clavicle. The epiphyseal center of ossification for the medial end of the clavicle appears about the 18th to 20th year, and does not fuse with the rest of the clavicle until about the 25th year. So, patients younger than 25 years may suffer an epiphyseal separation of the medial end of the clavicle when subjected to forces that might otherwise dislocate the sternoclavicular joint. This injury may be mistaken for a sternoclavicular joint dislocation, and it must be remembered that injury to the sternal end of the clavicle prior to the 25th year is more likely to be an epiphyseal separation of the sternal end of the clavicle than it is a sternoclavicular dislocation.

Techniques of reduction and splintage depend upon the direction of displacement, and are identical to those described for the corresponding sternoclavicular dislocation.

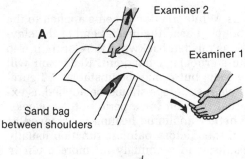

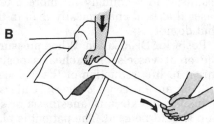

Fig. 3–15. Treatment of the sternoclavicular dislocation. *A,* posterior. *B,* anterior.

Fracture of the Sternal End of the Clavicle. This fracture is more likely to occur after the age of 25, and may result from forces similar to those that can dislocate the sternoclavicular joint. Again, techniques of reduction and splintage depend upon the direction of displacement, and are identical to those described for the corresponding sternoclavicular dislocation.

Indications for Orthopaedic Referral of Injuries to the Sternal End of the Clavicle. The individual who has suffered an injury to the sternal end of the clavicle should be referred to an orthopaedist under the following conditions:

1. When relocation of a posterior displacement cannot be maintained.

2. When predicted cosmetic results are unacceptable to the patient.

Fractures of the Scapula

Fractures of the *body* of the scapula usually are accompanied by other major injuries to the thorax. An automobile accident is the usual injuring event. These fractures of the body of the scapula do not require any special treatment, and often other more serious injuries will demand attention: multiple rib fractures with associated flail, hemothorax, pneumothorax, or myocardial contusion. The treatment of fracture of the body of the scapula is at most symptomatic splintage with a rib belt or sling.

Fractures of the scapula sometimes involve the *glenoid.* Since these fractures cross the articular surface of the glenohumeral joint, the displaced glenoid fracture, if left alone, will invariably lead to traumatic arthritis. A displaced glenoid fracture should be referred to an orthopaedist, as surgical reduction may be required.

A scapula may be fractured through its *neck* without injury to the articular surface of the joint. It is our opinion that unless the deformity and displacement are severe, symptomatic splintage with a sling will be quite sufficient to produce a good end result. Figure 3–16 diagrams the three forms of scapular fracture.

For all scapular injuries treated conservatively, as soon as pain permits, therapeutic exercises to prevent stiffening of the shoulder should begin. If the patient is

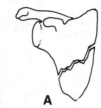 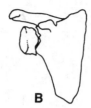 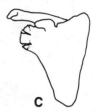

Fig. 3–16. Scapular fractures. *A*, body of scapula. *B*, neck of scapula with slight displacement. *C*, fracture of glenoid.

A   B   C

ambulatory, the regimen can begin with gravity-assisted pendulum exercises, and progress as pain permits. (See Figure 3–6.) If the patient is bedridden with other injuries, a physical therapist must help at the bedside with active assisted exercise when the patient's condition permits.

Dislocations of the Shoulder (the Glenohumeral Joint)

Dislocations of the shoulder are suffered most commonly as athletic injuries by vigorous young and middle-aged adults. A shoulder may dislocate anteriorly or posteriorly. Anterior dislocations are more common than posterior dislocations, and many posterior dislocations are missed on first visit to the primary physician.

Anterior Dislocations of the Shoulder. (See Figure 3–17.) This injury is produced by abduction and external rotation of the shoulder. The dislocated head of the humerus is anterior to the shoulder and may lie beneath the coracoid or more medially beneath the clavicle, or more laterally beneath the glenoid. Characteristic clinical features are the following:

1. The arm is held adjacent to the body with the elbow close to the body, adducted and externally rotated.

2. Any attempted movement of the shoulder provokes considerable pain, and the top of the shoulder is diffusely tender.

3. The normal smooth rounded contour of the shoulder, which is usually convex on its lateral side, is lost. With the humeral head displaced anteriorly, the lateral contour is sharply rectangular, and the anterior contour unusually prominent.

4. X-rays will show the dislocation and may also show any accompanying fracture.

Associated injuries and complications of anterior dislocations of the shoulder should always be looked for. These are of

two kinds:

1. One or more of three fractures may occur. The greater tubercle of the humerus may be fractured, with or without displacement, the attachment of the supraspinatus tendon to the greater tuberosity may be avulsed, and, particularly in the elderly, the neck of the humerus will be fractured. The next section in this chapter summarizes the nature of the fractures of the upper end of the humerus.

2. The second variety of complication is the injury to three nerves. The *axillary nerve* is the most likely to be injured. This nerve supplies the deltoid muscle. Injury to the axillary nerve may be detected by absence of contraction of the deltoid, or by hypesthesia over a small area at the level of the insertion of the deltoid which takes its sensory supply from the axillary nerve. As the patient with dislocation of the shoulder is in severe pain and is usually unable to abduct the shoulder, it is almost impossible to get the patient's cooperation to test for deltoid contraction, and the test for sensation may be the only assessment of axillary nerve function available to the practitioner. As there is a high incidence of injury to the axillary nerve, the practitioner should be very suspicious of this possible complication. The median and ulnar nerves are rarely injured. Injury to these nerves can be detected by examination of hand function. If the median nerve is injured, sensation to the thumb, index, and middle fingers will be impaired and opposition of the thumb to each of the fingers will be very weak, if not impossible. If the ulnar nerve is injured, sensation to the ring and fifth fingers will be impaired and abduction and adduction of the fingers will be very weak or impossible, and flexion of the metacarpophalangeal joints of the fingers with the proximal interphalangeal joints extended will be very weak or impossible. Review of me-

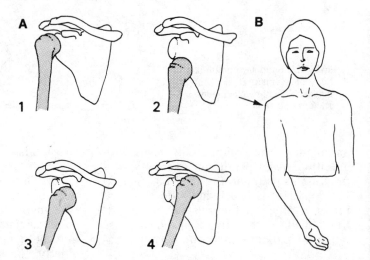

Fig. 3–17. Anterior dislocation of the shoulder. *A*, the positions: *1*, normal; *2*, subglenoid; *3*, subcoracoid; *4*, subclavicular. *B*, anterior view of patient's appearance. The round prominence of the shoulder has shifted anteriorly, leaving the lateral salient flat (*arrow*).

dian and ulnar nerve injuries is presented in greater detail in Chapter 6 and is summarized in Chapter 7.

Treatment. (See Figure 3–18.) The dislocation should be reduced at the earliest possible moment. Reduction may be accomplished with or without anesthesia, and we have found that in 80% of the cases, reduction may be obtained under sedation without anesthesia. We sedate the patient with 100 mg. of intravenous meperidine, and position the patient prone on the examining table, with the affected shoulder and arm hanging over the edge of the table. It is sometimes helpful to place a weight in the dependent hand. The patient may be left alone undisturbed for about 10–15 minutes, and as the muscle spasm is gradually overcome, the shoulder may relocate spontaneously. If after 15 minutes the shoulder has not relocated by itself, gentle traction and internal rotation upon the dependent arm may complete the reduction. Please note, however, that the trick is as much in relaxation as it is in traction. The tactful physician will coax the arm downward further than he will pull it.

In most cases, this method will bring about reduction of the dislocation. If it fails, however, we then position the patient supine, and sit or stand on the side of the injury, face to face with the patient. We then place the towel-swathed ball of our shoeless foot in the affected axilla and apply straight traction, as shown in Figure

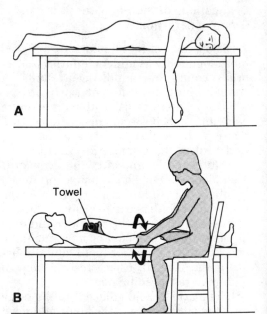

Fig. 3–18. Reduction of anterior dislocations of the shoulder. *A*, prone reduction method. After 10–20 minutes in the prone dependent position, gentle downward pulling action coupled with a few degrees internal and external rotation. *B*, Hippocratic maneuver. Straight traction on the arm, then gentle rotation (a few degrees external and internal during full traction).

3–18. Success of this maneuver may require more sedation or frank anesthesia. We have often succeeded after the slow addition of diazepam intravenously. Five to ten milligrams are usually sufficient. Occasionally in large individuals, we have used as much as 20 mg.

Regardless of method, the shoulder usually reduces with a click, after which x-rays must be obtained to be certain that reduction has been effected and no associated fracture missed, and contraction of the deltoid must be retested if the test was not reliable before reduction.

If this was the first episode of dislocation, the arm should be maintained for a period of about 3 weeks, with the shoulder internally rotated in adduction in the sagittal plane, or slightly anterior to it. This position of healing is obtained in a standard sling. Whether or not it is maintained depends upon the patient. We instruct our patients consciously to avoid abduction, external rotation, and extension. If they observe our instructions, they may safely remove the sling for bathing. In older individuals, to avoid the frozen shoulder, the maintenance of this position may be discontinued after a shorter period of time, while in younger patients, less vulnerable to stiffening, maintenance of this position may be extended to a period of 4 weeks. Though the point is debated, we have not found it necessary to maintain the position of healing longer than 4 weeks. In our experience, further immobilization does not reduce the incidence of recurrent dislocation.

After the 3 or 4 weeks in the position of healing, therapeutic exercises should be started. Particular attention must be paid to strengthening the subscapular muscle, and to restoring full range of motion to the shoulder. The subscapular tendon forms the anterior reinforcement of the capsule, and the strength of this muscle and the integrity of its tendon may be a crucial factor in prevention of recurrence. Subscapularis strengthening exercises are illustrated in Figure 3–19. Range of motion exercises have been described in the discussion of the myotendinous cuff syndrome. As compliance with the exercise program may decrease the vulnerability to recurrent dislocation, we almost invariably refer our patients to a tactful physical therapist.

Recurrent Dislocation. There is a high incidence of recurrence of anterior dislocation. This complication has been studied intensively, and factors determining the risk of recurrence have been identified:

1. Younger patients statistically seem to have a higher incidence of recurrent dislocation.

2. Improper maintenance of the position of healing may be one of the causes of recurrence, but the causative relationship has not been clearly proven. It has, however, been proven to our satisfaction that maintenance of this position beyond 3–4 weeks after reduction of a primary dislocation does not affect the rate of recurrence.

3. Primary dislocations produced by major trauma, if properly treated, seem to have less incidence of recurrent dislocation than those produced by a trivial trauma.

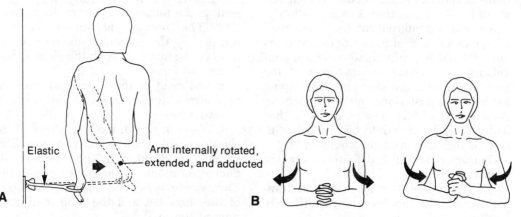

Elastic

Arm internally rotated, extended, and adducted

A

B

Fig. 3–19. Exercises for rehabilitation of shoulders injured by dislocation. *A*, adduction exercise for strengthening of the subscapularis and infraspinatus-teres minor. *B*, rotation exercises for strengthening the subscapularis (*right*) and infraspinatus-teres minor (*left*).

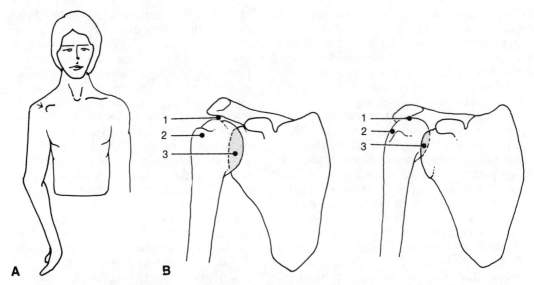

Fig. 3-20. Posterior dislocation of the shoulder. *A*, patient's appearance. Note that the shoulder is flat and the coracoid protrudes (*arrow*). *B*, three diagnostic features of anterior-posterior x-ray. *Left*, normal. *1*, upper border of head of humerus in normal lie. *2*, normal contour reveals greater tubercle. *3*, half-moon cresent of projected overlap. *Right*, posterior dislocations. *1*, head of humerus after dislocation, superior to normal lie. *2*, internal rotation hides the greater tubercle. *3*, half-moon cresent of projected overlap no longer apparent.

Recurrent dislocations may be *treated* with subscapularis strengthening exercises, but if dislocations continue to recur, surgical treatment is invariably necessary.

Posterior Dislocation of the Shoulder. Posterior dislocation of the shoulder is relatively uncommon and, unfortunately, it is commonly missed. When missed, a posterior dislocation may cause considerable residual disability. When the result of violence, the injuring violence is usually quite severe, and is directed against the shoulder of an arm that is in a position of adduction and internal rotation. However, a large percentage of posterior dislocations are suffered by individuals who are convulsing. The severe contractions of the muscles around the shoulder may rotate the humerus posteriorly out of the glenoid. As a matter of fact, any patient who has had a convulsion should be tested for injury or dislocation of the shoulder.

Characteristic clinical features are the following (See Figure 3-20):

1. The shoulder is very painful and immobile, and the shoulder joint is diffusely tender.

2. The arm is kept in a position of adduction and internal rotation.

3. Any attempt at external rotation, even to neutral position, causes considerable pain and is resisted.

4. With the humeral head posteriorly displaced, the coracoid process is abnormally prominent anteriorly, and a swelling or lump may be visible or palpable posteriorly.

5. Three abnormalities often appear in routine anteroposterior x-ray projection:

a. The normal smooth curved contour of the greater tubercle laterally may be absent as the humerus is internally rotated.

b. The normal half-moon crescent formed by the projected overlap of the head of the humerus with the glenoid may be absent.

c. The head of the dislocated humerus may appear to be displaced upward from its usual lie.

6. When in doubt, axillary views of the shoulder will confirm the diagnosis. This view is obtained with the shoulder abducted as much as possible to near 45°. The cassette is held on the superior aspect of the shoulder, and the tube is directed toward the axilla.

Any patient, particularly after a convulsion or very severe trauma, whose shoulder is held stiffly, with the arm in a position of adduction and internal rotation, must be suspect for a posterior dislocation of the shoulder.

Treatment. (See Figure 3–21.) If detected at the time of the injury, reduction of posterior dislocation may be easily accomplished, even without sedation. Leaving the arm as it lies, with traction applied along the axis of the arm, the shoulder is rotated externally, and at the same time, the head of the humerus may be pushed forward to relocate into the glenoid. Often the necessary forces may be so mild that both maneuvers can be effected by one operator. Once reactive muscle spasm has developed, sedation or anesthesia will be required. If enough time has elapsed for swelling to occur, reduction may be possible only with forces that will require counter traction. Counter traction is best provided by an assistant pulling on a towel that has been looped through the axilla. If necessary, a third operator will be required to push the head of the humerus forward. X-rays should be obtained after reduction, and should show the dislocation to be reduced. The arm should be splinted in a position of external rotation. The simplest method of splintage may be the use of an airplane splint, with the arm in abduction, and external rotation. Immobilization is maintained for a period of 3 weeks, after which therapeutic exercises should be started to strengthen the infraspinatus-teres minor and to restore range of motion to the shoulder. The infraspinatus-teres minor strengthening exercises are illustrated in Figure 3–19.

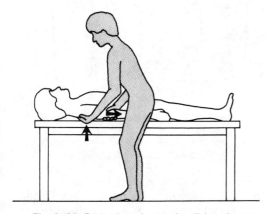

Fig. 3–21. Reduction of posterior dislocations.

Fractures of the Upper End of the Humerus

Fractures of the upper end of the humerus are quite common and occur particularly in the older-aged individual. With advancing age, osteoporosis develops, and simple falls can easily cause fractures in the upper end of the humerus. Combinations of these fractures with other fractures in the upper extremity that can be produced by similar mechanisms are common. For example, Colles fractures of the wrist, and fractures of the neck of the humerus may occur together. Fractures of the upper end of the humerus in younger patients are usually the result of major trauma. The very young patient may suffer an epiphyseal separation rather than a metaphyseal fracture at the neck of the humerus.

Classification of Fractures of the Upper End of the Humerus. (See Figure 3–22.) There are different classifications of fractures of the upper end of the humerus, some of which may be more complicated than others. However, we prefer the following classification, as it is practical and also incorporates much of the recent knowledge and analysis of these fractures.

1. Supraspinatus avulsions.
2. Fracture of the greater tubercle of the humerus without displacement.
3. Fracture of the greater tubercle of the humerus with marked displacement.
4. Fracture of the lesser tubercle. This fracture will sometimes accompany a posterior dislocation.
5. Fracture of the neck of the humerus without displacement, or firmly impacted, regardless of displacement (two-part fracture).
6. Fracture of the neck of the humerus with displacement, not impacted (two-part fracture).
7. Comminuted fractures of the neck of the humerus without displacement (three- or four-part fracture).
8. Comminuted fractures of the neck of the humerus with displacement (three or four-part fracture).

Characteristic Clinical Features of all Fractures are the Following:
1. The patient is generally an older-age

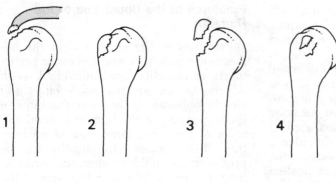

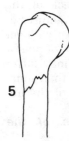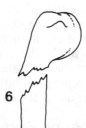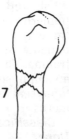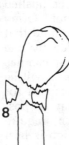

Fig. 3–22. Fractures of the upper end of the humerus. *1*, supraspinatus avulsion. *2*, fracture of the greater tubercle without displacement. *3*, fracture of the greater tubercle with marked displacement. *4*, fracture of the lesser tubercle. *5*, fracture of the neck without displacement, *6*, fracture of the neck with marked displacement. *7*, comminuted fracture without displacement. *8*, comminuted fracture with marked displacement.

individual who has fallen. It is generally assumed that many of these injuries are produced by a fall onto the outstretched hand, but more often than not, the patients cannot tell us how they landed.

2. The shoulder is often tensely swollen, ecchymotic, and diffusely tender.

3. Any attempt to move the shoulder causes increased pain.

4. X-rays of the shoulder obtained in the anteroposterior and across the chest lateral projections will demonstrate the fracture.

Treatment of Fractures of the Upper End of the Humerus. Fractures of the upper end of the humerus generally occur through a region of cancellous bone. Hence, healing of the fracture is usually no great problem, and as long as displacement is not great, the ultimate function may depend more upon the length of immobilization imposed on the patient and the tact of rehabilitation than upon the danger of malunion. Immobilization of the shoulder for a prolonged period of time, especially in the older-age individual, will lead inevitably to adhesions and a frozen shoulder. The treatment, therefore, in many moderately displaced fractures of the upper end of the humerus, with or without comminution, is splintage for comfort and active early movement as

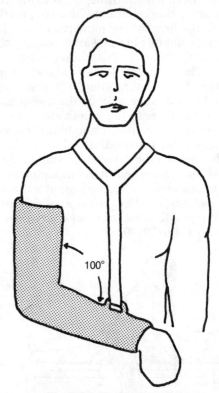

Fig. 3–23. The hanging arm cast.

soon as possible within the limits of the patient's tolerance. Comfortable splintage can be attained either with a sling, an arm immobilizer, or a Velpeau dressing. The

Table 3-1
Fractures of the Upper End of the Humerus

Type	Displacement	Clinical Features	Treatment
1. Fracture of the greater tuberosity and avulsions of the supraspinatus.	a. Wihout displacement.	Older-age patients. Pain in the shoulder. Movement painful.	1. Arm immobilized by sling immobilizer or Velpeau. 2. Begin active exercises as soon as possible, within a few days.
	b. With displacement.	Same.	1. Minimal displacement—treat as above. 2. Marked displacement—surgical treatment (orthopedic referral). 3. Avulsion of supraspinatus with displacement under the acromion—surgical treatment (orthopaedic referral).
2. Fracture of the lesser tuberosity.		Older-age patients. Pain in the shoulder.	Rule out posterior dislocation of the shoulder. Arm immobilizer, sling, or Velpeau until symptoms subside. Begin active exercises early.
3. Fracture of the neck of the humerus, two-part fracture.	a. Without displacement. b. Impacted in abduction or adduction.	Older-age patients. Pain and swelling of the shoulder region. Movements painful.	1. Velpeau, sling, or arm immobilizer for 2–3 weeks. 2. Begin active exercises early.
4. Fracture of the neck of the humerus, two-part fracture.	Marked displacement.	Older individuals. Considerable pain and swelling of the shoulder, ecchymosis, and shoulder movement painful.	1. If glenohumeral articulation is greatly disturbed—surgical treatment (orthopedic referral). 2. If glenohumeral articulation is not greatly disturbed—apply hanging arm cast, and begin active exercises early.
5. Comminuted fracture, neck of humerus, three- or four-part fracture.	a. Without displacement.	Older individuals. Considerable pain, swelling, ecchymosis, hematoma of shoulder, shoulder movement painful.	Arm immobilizer or sling or Velpeau. Start active exercises as soon as possible.
	b. With marked displacement.	Same as above.	*Conservative treatment.* Secure alignment by using hanging arm cast for 4–6 weeks. Start early pendulum exercises. When glenohumeral articulation is markedly disturbed, surgical treatment may be required (orthopaedic referral).

exercise regimen should begin with gravity-assisted pendulum exercises, and should progress as illustrated in Figure 3–6. If the regimen is pursued too timidly or too aggressively, pain and stiffness will increase. Hence, we usually request the assistance of a tactful physical therapist.

When the fracture is severely comminuted or markedly displaced, the ultimate position of the fragments becomes of some concern. When the greater tubercle or the supraspinatus insertion are markedly displaced, they must be reduced to restore normal rotator cuff function. When the displacement of a humeral neck fracture markedly disturbs the glenohumeral articulation, the fragments must be reduced to restore normal glenohumeral function and forestall a traumatic arthritis. These fractures often require surgical reduction and are best referred to an orthopaedist.

Marked displacements of the fracture of

the neck of the humerus which do not disturb the glenohumeral articulation, can often be improved by the traction of a hanging arm cast. Such improvement may allow greater restoration of ultimate range of motion, and may allow a greater degree of comfort early in convalescence. The use of a hanging cast requires complete understanding of the mechanism of the cast, and requires considerable cooperation on the part of the patient. As a matter of fact, the hanging cast has been discredited because its mechanism has been ignored in the application, and the patient's cooperation with the intent of the cast has not been obtained.

The Hanging Cast. The hanging cast is applied with the patient's elbow not at 90° as is usually and erroneously done, but at about 100° of extension. (See Figure 3–23.) The cast is well padded, but should not be too heavy, and is applied from the region of the axilla down to and including the hand. A ring should be created somewhere above the level of the wrist, and a cuff-and-collar sling created from stockinette should be applied through the ring. The position of the ring determines the direction of force at the fracture line. The de-

sired position corrects the angulation; other positions will either maintain or overcorrect the angulation. The desired position is discovered by trial and error, using x-ray to monitor the effect of the traction force upon the angulation. For comfort, a piece of felt should be placed in the stockinette where the sling passes over the patient's neck. The ring and the sling should be placed so that the elbow will lie at the side of the body, and the hand just in front of the navel.

It must be understood that this treatment employs the weight of the arm and the cast as a continuous traction force to align the fragments in position. Patients should be made to understand this principle and the fact that it will work only if they are on their feet or sitting. They should sleep in a more or less upright position.

These fractures bleed, and dependent swelling in the cast and arm may dangerously compromise the circulation. Patients must be taught the signs and symptoms of circulatory strangulation.

The fractures of the upper end of the humerus, their clinical features, and their treatment, are summarized in Table 3–1.

CHAPTER 4

The Shaft of the Upper Arm

Disorders of the shaft of the upper arm occur less commonly than do disorders of the shoulder, elbow, and wrist. However, primary care physicians should become quite familiar with four disorders: radial nerve palsy, deltoid tendinitis, rupture of the tendon of the long head of the biceps, and fracture of the shaft of the humerus.

Essential Anatomy

(See Figure 4–1.) The following points of anatomy are critical to an understanding of the disorders of the shaft of the upper arm:

The *radial nerve* enters the arm from the axilla posterior to the humerus and spirals distally along the humerus, between the medial and lateral heads of the triceps muscle, in what is called the radial groove. In the distal arm, it penetrates the lateral intermuscular septum, and enters the forearm between the brachioradialis and the biceps. The nerve is particularly vulnerable to injury at two points: as it spirals around the midshaft of the radius posterolaterally, and as it enters the forearm between the brachioradialis and the biceps. The radial nerve innervates the extensors of the wrist and the extensors of the fingers, and shares with the median and ulnar nerves the sensory supply to the dorsum of the hand and fingers. The space on the dorsum of the hand, between the thumb and the index finger is supplied by the radial nerve alone. Loss of the ability to extend the wrist and the fingers and loss of sensation over the dorsum of the web between the thumb and index finger are characteristic of injury to the radial nerve above the elbow.

The *ulnar nerve* courses posterior to the brachial artery along the medial aspect of the upper arm. While superiorly, it lies in the anterior compartment, about the middle third of the arm it pierces the medial intermuscular septum to course through the posterior compartment, around the medial epicondyle of the humerus, to enter the dorsomedial forearm. The ulnar nerve supplies the intrinsic muscles of the hand, except for the short muscles that constitute the thenar eminence which are supplied by the median nerve. The inability to abduct and adduct the fingers with the fingers in extension, and the inability to flex the metacarpophalangeal joints with the interphalangeal joints in extension, and sensory loss over the palmar aspect of the fifth finger and ulnar aspect of the hand are characteristic of an ulnar nerve injury.

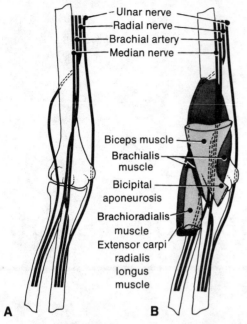
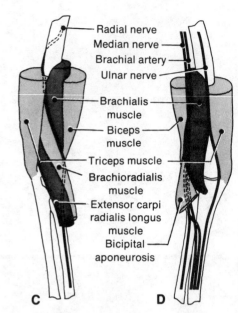

Fig. 4–1. Relationships of nerves in arm and elbow. *A.* Anterior view, nerves alone. *B.* Anterior view with muscles at the elbow. *C.* Lateral view. *D.* Medial view.

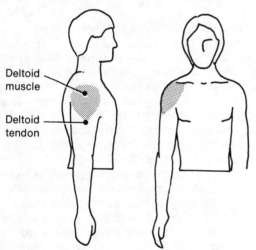

Fig. 4–2. The deltoid muscle and its insertion.

The *median nerve* courses anterior to the brachial artery along the medial aspect of the upper arm. Somewhere in the distal half of the upper arm, it crosses the brachial artery, to pass through the antecubital space, medial to the brachial artery, and deep to the biceps tendon. The median nerve innervates the muscles of the flexor aspect of the forearm, and the short muscles that constitute the thenar eminence: the opponens pollicis, the abductor pollicis

brevis, and the superficial head of the flexor pollicis brevis. These muscles flex the wrist and the fingers, and flex and oppose the thumb. Loss of the ability to oppose the thumb is uniquely characteristic of median nerve injury.

Note that the brachial artery and the ulnar and median nerves are separated from the humerus by the brachialis muscle and the medial head of the triceps muscle, while the radial nerve lies directly upon the posterior and lateral surfaces of the upper and middle thirds of the humerus.

The *deltoid muscle* attaches to the deltoid tubercle on the lateral surface of the upper third of the upper arm, anterior to the lateral head of the triceps. (See Fig. 4–2.)

The relationships of the tendon of the long head of the biceps were described in the previous chapter. The long head of the biceps shares responsibility for elbow flexion with the short head of the biceps, the brachialis, and the brachioradialis.

The Four Disorders

Radial Nerve Palsy

As will be discussed subsequently, the radial nerve can be injured by a fracture

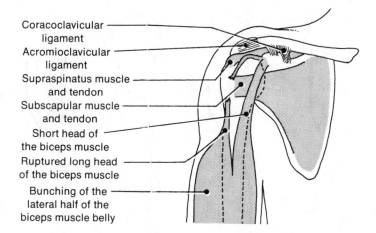

Coracoclavicular ligament
Acromioclavicular ligament
Supraspinatus muscle and tendon
Subscapular muscle and tendon
Short head of the biceps muscle
Ruptured long head of the biceps muscle
Bunching of the lateral half of the biceps muscle belly

Fig. 4–3. Rupture of the long head of the biceps.

of the shaft of the humerus, by a fracture of the lateral humeral condyle, or proximal head of the radius, or by a dislocation of the radiohumeral joint. This paragraph refers to an entrapment neuropathy, sardonically termed the Saturday night palsy. Classically, the term refers to a syndrome of radial nerve dysfunction caused by prolonged pressure on the nerve at the elbow, which results when the arm is draped over the back of a chair for hours. Individuals acutely intoxicated by a Saturday night tavern binge have fallen asleep in this position and awakened hours later with a radial palsy, hence the origin of the name. Individuals presenting to us with morning radial palsy have seemed to us to have sustained the palsy more commonly from pressure on the radial nerve as it lies along the posterior and lateral humerus in its upper and middle thirds. They have often been able to tell us that they have awakened lying on the affected side in an attitude that might well press firmly upon the posterior and lateral aspects of the arm. Usually, enough function remains in the face of these palsies, so that there is no danger of stiffness developing during convalescence, and treatment may be confined to a reassuring explanation and instructions to avoid positions that entrap the nerve.

Deltoid Tendinitis

Occasionally, individuals presenting with pain suggestive of a musculotendinous cuff pain syndrome will, on careful evaluation, prove to be suffering from deltoid tendon pain.

The characteristic clinical features are the following:

1. Onset most commonly in adults of middle age and older.

2. *Rarely* the history of a direct contusion, sudden abduction strain, or a prolonged effort requiring repeated abduction movements to which the patient is not conditioned.

3. Pain felt in the deltoid and down the lateral aspect of the arm. The longer the duration and greater the severity of the pain, the more likely is the entire arm to ache and develop paresthesias.

4. Pain increased by resisted abduction, but rarely is the range of motion as restricted as it is by musculotendinous cuff pain.

5. Unique tenderness directly over the deltoid insertion to its tubercle, on the lateral surface of the humerus.

Treatment. 1. Exercise. Avoidance of strongly resisted abduction, but active range of motion exercises as illustrated in Figure 3–6, to progress as pain allows.

2. Drugs. Anti-inflammatory drugs may be helpful, particularly when signs of inflammation are visible. We prescribe anti-inflammatory drugs by the same protocol which we described for the musculotendinous cuff pain syndrome.

3. Physical modalities. When inflammation is visible, we recommend ice, when not visible, we recommend a trial of heat or ice. The patient should choose which is more analgesic. The occasional individual

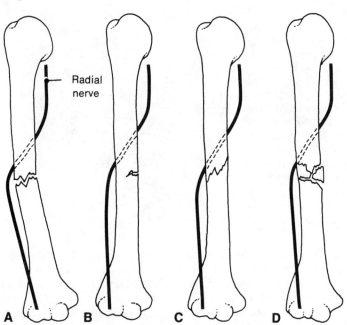

Radial nerve

Fig. 4–4. Fractures of the humerus. *A.* Transverse complete. *B.* Transverse incomplete. *C.* Oblique undisplaced. *D.* Comminuted.

A   B   C   D

more analgesic. The occasional individual may report dramatic relief from a physical therapist's application of ultrasound or diathermy. Usually those modes seem to us no more beneficial than heat or ice.

4. Local injections. One cubic centimeter of a corticosteroid injected directly into the deltoid tendon will often yield a complete and rapid remission.

Rupture of the Tendon of the Long Head of the Biceps

The previous chapter discussed the degenerative inflammation of the tendon of the long head of the biceps. These paragraphs will discuss the occasional ultimate result of that degeneration—rupture of the tendon. (See Figure 4–3.)

Characteristic clinical features are as follows:

1. An adult of middle age or older, who may or may not have experienced episodes of musculotendinous cuff pain in the past, will report a sudden and usually painful popping sensation in the upper arm or shoulder during a lifting effort.

2. The biceps bulges peculiarly in the lower third of the arm, and an unusual concavity is evident on the medial aspect of the upper third, witnessing to the distal retraction of the long head of the biceps.

3. The arm may ache for several days following the rupture, and abduction and rotation movements of the shoulder may increase the pain.

4. The bicipital groove may be tender for several days after the rupture.

5. Ecchymoses often appear about the elbow several days after the rupture.

6. The strength of elbow flexion is little impaired, and with exercise, can be fully restored. This favorable functional prognosis is not so mysterious when one considers that the brachioradialis, the brachialis, and the short and long heads of the biceps all contribute to the strength of flexion.

Treatment. The favorable functional prognosis must be emphatically explained to the patient. When predictions and the cosmetic defect are acceptable to the patient, conservative treatment can proceed. Conservative treatment consists of:

1. Range of motion, icing, and occasional anti-inflammatory medication to encourage rapid remission of any resulting musculotendinous cuff pain.

2. Eventual resisted elbow flexion exercises to build the remaining muscle groups to a point that substitute fully for the lost function of the long head of the biceps.

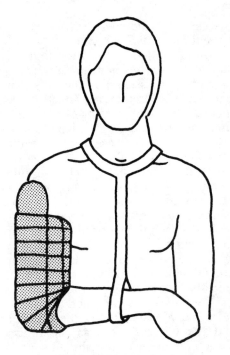

Fig. 4–5. Sugar tong splint.

When predictions or the cosmetic defect are not acceptable to the patient, referral to an orthopaedist for consideration of surgical repair may be required.

Fracture of the Shaft of the Humerus

Fracture of the shaft of the humerus may be transverse, oblique, comminuted, complete, or incomplete. (See Figure 4–4.) Alignment and apposition are usually satisfactory when the arm is dependent, but occasionally displacement is unacceptably marked. If not a pathologic fracture, it is the result of rather severe forces, either direct blunt impact, or a levering force directly to the humerus, such as would occur were a heavy weight to strike the elbow of an arm that was resting with the midshaft of the humerus upon a railing. The incidence of neurovascular injury accompanying fracture of the shaft of the humerus is high. As explained in the paragraphs concerning the essentials of anatomy, the radial nerve is particularly vulnerable.

Characteristic clinical features are the following:

1. The injury is usually sustained on the job by those who work with heavy equipment, or in an auto accident.

2. The arm is visibly swollen and cannot be used.

3. When the fracture is complete, heavy bony crepitus will be felt in the midshaft of the humerus with any manipulation of the arm. When the fracture is incomplete, the midshaft of the humerus will be exquisitely tender.

4. A few days after the injury, ecchymoses and edema will appear about the elbow and the forearm.

5. Anteroposterior and lateral x-ray projections will confirm the presence and nature of the fracture.

Treatment. **Initial Evaluation.** The presence of a strong radial pulse should be confirmed, and when absent, an orthopaedic consultation should be obtained immediately. If a strong radial pulse is confirmed, function of the radial, ulnar, and median nerves should be assessed. Should evidence of a peripheral nerve dysfunction be demonstrated, the fracture should be splinted as discussed in the next paragraphs, and the patient should be referred to an orthopaedist within a few days at most. The radial nerve is by far the most likely to be injured. It is generally agreed that immediate surgical exploration is not necessary in cases of radial nerve palsy accompanying fractures of the humerus, as in a large percentage of cases, it is merely a contusion of the radial nerve, rather than total transection, and return of radial nerve function can be looked for within 4 weeks. The first muscle innervated by the radial nerve is the brachioradialis which helps to flex the elbow. Innervated next are the extensor carpi radialis longus and brevis which are extensors of the wrist. The physician looks for return of function in these muscles within 6 weeks. If, however, function of these muscles does not return in six weeks, then exploration of the radial nerve must be considered. It is the best policy for the primary practitioner always to refer a patient with radial nerve palsy to an orthopaedist for further follow-up and treatment.

Immobilization. The undisplaced fracture may be immobilized by the so-called sugar tong splint. (See Figure 4–5.) This is applied by first padding the entire extremity with Sof-rol or sheet wadding, and then carrying a long plaster splint from the shoulder on the lateral side down the lateral aspect of the upper arm, around the elbow with the elbow flexed, and then up along the inner aspect of the arm to the axilla. This splint can be reinforced by anterior and posterior splints if necessary, to effect a stable immobilization, and bias stockinette bandage or Ace bandage is applied snugly around the splinted arm. Once the plaster has set, with the elbow at 90° of flexion and in midrotation, with the thumb upward, plaster may be then carried onto the forearm, should the immobilization still appear insufficiently stable.

If the fracture of the humerus is incomplete, an arm immobilizer, with or without Velpeau dressing will be adequate.

If the fracture is grossly displaced or comminuted, one of two methods of treatment may be pursued. Under anesthesia, an attempt may be made to manipulate the fracture, and the same form of external splintage as described above may be applied. A second, simpler, and probably safer method is to apply the hanging arm cast. The principles and application of the hanging arm cast were described in the previous chapter under "Treatment of Fractures of the Upper End of the Humerus."

Evaluation after immobilization. Cases have been reported of humeral shaft fractures which presented with normal radial nerve function, only to lose radial nerve function during reduction or application of a cast. Such a development clearly indicates that the radial nerve has been impaled or caught between the fracture fragments and is an indication for immediate surgery. Radial nerve function must be reassessed after application of the plaster and the patient referred immediately to an orthopaedist if the function has been lost.

Rehabilitation. This fracture is very slow to heal and is very vulnerable to delayed union and non-union. Rarely can the first stage of clinical union be expected before 4 months or strength sufficient to allow resisted exercises before 6 months or final radiologic union before 1 year. Gravity-assisted pendulum exercises of the shoulder should be started when the patient is walking about without pain. Range of motion of the wrist and fingers should be started immediately and gripping exercises should be started when the pendulum exercises are started. Movement of the hand and fingers can continue throughout the day. The pendulum exercise should be performed for 5 minutes at least four times daily.

When the first stage of clinical union is evident and bridging callus is visible on x-ray, gravity-resisted exercise can begin. We are reluctant to add weights until callus is dense and new bone bridges part of the fracture line. We begin with 5 pounds and augment by 5 pounds each month. Should pain return in the fracture site, we stop the use of weights and resume with the next lower weight when the pain subsides. We advise the curl, the chest press, and the vertical press as the return of range of motion of the shoulder permits.

The entire rehabilitation should be supervised by a physical therapist if available.

We x-ray a fracture at 2 and 4 weeks to assess maintenance of the position. Thereafter, we x-ray when the first signs of clinical union are evident and bimonthly until rehabilitation is complete. Recurrence of pain is reason for an interim x-ray. We assess for the first stage of clinical union after the 4th month. To do so, we remove the splintage and gently attempt to move the fracture site with one hand above and one below the fracture and the thumbs on the fracture. We define the first stage of clinical union as that degree of healing which painlessly resists movement when the fragments are gently stressed. "Gentle" is hard to define, but is perhaps that force necessary to almost break a full-length standard wooden pencil.

Summary of Treatment of Fractures of the Shaft of the Humerus. Incomplete and Undisplaced Fractures. Immobilize with an arm immobilizer, Velpeau dressing, or sugar tong splint until examination confirms the first stage of clinical union, and x-ray shows bridging callus.

Complete Fracture in Good Alignment and Opposition. Immobilize with a sugar tong splint until examination confirms the first stage of clinical union, and x-ray shows bridging callus. More rigid fixation may be obtained by adding anterior and posterior splints and extending the splintage to include the forearm.

Comminuted and Displaced Fractures. Reduce under anesthesia and apply sugar tong splintage, or more easily and probably more safely apply a hanging arm cast. Again, immobilization should be continued until exam confirms the first stage of clinical union, and x-ray shows bridging callus.

Radial Nerve Dysfunction before Manipulation or Splintage. The immediate treatment should be as specified as above, and the patient should then be referred promptly to an orthopaedist.

Radial Nerve Dysfunction Appears After Manipulation or Splintage. The patient must be immediately referred to an orthopaedist, as the radial nerve may be caught between the fracture fragments and require immediate exploration.

CHAPTER 5
The Elbow Joint

Essential Anatomy

The lower end of the humerus is a complex articular surface: a rounded sphere, the capitulum, facing anteriorly and inferiorly on the lateral side, and a pulley-like groove, the trochlea, curving from anterior to posterior on the medial side. (See Figure 5-1.) The capitulum and a concave disc, the head of the radius, form the radiohumeral articulation. The unique movement of this articulation is axial rotation of the radius which permits pronation and supination of the forearm. The trochlea and the trochlear fossa of the ulna form the ulnohumeral articulation. The trochlear fossa is bounded by two pillars, one anteriorly called the coronoid process of the ulna, and the other posteriorly called the olecranon of the ulna. Its articular surface bears a convex ridge which fits into the pulley-like trochlea of the humerus. The ulnohumeral articulation permits flexion and extension of the elbow.

When the elbow is completely flexed, the coronoid process fits into a small concavity in the lower end of the anterior surface of the humerus called the coronoid fossa, and when the elbow is completely extended, the olecranon process fits into a large shallow concavity in the lower end of the posterior surface of the humerus, called the olecranon fossa. Posteriorly, the trochlea extends obliquely upward and medially, such that when the forearm is completely extended, it is not in line with the upper arm, but deviates to form the normal valgus carrying angle of the arm. On the average, the valgus carrying angle in women is greater than that in men.

A narrow junction between the head and the shaft of the radius is called the neck of the radius. Surrounding the head and neck of the radius is the annular ligament. It attaches to the anterior and posterior margins of a shallow groove on the lateral surface of the ulna at the level of the coronoid process, called the radial notch. This annular ligament stabilizes the rotation of the radius upon the capitulum. (See Figure 5-2.) As the head of the radius overhangs the neck, at least after the age of 5 years, that portion of the annular ligament which surrounds the neck effectively resists forces that would otherwise pull the radial head through the ring of the ligament out of articulation with the capitulum.

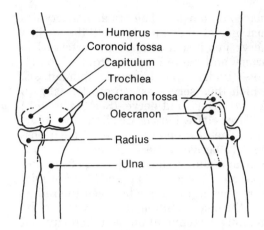

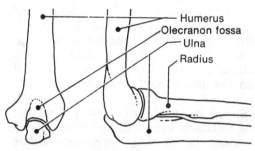

Fig. 5-1. The elbow joint. *A*, anterior view. *B*, posterior view. *C*, posterior view, 90° flexion. *D*, lateral view.

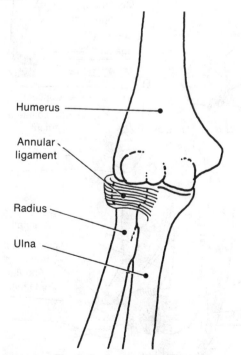

Fig. 5-2. Annular ligament.

The articular capsule of the elbow joint encloses the articular surfaces. It makes its proximal attachment to the superior margin of the coronoid fossa on the anterior surface of the humerus, and to the superior margin of the olecranon fossa on the posterior surface of the humerus, and it makes its distal attachments to the margins of the trochlear fossa of the ulna, and to the annular ligament surrounding the head and neck of radius. (See Figure 5-3.) While the capsule is thin anteriorly and posteriorly, reinforcing bands of ligaments thicken it on its lateral and medial sides. The medial ligament, which is also called the ulnar collateral ligament, is a thick triangular reinforcement which is attached to the medial epicondyle proximally, and to the margin of the articular surface of the trochlear fossa distally, and to the coronoid process anteriorly. The lateral ligament, which is also called the radial collateral ligament, is a thick band which is attached to the lateral epicondyle of the humerus proximally and to the annular ligament of the radius distally. (See Figure 5-3.)

The radial nerve pierces the lateral intermuscular septum to enter the anterior compartment of the arm in its lower third. There it lies in a groove between the brachialis muscle medially and the brachioradialis and extensor carpi radialis longus laterally. Within that groove, it enters the elbow in front of the lateral epicondyle of the humerus. (See Figure 4-1.)

The ulnar nerve pierces the medial intermuscular septum to enter the posterior compartment of the arm in its lower third. There it lies upon the medial border of the triceps muscle. From that lie upon the triceps, it enters the elbow behind the medial epicondyle where it is easily palpated as a subcutaneous structure. The three bellies of the triceps muscle fuse to form their common tendon at the back of the elbow. At that point, the tendon reinforces the posterior capsule of the joint before taking insertion upon the olecranon. (See Figure 4-1.)

The median nerve accompanies the brachial artery down the anterior compartment of the arm in the groove between the brachialis and the biceps muscles. In the lower third of the arm, the median nerve crosses from a position anterolateral to the artery to a position medial to the artery. Both enter the front of the elbow lying upon the brachialis muscle. The brachialis muscle is the large muscle that takes broad insertion from the anterior surface of the lower two-thirds of the humerus and inserts upon the coronoid process of the ulna. As it crosses the front of the elbow, it reinforces the anterior capsule of the elbow joint. The biceps muscle is a double-bellied muscle of similar size which lies in front of the brachialis muscle. At the upper border of the elbow joint, the two bellies of the biceps fuse to form the biceps tendon laterally and the bicipital aponeurosis medially. The tendon takes insertion upon the radial tuberosity just distal to the radial neck, and the bicipital aponeurosis remains a superficial structure inserting upon the deep fascia on the medial aspect of the forearm at the lower border of the elbow joint. The tendon of the biceps can be easily palpated on the front of the elbow when the muscle is placed on tension. The brachial artery lies just medial to this tendon, and the median nerve lies just medial to the artery. The artery and nerve cross in front of the elbow under the bicipital aponeurosis, which thus serves as a protective sheath for the artery and nerve. (See Figure 4–1.)

Three elbow bursae are clinically important. The *olecranon bursa* is situated posteriorly between the skin and the olecranon, and allows smooth gliding of the skin upon the triceps tendon. The *bicipitoradial bursa* lies in the angle between the radius and the biceps tendon, just proximal to the tendon's attachment on the tuberosity and allows smooth gliding of the tendon upon the surface of the bone. The *radiohumeral bursa* lies on the lateral aspect of the elbow, over the articulation between the radius and the capitulum. It allows smooth gliding between the radiohumeral joint and the lateral collateral ligament. (See Figure 5–4.)

Superficial to the attachment of the lateral collateral ligament, the posterior surface and the tip of the lateral epicondyle

Fig. 5–3. Articular capsule of the elbow joint. *A*, anterior view. *B*, medial view. *C*, lateral view.

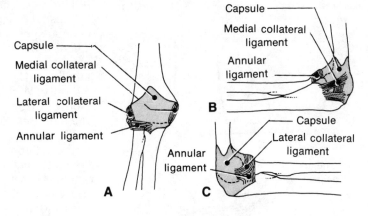

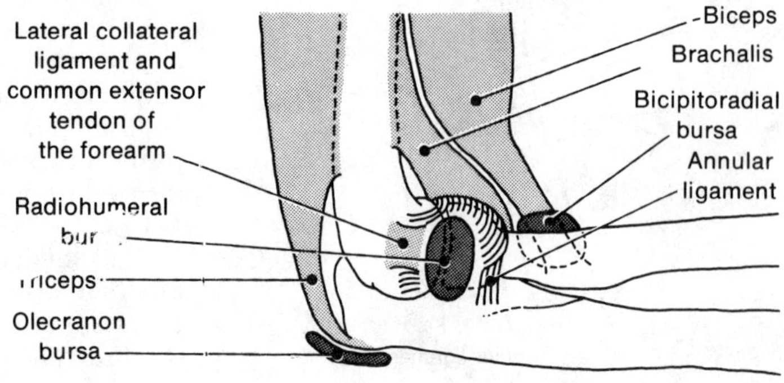

Fig. 5–4. Three elbow bursae. The lateral collateral ligament, and common extensor tendon have been reflected away to expose the radiohumeral bursa.

give origin to the extensor muscles of the forearm. Superficial to the attachment of the medial collateral ligament, the anterior surface and the tip of the medial epicondyle give origin to the flexor muscles of the forearm.

Soft Tissue Diseases of the Elbow

Tennis Elbow

The so-called tennis elbow is one of the commonest musculoskeletal ailments. It is thought to be the result of repeated unrecognized trauma. Contrary to its name, while the backhand drive and the wrist whip of the overhand serve in tennis may cause injury to the fibers on the lateral aspect of the elbow, the problem is not unique to tennis players. Golfers whose leading arm during the swing is held with the forearm pronated, and workers who must wield heavy weights like hammers with the forearm pronated, or who—using tools like screwdrivers—must repeatedly rotate their forearms against strong resistance, are at least if not more likely to develop the problem.

Definitive of the clinical syndrome are the following symptoms and signs:

1. Pain is felt in the lateral aspect of the elbow joint, and when intense or long-standing, will refer into the extensor aspect of the entire forearm.

2. As the condition tends for long periods to be mild and to remit with rest, patients often present initially complaining of a long-standing problem.

3. Except in the severest examples, active and passive movements are complete, but are often accompanied by pain.

4. Eventually, nearly all who suffer the condition begin to limit their use of the arm, even to the point where they may change their methods of eating and dressing.

5. Lifting is distinctly more painful when the forearm is pronated rather than supinated. With the forearm in supination, the structures on the lateral aspect of the elbow are obviously less stressed.

6. It is probably the chronicity of pain which causes many who suffer the condition to seem irritable and intolerant.

7. X-rays are usually normal, but may reveal small calcific deposits adjacent to the lateral epicondyle. These are compatible with chronic irritation of the common extensor tendon and/or lateral collateral ligament.

While the exact pathophysiology has not been certainly defined, other findings than the above suggest that this common syndrome results from one of three pathologic processes, each or all of which may result from the repeated unrecognized traumas assumed to be the original cause.

1. Lateral epicondylitis. Tenderness directly over the lateral epicondyle, the site of attachment of the common extensor tendon and lateral collateral ligament, implies to many that the syndrome is resulting from the inflammatory reaction which follows a partial tear of the common extensor tendon or lateral collateral ligament.

2. Radiohumeral bursitis. Tenderness directly over the radiohumeral bursa implies to many that the syndrome is resulting from inflammation of the bursa.

3. Annular ligament strain. Tenderness directly over the annular ligament at the head and neck of the radius and exquisite pain on pronation-supination movements imply to many the inflammatory reaction which follows a partial tear of the annular ligament.

Treatment. While, as in much of medicine, the exact pathologic processes that result in this syndrome are not certainly defined, there is, nonetheless, a course of conservative treatment which may improve symptoms.

When the syndrome is characterized by tenderness over the lateral humeral epicondyle exclusively, when the pain does not cause the patient to immobilize the arm, and when the patient wishes to continue his activities, a combination of caution and local stimulation will often yield a satisfactory remission within a few weeks. We have not compared the frequency of these remissions with the frequency of remissions among those who are not treated.

1. During the activity, a canvas strap should be worn tightly about the upper forearm. (See Figure 5-5.) For unclear reasons, such a binding will permit some

workers, tennis players, and golfers to continue their work or their sport without great inhibition and without a worsening of the syndrome. However, the greatest or most prolonged stresses must be avoided as well: the heaviest hammers should be let alone; the tightest screws delegated to

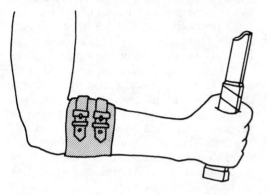

Fig. 5–5. Supporting strap for mild tennis elbow.

the other arm or to a fellow worker; lifting anything heavier than one's tools should not be done with the forearm in pronation; long drill on the driving range and long drill with backhand strokes or serving should be avoided.

2. Several times daily, ideally every hour or two, the patient should massage the tender epicondyle firmly enough to cause pain. The massage should continue for at least 1 minute. Immediately following the massage, the patient should stretch the common extensor tendon by maximum volar flexion of the wrist with the elbow fully extended and the forearm fully pronated. The stretching position should be rhythmically set and released for at least 1 minute. (See Figure 5–6.)

3. As often as the patient's schedule allows, ice or heat may be applied to the lateral aspect of the elbow for 15–30 minutes. The patient should try both modali-

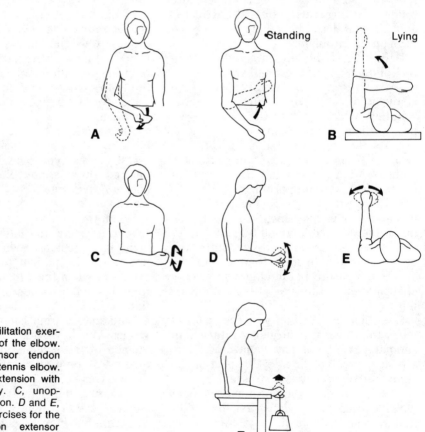

Fig. 5–6. Rehabilitation exercises for disorders of the elbow. *A,* common extensor tendon stretching for mild tennis elbow. *B,* acute flexion/extension with and against gravity. *C,* unopposed forearm rotation. *D* and *E,* range of motion exercises for the wrist. *F,* common extensor strengthening exercise.

ties and stick with the one which seems to yield the greatest comfort.

When the syndrome is characterized by tenderness over the radiohumeral bursa, or over the annular ligament, with or without epicondylar tenderness, or when the pain does cause the patient to immobilize the arm, or when the problem is long-standing and the patient's complaint most urgent, the treatment must emphasize rest and accept the consequent disability.

1. The forearm should be kept immobilized either voluntarily by the patient with the help of a sling, or by a posterior plaster splint removable by the patient for baths. A splint should be applied to hold the elbow at 90° flexion, the forearm in moderate supination, and the wrist in moderate dorsiflexion. This position is often the most comfortable and probably affords greatest ease to the radiohumeral bursa and annular ligament as well as to the common extensor tendon.

2. All modalities of heat or cold and the office use of ultrasound may appear to give benefit. Ice must be used if inflammation is evidenced by local swelling or heat. Otherwise, either may benefit. The patient must use whichever is the most comforting. Ultrasound may be tried unless signs of inflammation are marked, but should be discontinued if pain worsens after it.

3. Anti-inflammatory medication may be tried. Aspirin grains 10–15, given 3–4 times daily should be used until tinnitus or dyspepsia appears. The dosage should then be decreased until tinnitus disappears. Dyspepsia can sometimes be relieved by the concomitant addition of antacids. Phenylbutazone 100 mg. may be given 2–4 times daily for 1 week at a time. A complete blood count must be obtained at the outset and before any resumption in dosage. Any evidence of a decrease in red blood cells, neutrophils, or platelets contraindicates a repeated dosage of phenylbutazone. Dexamethasone 0.04 mg./kg. daily or prednisolone 0.3 mg./kg. daily may be given for 1 week and then tapered over 1 week.

4. A corticosteroid may be injected into each tender area, whether the lateral epicondyle, the radiohumeral bursa, or the annular ligament; 0.5 cc. of any intra-articular corticosteroid is appropriate. It has been our observation that radiohumeral bursitis responds to cortisone injection more satisfactorily than do the other two entities. Whether and when to inject depend largely on the patient's choice. Particularly in cases of presumed radiohumeral bursitis, we advise our patients that injection is somewhat more likely to benefit than are the systemic anti-inflammatory medications.

When this regimen fails to yield a satisfactory remission, the elbow may have to be immobilized for a continuous period of 6–8 weeks. We effect this immobilization with a long-arm cast with the elbow at 90°, the forearm in moderate supination, and the wrist in moderate dorsiflexion. Following immobilization, exercises must begin to restore range of motion to the elbow and wrist, and to strengthen the muscles of the forearm, and particularly the attachment of the common extensors to the lateral humeral epicondyle. To restore range of motion, we teach active gravity-assisted and -resisted flexion and extension exercises of the elbow, active unresisted rotation exercises of the forearm, and active gravity-assisted and -resisted flexion and extension exercises of the wrist. Once mobility is restored, we teach weight-resisted extension exercise of the wrist. We begin with 1–3 pounds resistance, depending upon the native strength of the individual, and augment by 1 pound/week to 5–20 pounds, again depending upon the native strength of the individual and vigor of activity intended after full rehabilitation. (See Figure 5-6.)

Should the syndrome recur during rehabilitation after the 6–8 weeks immobilization, or should it recur shortly after resuming desired activities, the primary clinician may feel obliged to refer the patient to an orthopaedist.

Pitcher's Elbow

Repeated unrecognized injuries similar to those presumed to cause the tennis elbow can cause the pitcher's elbow on the medial side. Consistent with its name, the syndrome quite commonly afflicts baseball pitchers. Laborers whose work require heavy pulling may develop the same syndrome. Here on the Northwest Coast, we occasionally see professional fishermen who complain of the problem. Perhaps their injury occurs while pulling heavy nets or lines. The pathology is thought to be a sprain of the medial collateral ligament or a strain of the common flexor tendon, where they attach to the medial epicondyle.

Principles of treatment are identical to those outlined for lateral humeral epicondylitis. If the elbow is to be immobilized, however, it is done with the elbow at 90°, the forearm in moderate pronation, and the wrist in moderate volar flexion.

Articular Degenerations Which Mimic Tennis Elbow and Pitcher's Elbow

The forces which can produce the elbow fractures discussed later in this chapter, and the repeated relatively violent joint play that necessarily accompanies certain athletic activities (classically, overhand pitching), besides the other injuries and wear and tear they produce, can also inflict considerable damage to the articular cartilage of the radiohumeral, and ulnohumeral joints. The pain which results from these cartilage injuries and the associated reactive synovitis adjacent to the injuries will mimic the characteristics of tennis elbow and pitcher's elbow: Radiohumeral injury will mimic tennis elbow, and ulnohumeral injury will mimic pitcher's elbow. Like most cartilage injuries, these tend to produce persistent pain syndrome, which may yield only to a termination of all wearing activities. These problems may be most prevalent in North American culture among Little League pitchers and middle-aged skilled laborers.

Two clinical characteristics help to distinguish these problems from tennis elbow and pitcher's elbow:

1. Usually the joint line is tender.

2. Usually axial compression of the joint produces pain. An abduction force applied to the extended elbow will compress the radiohumeral joint, and an adduction force will compress the ulnohumeral joint.

The occasional patient will complain of painful snapping or even jamming which will suggest the presence of a loose body and turn the practitioner's attention to the joint itself.

X-rays may show the bony changes of a malunited condylar or radial head or neck fracture, and the bony changes characteristic of long-standing degenerative arthritis. (See Chapter 18.)

As these problems tend to be most resistant to conservative treatment, often require surgery, and often gravely affect a young athlete's aspirations or a working person's career, we recommend that patients so afflicted be referred to an orthopaedist.

Bicipitoradial Bursitis

In primary practice, this disorder is encountered somewhat less often than pitcher's elbow, and much less often than tennis elbow, though it may be encountered as often as that variant of tennis elbow presumed to be radiohumeral bursitis.

Definitive of the clinical syndrome are the following symptoms and signs:

1. Pain is referred down the flexor aspect of the forearm and up the biceps muscle.

2. Flexion and supination, particularly against resistance, will aggravate the pain.

3. Deep palpation between the biceps tendon and radial neck will provoke unique tenderness. (See Figure 5–7.)

4. Signs of inflammation are usually *not* visible.

5. X-rays are normal.

Treatment. 1. The arm should be immobilized in a sling or a posterior splint with the elbow at 90° and the forearm in midrotation with the thumb up.

2. Ice pack or heat may be applied, whichever gives more comfort. The chosen modality may be used as often and for as long as desired.

3. Anti-inflammatory medications may be tried. Drugs and dosages are as described for tennis elbow.

4. A corticosteroid may be injected into the region of the bursa; 1 cc. of any intra-articular corticosteroid is appropriate. Often, whether or not to inject depends on the patient's choice. If the decision is left to us, we advise that a course of an oral

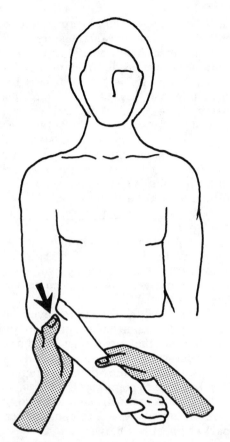

Fig. 5–7. Point of tenderness associated with bicipitoradial bursitis. Arm in 30° flexion.

anti-inflammatory agent, with immobilization and thermal modalities, be tried first, for at least 1 week.

Olecranon Bursitis

In primary practice, this disorder is encountered about as often as is the tennis elbow. It presents in one of two forms:

A Painless Cystic Swelling, not Visibly Inflamed, and at Most Only Slightly Tender. This painless swelling represents an increase in transudate produced by a synovium changed by the effects of chronic irritation. Among the changes which the synovium undergoes is the development of villous projections of reticular connective tissue lined by synovium. Some of these projections separate off from the bursal lining, and lie free in the bursal space, where they are palpable as hard moveable kernels which have been called rice bodies. Fluid aspirated from

such a bursa is usually clear, straw-colored, and more serous than mucoid in consistency.

Treatment. 1. Patients are often fairly alarmed by the swelling, and an explanation of the benign if annoying process can be most reassuring.

2. After an intradermal and subcutaneous infusion with a local anesthetic, a No. 18 needle on a 10-cc. syringe is introduced into the bursal space, and all fluid is aspirated. The needle should not enter the point of the elbow, as friction and stretching at the point of the elbow can irritate the needle tract so as to create a persisting sinus tract. We introduce the needle laterally and in zigzag fashion to prevent the puncture through the bursa wall from remaining in line with the puncture through the skin. (See Figure 5–8.)

3. If the fluid is clear, as it usually is, the syringe is removed from the needle, leaving the needle in the bursa; a second syringe preloaded with 1 cc. of any intra-articular corticosteroid is attached to the needle, and its contents are expressed into the bursal cavity. The needle and syringes can be easily separated and attached if the hub of the needle is held with a hemostat.

4. The elbow is wrapped with an Ace bandage to compress the bursa and somewhat limit elbow motion.

5. The patient is advised to find means to avoid pressure on the olecranon in future.

6. Recurrences are treated in the same way. When fluid accumulates repeatedly, some patients come to accept it and do not return for treatment, others importune for a cure. For the urgent, an excision of the bursa may be necessary.

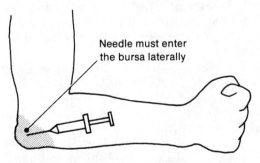

Needle must enter the bursa laterally

Fig. 5–8. Aspiration and/or irrigation of the olecranon bursa space.

***A Painful Cystic Swelling, Visibly In-
flamed and Quite Tender.*** This painful
swelling represents an acute inflammation
of the bursa, reflecting one of at least three
processes:

1. Trauma. A sharp blow to the point of
the olecranon can contuse the bursa, causing it to bleed into the bursal space, and to
become inflamed. The diagnosis is made
when aspiration removes blood.

2. Infection. Its superficial location and
the communication of its lymphatics with
those of the overlying skin are the anatomic basis of the bursa's peculiar vulnerability to infection. Not infrequently, a minor abrasion over the point of the elbow
will become complicated by an infectious
olecranon bursitis. The diagnosis must be
presumed when aspiration removes
cloudy fluid. The diagnosis is confirmed
when bacteria are detected on Gram stain,
or colonies are recovered on culture me-
dium.

3. Cryptogenic. Somewhat less common
than the acute bursitis of injury or infection is a bursitis of unknown cause, often
but not always associated with an elevated
serum uric acid. This occasional association with an elevated serum uric acid has
led to speculation about a pathogenic relationship of this bursitis to the gouty
diatheses, even though the bursitis does
not necessarily occur in company with
gouty arthritis, even though the bursal
fluid does not contain uric acid crystals,
and even though an identical picture occurs in association with normal serum uric
acid. The major defense of this speculation
is the increased incidence of cryptogenic
olecranon bursitis in those whose serum
uric acids are elevated.

Treatment. 1. A painful visibly inflamed bursitis must be aspirated.

2. The nature of the fluid obtained determines the next step.

a. Bloody. All the blood is removed, and
a sample is cultured for bacteria.

b. Cloudy. All the fluid is removed, and
a sample is Gram stained and cultured for
bacteria. At this point, we habitually add
a step which is not standard. We leave the
needle in place, remove the aspirating syringe, attach a syringe containing 10 cc.
aqueous penicillin made to a concentration

of 10,000 units/cc., and express its contents
into the bursal space and reaspirate it three
to four times. After the last aspiration, we
withdraw the needle, leaving the bursal
space empty. If the patient is sensitive to
penicillin, we use 10 cc. of an aqueous
neomycin solution made to a concentration of 1 mg./cc. When the culture results
are received, appropriate systemic antibiotics are given, and the antibiotic irrigation is repeated every time the bursa refills,
until the fluid is sterile, and signs of acute
inflammation have disappeared. Rarely
have we been forced to incise and drain
the bursa. When forced to do so by failure
of our preferred method, we make the
incision laterally, not over the point of the
elbow. As explained above, wounds over
the point of the elbow can become persistent sinus tracts.

c. Clear. All the fluid is removed, and 1
cc. of any intra-articular corticosteroid is
injected into the bursal space by the technique described for painless bursitis.

3. In all cases, the elbow is wrapped in
Ace bandage to compress the bursa.

4. Patients are instructed to avoid pressure on the elbow and to apply either ice
packs or heat as follows:

a. Traumatic bursitis. Ice packs for at
least 2 days, then ice or heat as desired for
comfort.

b. Infectious. Heat unless pain is severe
and the patient finds ice to be more comforting.

c. Cryptogenic. Heat or ice, whichever
is more comforting.

5. Most acute bursitis will yield to these
treatments within 1–2 weeks. However,
traumatic and cryptogenic bursitis may become tenacious in the painless form, in
which case the alternatives of Step number 6 in the treatment of painless bursitis
(see above) must be considered. When infectious bursitis does not yield to systemic
antibiotics and local antibiotic irrigations,
the bursa must be opened widely to facilitate constant drainage, or the bursa must
be excised and the wound packed open.
The incision in either case is made lateral
to the olecranon to avoid any possible injury to the ulnar nerve, and to avoid a
painful scar over the tip of the olecranon.
Appropriate systemic antibiotics are continued.

Nerve Entrapment Syndrome

Congenital bands and congenital or acquired valgus or varus carrying angles at the elbow can entrap any of the three nerves which cross the elbow into the forearm, and produce the dysesthesias and weakness characteristic of the three neuropathies of the forearm and hand. The radial, median, and ulnar nerve syndromes are reviewed in the context of the supracondylar fracture. (See below.) The same syndrome can result from entrapment in the absence of injury. When an entrapment syndrome is recognized, we recommend that the patient be referred to an orthopaedist as surgical treatment is often necessary.

Fractures and Dislocations at the Elbow

Many fractures and dislocations at the elbow are severe injuries which threaten serious disability and should be referred when possible to an orthopaedist. However, the emergency treatment of any such injury may fall to a primary physician whose acts or omissions may determine whether there will be a gratifying recovery or a permanent disability. Other fractures and dislocations at the elbow are best treated definitively by the primary physician. This section will describe most of the injuries and recommend the level of responsibility which the primary physician should assume for each. Potential complications have been alluded to in context, but definitive discussions of the two crippling complications of severe elbow injuries have been deferred to the end of this section.

Nursemaid's Elbow (Pulled Elbow)

This injury is an axial subluxation of the radial head away from the capitulum, through the annular ligament. (See Figure 5-9.) The shape of the radial head during infancy allows for this injury and accounts for its almost exclusive prevalence among children between 18 months and 3 years of age. (See above under "Essential Anatomy.") Abrupt axial forces and abrupt pronating forces can produce this subluxation.

The injury takes its name from its classic etiology: A nursemaid's sudden jerk on the extended arm of a toddler in her charge when lifting the child over a curb or some other obstruction in its path. The children brought to us have sustained the injury from such a jerk, but equally frequently from some force applied during a fall. We suspect that some toddlers falling from a piece of furniture will hold on with one arm, thus jerking the elbow as they interrupt the fall. We suspect that other children fall onto an arm in such a way as to pronate it forcefully.

Characteristic clinical features are the following:

1. A toddler who has been jerked upward by an arm, or has fallen, cried immediately for several minutes, stopped, and continued to move about, even played, but kept the injured arm motionless at its side, and cried again whenever it tried to use the arm.

2. The arm appears normal.

3. If an examiner has won the trust of the child, gentle palpation will elicit crying and withdrawal only when applied over the radiohumeral joint, and passive movements elicit crying only when the manipulation is applied to the elbow.

4. An x-ray will be normal. We no longer x-ray this injury. After several encounters with this injury, the practitioner will find that the facts of history and physical exam alone will allow a presumptive diagnosis.

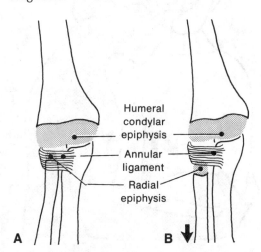

Humeral condylar epiphysis

Annular ligament

Radial epiphysis

Fig. 5-9. Nursemaid's elbow. *A,* normal articulation. *B,* radiohumeral subluxation.

5. The definitive diagnosis is made by the maneuver which effects the cure.

Treatment. We attend closely to the history. Unless we perceive other reasons to suspect child abuse, we deal with the adults in the best of humor—many of them already feel pathetically clumsy and crude. We examine and treat the child where he is—whether in the adult's lap or standing in the middle of the room. (See Figure 5-10.) We kneel or sit face to face with the child, gently bring the forearm to 90° and support it there with one hand, while palpating the entire arm with the other. We support the right arm with our right hand, and the left arm with our left hand. When satisfied of no visible or palpable deformities or crepitations, and of the unique tenderness over the radiohumeral joint, we perform the reduction. The examining hand grips the elbow gently with the thumb over the radiohumeral joint. The supporting hand effects the manipulation by rotating the forearm first into full pronation, then into full supination. Reduction will be perceived as a click by the examining hand near the end of supination. The examination and reduction take less than 30 seconds. The child will not attempt to withdraw the injured arm, but will cry

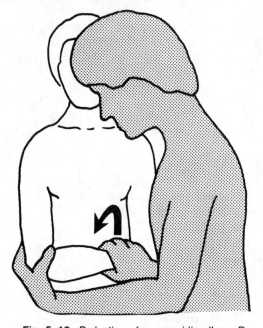

Fig. 5-10. Reduction of nursemaid's elbow. Rotate from full pronation to full supination.

bitterly during and often for several minutes after the reduction. We often leave the room at this point, assuring the parents affably of a gratifying result. Upon our return 10-15 minutes later, the child is usually using the arm for play or for putting on a coat, and the adults are utterly relieved. Nothing further need be done, except to explain the mechanism of the injury to the adults. The child need not be restricted in any way.

Supracondylar Fracture

This fracture is one of the injuries to the elbow that is fraught with complications and the danger of permanent disability. It is usually sustained by young children between the ages of 5 and 8 years, as the result of a fall on an outstretched hand. The fracture is either transverse or short oblique, through or just at the upper border of the olecranon fossa. (See Figure 5-11.) Displacement is often gross. The distal fragment has usually been displaced posteriorly. Rarely, it has been displaced anteriorly, perhaps by forces directed through a hyperextended elbow. In addition to posterior or anterior displacement, the distal fragment is usually displaced medially or laterally as well. Consideration of the anatomy of the elbow and the pathophysiology of fractures will suggest the neurovascular complications that will result immediately or within the first several hours after injury. When, as is most common, the distal fragment has been displaced posteriorly, the distal end of the proximal fragment may impale the median nerve, the brachial vessels, or the radial nerve. Arterial rupture, venous rupture, or median nerve or radial nerve laceration or contusion may result. Injury to the artery, short of rupture, may induce a reactive arterial spasm. Increased tissue pressure from bleeding and transudation may create a tourniquet effect, initially obstructing venous outflow and eventually obstructing arterial inflow. Untreated, the vascular dysfunctions can lead to Volkmann's ischemic contracture, see below under "Two Major Complications of Severe Elbow Injury," or to frank gangrene. When, less commonly, the distal fragment has been anteriorly displaced, particularly if

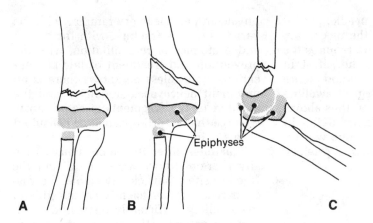

Epiphyses

Fig. 5-11. Supracondylar fractures of the humerus. *A*, transverse. *B*, oblique. *C*, lateral view, showing most common angulation.

also laterally displaced, the ulnar nerve may be contused or lacerated. This complication is the least common.

As soon as a supracondylar fracture is suspected, or an elbow injury is seen to have resulted in any swelling, a meticulous examination of neurovascular function must be made.

1. Vascular. The radial pulse must be sought. If it cannot be found, dysfunction of the brachial artery must be suspected. Whether the pulse can be found or not if nail beds are cyanotic and capillary return sluggish, and if motion of the fingers is painful and restricted, dysfunction of the brachial artery must be presumed.

2. Median nerve. If the patient cannot actively flex the fingers or the wrist, or if the thumb, index, middle, and radial half of the ring fingers are dysesthetic, injury to the median nerve must be presumed.

3. Radial nerve. If the patient cannot extend the fingers or the wrist, or if the dorsal web between the thumb and the hand is dysesthetic, injury to the radial nerve must be presumed.

4. Ulnar nerve. If the patient cannot actively adduct and abduct the straightened fingers or flex the metacarpophalangeal joints with the proximal and distal interphalangeal joints straightened, or if the fifth finger is dysesthetic, ulnar nerve injury must be presumed.

Evidence of vascular dysfunction is cause for immediate involvement by an orthopaedist or vascular surgeon. Evidence of neural dysfunction, is cause for same-day referral to an orthopaedist.

Treatment. **All Patients must be Admitted to a Hospital.**

Emergency Treatment. While awaiting hospitalization and reduction of a fracture, a posterior plaster splint should be applied and held in place with a lightly wrapped Ace bandage or bias stockinette. Wrappings should not extend across the front of the elbow. The elbow should be at an angle which does not obliterate the radial pulse—the greater the flexion, the greater the tissue pressure at the elbow. We recommend that splints be applied with the elbow in about 30° of flexion or less if the pulse is weak even at that shallow angle. (See Figure 5-12.) For greater stability, once the splints are in place, the elbow may be flexed further, if the radial pulse remains strong.

Reductive Treatment. Traction in bed is the treatment of choice. With the patient supine, the shoulder abducted to 90°, and the elbow semiflexed to the ceiling, adhesive traction tapes are applied to the medial and lateral aspects of the upper arm, and straight traction is applied along the axis of the humerus by a 3-pound weight, and adhesive traction tapes are applied to the forearm with straight traction applied to the forearm by a 1-pound weight. (See Figure 5-13.) When the distal fragment is posteriorly angulated, a 1-pound weight may be added over the fracture site. The recommended weights are average for preschool children. Larger children and adults require proportionately heavier weights. Traction to the upper arm may be applied more effectively through a Kirschner wire, or—lacking that—a No. 18 needle, passed from side to side through the olecranon. While this method of traction requires the least handling and is thus the safest in inexperienced hands, a method more likely to combat the problem of swelling places the arm 90° in front of, thus above, the supine patient. (See Figure 5–13.) In many cases, these methods alone will reduce the fracture, but unless a primary physician becomes very familiar with the varieties of this fracture, with the course and principles of rehabilitation, with the prevention and treatment of late complications, and unless he knows there is no imminent neurovascular danger, and the position of the fragments is satisfactory, we urge that an orthopaedist be consulted at this point.

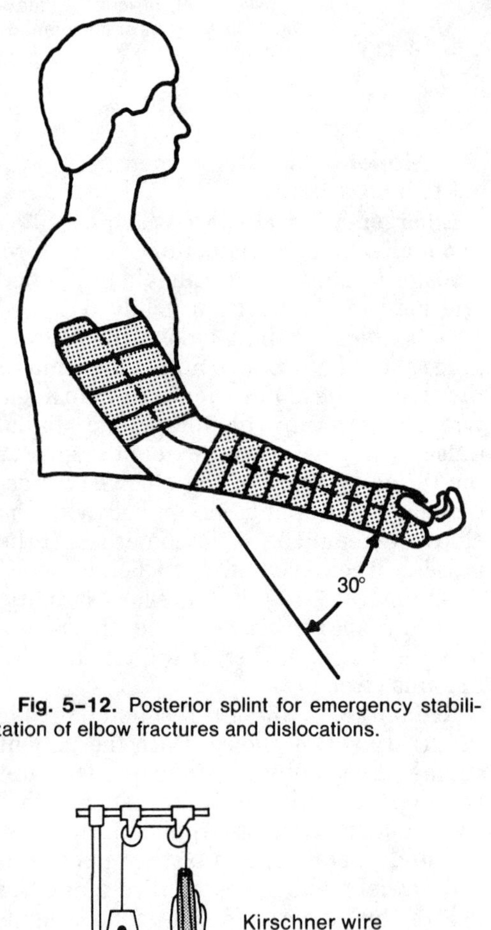

Treatment after the Acute Phase. Usually after one to two weeks in traction, the fracture site is sufficiently stable, the vascular recovery sufficiently advanced, and the swelling sufficiently decreased to allow the patient to be up and about with the arm in a posterior plaster splint. *At no time during the first 1–3 weeks following injury should a circular cast ever be applied to elbow injuries,* and even in a posterior splint, the front of the elbow should have no wrappings applied to it. The splint is applied with the arm in relaxed supination. Parents of a child must be instructed to examine for vascular impairment and to do so several times daily throughout the period of immobilization. Anteroposterior (AP) and lateral x-rays are taken 1 week after discharge. If the position is acceptable (at least 50% apposition, no lateral or medial angulation, and no more than 15° of anterior or posterior angulation), further x-rays need be made only to evaluate an increase in pain or upon a disruption of the splint, and after 6 weeks, when the splint is removed and the fracture is examined for stability. If after 6 weeks the fracture is clinically stable and x-rays

Fig. 5–12. Posterior splint for emergency stabilization of elbow fractures and dislocations.

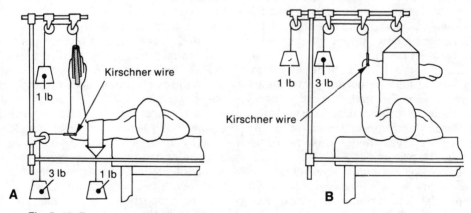

Fig. 5–13. Traction reduction/immobilization of supracondylar fractures of the humerus.

show bridging callus, rehabilitation may begin.

Rehabilitation. If at all possible, a tactful physical therapist should supervise the rehabilitation. Like the shoulder, only more so, the convalescing elbow is endangered by too strenuous or too cautious exercise. A child left to herself will do better than one forced to do painful exercises, but the child doing just the right exercises will do better than both. At first, exercises are prescribed to restore a full range of motion. These are active elbow flexion and extension, performed with and against gravity, and active unresisted forearm rotation. (See Figure 5–6.) Once active range of motion is painless, even if still somewhat restricted, weights may be added, *not for stretching*, but for muscle-building. Should the use of weights increase pain, they must be discontinued until active range of motion again becomes painless.

Fractures of the Articular Surface of the Condyles

These fractures are variations of five basic forms. (See Figure 5–14.)
1. Fracture of the capitulum alone.
2. Fracture of the trochlea alone.
3. Transverse intercondylar fractures separating off the capitulum and trochlea as a piece.
4. T-shaped intercondylar fracture, separating off the capitulum and trochlea as separate pieces.
5. Vertical or spiral fracture of either condyle, most usually the lateral condyle.

These fractures almost invariably distort the articular surface of the elbow, and unless the fragments are accurately reduced, a permanently disabled elbow will result. These fractures are most likely to be sustained by preschool children. The condyles of preschool children are cartilagenous and as such do not show on x-ray pictures. No wonder that the fractures are often missed. The primary practitioner's responsibility is not to miss them.

Characteristic clinical features are the following:
1. The injury has usually resulted from a fall onto the outstretched arm.
2. Any elbow movement provokes pain.
3. The injured elbow generally appears swollen in comparison with the uninjured elbow. Such swelling is harder to perceive in a plump toddler.
4. X-ray will occasionally show a fleck of bone separated from the metaphysis, and if the x-ray is of excellent soft tissue quality, it will always show a "positive fat pad sign." Normally, the inner plane of the triceps and brachialis muscles can be seen to lie close to the intercondylar bone. Whenever the joint is distended by blood or other fluid, these planes will be pushed away with the joint capsule from the intercondylar bone. Careful comparison of lateral views of both elbows will allow the practitioner to recognize the fat pad sign. (See Figure 5–15.) It must be stressed that only x-rays of superb quality will allow detection of a fat pad sign.
5. Whenever a preschool child appears to have injured an elbow, and the diagnosis cannot be made by physical examination or x-ray, a condylar fracture should be presumed, the elbow should be immobilized in a posterior splint, and an x-ray examination repeated in 1–2 weeks. By that time, the pathology of healing will have produced the bone resorption and calcium deposition that will allow the diagnosis to be made by x-ray.

The neurovascular complications, the critical importance of early and repeated neurovascular examination, and the neu-

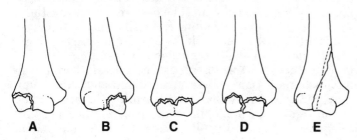

A   B   C   D   E

Fig. 5–14. Fractures of the articular surfaces of the condyles, anterior view. *A*, fracture of the capitulum. *B*, fracture of the trochlea. *C*, transverse intercondylar fracture. *D*, T-shaped intercondylar fracture. *E*, spiral fracture.

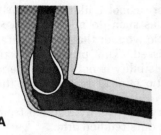 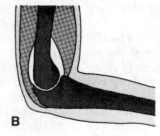

A   **B**

Fig. 5–15. Diagrammatic illustration of the fatpad sign. *A,* normal soft tissue x-ray of elbow, lateral projection. *B,* soft tissue x-ray of elbow with fluid in joint, lateral projection.

rovascular indications for referral to a vascular surgeon or an orthopaedist are the same as outlined for supracondylar fracture.

Treatment. 1. The rare fracture which is not displaced and is uncomplicated by neurovascular dysfunctions should be treated definitively by the primary physician by immobilization in a posterior splint, with the elbow as near 90° as circulation allows, and with the forearm in supination. Fractures sustained by preschool children and initially not visible by x-ray are usually undisplaced. The repeat x-rays recommended above will decide the issue.

2. All displaced fractures should be reduced by an orthopaedist in hospital. The primary physician should immobilize the injured arm in a posterior plaster splint, admit the patient to a hospital, and request an orthopaedist's prompt services.

3. Whether an undisplaced fracture which is definitively treated by the primary physician, or whether a displaced fracture only temporarily splinted by the primary physician, strict circulatory precautions must be observed, as outlined for the supracondylar fracture.

4. The principles of rehabilitation are identical to those outlined for the supracondylar fracture.

Fractures of the Medial Epicondyle

These fractures represent an avulsion of the epicondylar attachment of the flexor-pronator muscles in the forearm. Forceful elbow abduction and/or wrist dorsiflexion tend to cause this fracture. Rarely, direct tangential forces may cause it. The fracture will present in any of three degrees of displacement (See Figure 5–16.):

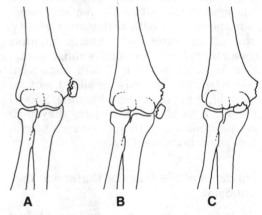

A   **B**   **C**

Fig. 5–16. Fractures of the medial epicondyle. *A,* minimal displacement. *B,* marked displacement. *C,* displacement into the joint.

1. Minimal displacement with all alignment satisfactory.

2. Distal displacement toward the joint line.

3. Displacement into the joint, between the articular surfaces of the trochlea and the ulna.

The reader will recall that the ulnar nerve courses immediately behind the medial epicondyle. The events of this injury will occasionally contuse and rarely lacerate the ulnar nerve as it rounds the elbow. As soon as this fracture is recognized, a meticulous evaluation of ulnar nerve function must be performed. The dysfunctions resulting from ulnar nerve injury at the elbow have been summarized above under "Supracondylar Fracture."

Treatment. 1. The primary care physician should treat definitively the minimally displaced fracture. The arm should be immobilized in a posterior plaster splint with the elbow as near 90° as circulation allows, the forearm pronated, and the wrist slightly flexed. (See Figure 5–17.) This position relaxes the muscles which attach to the epicondyle, thereby decreasing the likelihood of any further displacement. *During and after application of the splint, the same care to preserve the circulation must be observed as was outlined above under "Treatment" for "Supracondylar Fractures."*

2. If the fracture fragment has been displaced toward the joint line, but has not entered it, the primary physician should attempt a reduction. With the elbow slightly flexed, the flexor-pronator muscles of the forearm are relaxed by pronating the forearm and flexing the wrist. With the extremity held in this position, the operator attempts to push the displaced fragment upward to its position on the condyle, with his thumb. (See Figure 5–18.) The position of pronation and wrist flexion must be maintained from that point on. Upon completing the reduction attempt, an x-ray should be taken. If a reduction has been accomplished, the arm should be immobilized with the elbow as near 90° as circulation allows, and with the forearm in its position of pronation and wrist flexion.

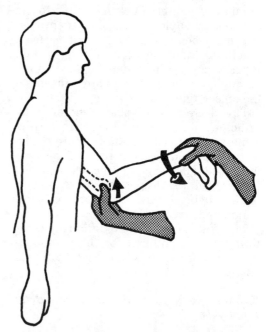

Fig. 5–18. Closed reduction of the displaced fracture of the medial epicondyle.

3. If a fracture fragment has been displaced into the joint, the arm should be splinted as for the undisplaced fracture, and the patient should be admitted to a hospital, and an orthopaedist's prompt services should be requested.

4. When ulnar nerve dysfunction is evident, and the fracture fragment is undisplaced at the outset or has been reduced by the primary physician, function may well return within a few days. It is quite proper for a primary physician to immobilize the arm as described above, and to watch for return of function for 3 days. If function returns, the primary physician should continue his treatment. If function does not return, the primary physician must refer his patient to an orthopaedist. Exploration of the nerve and anterior transposition may be required.

5. The principles of rehabilitation are identical to those outlined for the supracondylar fracture, though full rehabilitation is often attained much sooner.

Fracture of the Lateral Epicondyle

This fracture is fairly rare. Full elbow extension, full forearm pronation, and full wrist flexion are necessary for the trans-

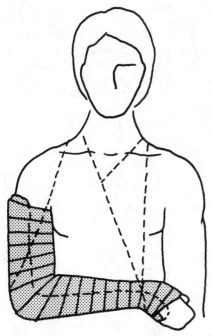

Fig. 5–17. Immobilization of reduced medial epicondyle fracture.

mission of indirect avulsing forces to the lateral epicondyle. Our involuntary protective movements tend to prevent us from assuming these positions during a fall. Equally rarely, direct avulsing forces may be applied by a glancing blow tangent to the epicondyle.

The degrees of displacement and the principles of treatment and referral are the same as described for the fracture of the medial epicondyle. However, in the case of the lateral epicondyle, the nerve at risk is the radial, and the position for relaxation of the attached muscles is forearm supination and wrist extension.

The principles of rehabilitation are identical to those outlined for the supracondylar fracture, though full rehabilitation is attained much sooner.

Fracture-Separation of an Epicondylar Epiphysis

Fracture-separation of an epicondylar epiphysis is rare in preschool children. When a fleck of displaced metaphysis suggests an epicondylar fracture separation, it should be presumed to represent a condylar fracture separation until proven otherwise by follow-up x-rays.

Fracture of the Head and Neck of the Radius (See Figure 5–19)

Children generally sustain a fracture of the neck of the radius, while adults sustain a fracture of the head of the radius. Too often, these fractures have been missed and attributed to "muscle strain or elbow sprain." The clinical characteristics of either fracture are as follows:

1. Pain will be felt in the extensor aspect of the forearm.
2. By comparing the two elbows, the examiner will usually distinguish a swelling of the injured elbow.
3. The patient will hold the elbow in slight flexion, and the forearm in pronation.
4. AP and lateral x-rays of the elbow will identify the fracture.

Most fractures of the neck of the radius are undisplaced or very minimally compressed or angulated (5° or less). These fractures need no reduction, and should be immobilized as described below. Any angulation greater than 5° should be reduced as described below.

Fractures of the head of the radius are varieties of three forms:

1. A crack into the joint line without displacement of its articular margins.
2. Fracture of a segment of the circumference of the radial head disrupting the articular surface by variable degrees of axial displacement.
3. A comminuted fracture of the head of the radius, generally distorting the articular surface.

Treatment. The object of treatment of these fractures is the restoration of a smooth radial articular surface, aligned complementary to the surface of the capitulum. If this object cannot be achieved, better function will result if the head of the radius be excised than if it be left to create a malfunctioning joint. The primary physician should proceed as follows:

Fractures of the Neck.

1. If the fracture is undisplaced or minimally displaced, the arm should be immobilized in a posterior plaster splint, with

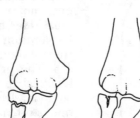

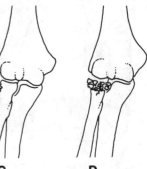

Fig. 5–19. Head and neck fractures of the radius, anterior view. *A*, fracture of neck in acceptable apposition and alignment. *B*, fracture into the joint without displacement. *C*, fracture of a segment of the disc of the radius unacceptably displaced. *D*, comminuted fracture of the head of the radius.

A   B   C   D

forearm fully supinated and the elbow as near 90° as circulation allows. Pain causes the patient to resist supination. Regional anesthesia, with or without sedation, will usually permit the maneuver. Just distal to the lateral epicondyle on the dorsum of the forearm, the radial head is a superficial structure. A needle passed down to bone from a point 2–3 cm. distal from the lateral epicondyle on the dorsum of the forearm can be made with some exploration to enter the fracture hematoma. At that point, 5–10 cc. of a local anesthetic are injected. Occasionally, a regional intravenous block may be required. See Chapter 16 for a discussion of the virtues and dangers of the different modes of regional anesthesia.

2. If displacement is unacceptable—loss of apposition or angulation greater than 5°—closed reduction must be attempted. After anesthesia as described, the elbow is fully extended, and the forearm fully supinated. While one operator applies strong traction at the wrist, the other operator applies force at the fracture site, directed appropriately to effect a reduction. After completing the attempt, the operators keep the forearm supinated, with the elbow extended or at 90°, as is easiest, and AP and lateral x-rays are taken. If reduction has been achieved, the arm is immobilized in a posterior plaster splint with the elbow as near 90° as circulation allows, and with the forearm fully supinated. If reduction has not been achieved, the arm is splinted as above, and the patient is referred on the same day to an orthopaedist.

Fracture of the Head.

1. If a fracture into the articular surface is undisplaced, or if a fracture of a segment of the disc of the radius is incomplete, splintage as above is proper.

2. If a fracture of a segment of the disc of the radius is complete and minimally displaced, satisfactory reduction may be obtained simply by full supination of the forearm. After this maneuver, x-rays are repeated. If a smooth articular surface has been restored, reduction is acceptable, and the arm should be immobilized as above. If a smooth articular surface has not been restored, the arm should be immobilized as above, and the patient referred on the same day to an orthopaedist. Open reduction may be necessary.

3. If the fracture is comminuted, and the articular surface is generally distorted, the arm should be immobilized in a posterior plaster splint in a position of comfort, the patient should be admitted to a hospital, and an orthopaedist's prompt services should be requested. Excision of the head of the radius may be necessary.

Principles of rehabilitation of both radial neck and radial head fractures are identical to those outlined for the supracondylar fracture, though full rehabilitation is often achieved much sooner.

Fractures of the Olecranon

These fractures are comparatively uncommon and are of two forms (See Figure 5–20.):

1. Avulsions of the attachment of the triceps tendon occurring when the triceps is resisting sudden great force with the elbow in slight or moderate flexion.

2. Transverse fractures through the body of the olecranon, occurring when the patient falls directly onto the olecranon of the flexed elbow.

Either fracture may be greatly or not at all displaced.

Treatment. 1. If the fracture is incomplete and undisplaced, the primary physician should immobilize the arm in comfortable flexion with a posterior plaster splint. The forearm splint may be applied loosely enough to permit forearm rotation

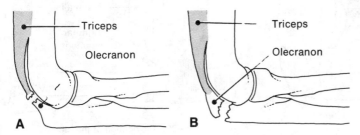

Triceps

Olecranon

Triceps

Olecranon

A   **B**

Fig. 5–20. Fractures of the olecranon. *A*, lateral view. Avulsion fracture of the tip of the olecranon. *B*, lateral view. Transverse fracture through the body of the olecranon.

as the patient desires. This immobilization should be maintained for 4–6 weeks before beginning rehabilitation.

2. If the fracture is complete and undisplaced, or only slightly displaced, the primary physician should immobilize the arm in a posterior plaster splint with the elbow at 30° flexion. This immobilization should be maintained for 4–6 weeks before beginning rehabilitation. At 30° flexion, the triceps muscle is relaxed, and the likelihood of further displacement of the fracture fragment is thereby decreased.

3'. If the fracture is complete, and moderately or markedly displaced, the primary physician should splint the arm in a posterior plaster splint, with the elbow in a position of comfort, admit the patient to a hospital, and request an orthopaedist's prompt services. Open reduction and internal fixation may be required.

4. The principles of rehabilitation are identical to those outlined for the supracondylar fracture, though full rehabilitation is often achieved much sooner.

Fractures of the Coronoid Process

An avulsion fracture of the coronoid is not rare and often is discovered when patients present with what they infer to be a sprained elbow. A sudden strong contraction of the brachialis muscle against heavy resistance can avulse its coronoid attachment. This fracture appears on x-ray as a bone chip separated a few to several millimeters from the tip of the coronoid process. (See Figure 5–21.)

Treatment. 1. Adequate reduction is nearly always obtained with the elbow flexed as near to 90° as circulation allows. Up to 5 mm. separation is acceptable.

2. If reduction is acceptable, the primary physician should immobilize the arm in a posterior plaster splint with the elbow as near 90° as circulation allows, and with the forearm in supination. Immobilization should continue for 4–6 weeks. If reduction is not acceptable, the arm should be made comfortable in a sling and an orthopaedist's services requested.

3. The principles of rehabilitation are identical to those outlined for supracondylar fracture, though full rehabilitation is often achieved much sooner.

A fracture of the body of the coronoid may accompany posterior dislocations of the elbow. This fracture is discussed in the section following.

Dislocations of the Elbow

This injury is usually sustained by young adults. The dislocation is usually posterior, and may be either lateral or medial as well. (See Figure 5–22.) The coronoid process is often but not always fractured. The radial head and either or both condyles are rarely fractured. Neurovascular injuries are less likely to complicate dislocation than to complicate condylar and supracondylar fractures, but they must be diligently looked for. The most likely form of neurovascular injury in association with the elbow dislocation will result from the circulatory impairment

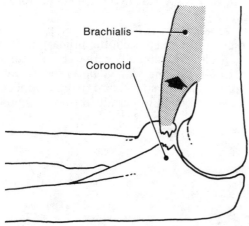

Fig. 5–21. Medial view. Avulsion fracture of the tip of the coronoid process.

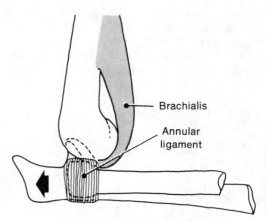

Fig. 5–22. Dislocation of the elbow.

produced by increasing tissue pressure, as blood and transudate accumulate in injured soft tissues.

Treatment. 1. After x-ray examination for associated fractures, if the humerus is intact, the primary physician should attempt to reduce the dislocation. Moderate sedation with Meperidine and diazepam as employed during reduction of glenohumeral joint dislocations will usually result in sufficient relaxation to allow a reduction. See pages 38–39 of Chapter 3. Reduction is effected by straight traction in the axis of the humerus upon the partially flexed forearm, with one hand anterior to the elbow and one on the posteriorly displaced olecranon. Countertraction from the axilla will usually be necessary. (See Figure 5–23.)

2. If the coronoid is fractured, a followup x-ray should be made to insure that the loose fragment has not been drawn into the joint, and that with the elbow as near 90° as circulation allows, it is nearly apposed to the body of the coronoid. If its position is acceptable, further treatment is identical to that for the uncomplicated dislocation. If unacceptable, an orthopaedist's services must be requested.

3. If the radial head is fractured, it must be treated as described above under "Fracture of the Head."

4. If either or both condyles are fractured, the services of an orthopaedist should be requested immediately. Only if an orthopaedist is unavailable and the circulation to the forearm is impaired should the primary physician attempt to reduce this combined fracture dislocation. The reduction manipulation is the same as that described in paragraph 1 above. Otherwise, the arm should be immobilized as it is in a posterior plaster splint, and the patient admitted to a hospital to await the services of the orthopaedist. The arm should be elevated, and the circulation evaluated at least every 30 minutes.

5. Once the uncomplicated dislocation is reduced, the arm should be immobilized in a posterior plaster splint, with the elbow as near 90° as circulation will allow, and with the forearm in moderate supination. This position should be maintained for 4 weeks.

6. The principles of rehabilitation are identical to those outlined for the supracondylar fracture.

Congenital and Acquired Deformities

Occasionally, injured patients will be encountered whose physical and x-ray findings are inconsistent with each other and with the history of the injury. Generally, these dilemmas arise when a deformity antedates an injury. Acquired deformities are probably more common than congenital deformities. In general, the deformities are these:

1. Congenital malformations of the condyles, the radial head, or the trochlear fossa of the ulna.

2. Malunited condylar fractures missed in preschool years.

3. Old displaced epicondylar fractures.

4. Malunited radial head or neck fractures.

5. Persistent subluxations of the radial head, missed in infancy, and now irreducible except by surgery, due to the normal overgrowth of the radial head.

When these dilemmas arise, orthopaedic interpretation is generally required.

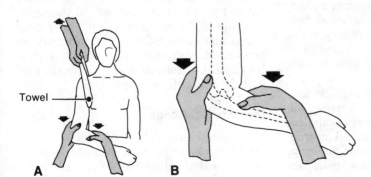

Towel

A   **B**

Fig. 5–23. Reduction of elbow dislocation.

Two Major Complications of Severe Elbow Injury

Volkmann's Ischemic Contracture

This most calamitous of complications results from overlong impairment of blood supply to the muscles of the forearm. If ischemic too long, the muscles die, undergo autolysis, and are eventually replaced by fibrous tissue. The ultimate result is complete paralysis and grotesque flexion deformity of the fingers and wrist.

Severe elbow injuries can produce this complication in three ways:

1. The brachial artery can be disrupted by laceration or by contusion and eventual thrombosis. These disruptions prevent inward blood flow adequate to nourish the muscles.

2. A contused brachial artery can develop an intense arteriospasm in reaction to its injury—so intense as to prevent inward blood flow adequate to nourish the muscles.

3. As blood and transudate accumulate in and around the elbow, tissue pressure rises until venous return is obstructed. As venous return diminishes, the rate and pressure of transudation increase until tissue pressure is eventually as great as precapillary pressure, and at this point inward blood flow to the muscles ceases. As any flexion of the elbow increases the tissue pressure at the elbow, there is a degree of flexion beyond which this deterioration of circulation is very likely to occur.

Not only severe elbow injuries are vulnerable to this complication. Any injury treated with a long arm cast with the elbow in flexion can result in this complication. All that is required is that the cast be applied with a tightness close to venous pressure, and that continued bleeding or transudation swell the arm against a rigid cast until venous pressure is exceeded. Shortly thereafter, the precapillary pressure will be approached, and circulation will become inadequate for muscle survival.

Hence, no elbow injury should be immobilized in a rigid circular dressing; all elbow injuries should be closely watched for circulatory impairment; and all injured extremities treated by a circular dressing, particularly a long arm cast must be closely watched for circulatory impairment.

The signs and symptoms of circulatory impairment are the following:

1. The patient complains of severe intractable pain in the forearm and fingers, worsened by any attempt actively or passively to extend the fingers. This complaint is the earliest sign. In time, signs 2–4 appear.

2. The fingers are swollen and cyanotic or pale.

3. While pressure on the nail plate of the normal finger will induce blanching of the nail bed, followed by a return of the pink color upon release, similar pressure in a setting of circulatory obstruction may further blanch a cyanotic or pallid nail bed, but release will *not* result in rapid appearance of a normal pink color.

4. The patient will acknowledge paresthesias and hypesthesias in the fingers.

Should any of these signs appear, all constrictive dressings should be removed or at least loosened. A cast may be slit and the slit levered open enough to relieve the symptoms and signs of circulatory insufficiency. When a widened slit yields inadequate release, the cast must be bivalved, and soft wrappings cut through as well. When these measures prove inadequate, all dressings must be removed and the elbow fully extended. If even these measures yield no relief, immediate surgical intervention is mandatory: either in the form of a fasciotomy or vascular repair, or both.

Pain in a cast can never be ignored or treated with analgesics until circulation is proved by careful examination to be inadequate: warm fingers and pink nailbeds with brisk capillary return, no more than tolerable increase in pain with persistent active finger motion, and normal sensation in some if not all fingers (e.g., early convalescence from a Colles fracture may be associated with some median nerve dysfunction, but sensation in the fourth and fifth fingers will be normal).

Myositis Ossificans

A later complication of elbow injury which can be crippling if improperly managed is calcification and eventual ossification in injured muscles and deep fascia. At any point during rehabilitation, the condition may reveal itself by increase in pain and a decrease in range of motion. If in the early stage of calcification all passive stretching exercise be discontinued, and the extent of motion during active exercise be decreased, the calcium may resorb, and ossification be prevented. Any ossification that occurs cannot be reversed. Bone in muscle and deep fascia will obviously weaken and limit elbow motion.

Hence, a persistent increase in pain during rehabilitation demands a decrease in the vigor of the active exercise program, and a cessation of any passive exercise. Upon the appearance of calcification, we advise that an orthopaedist be involved.

CHAPTER 6

The Forearm, Wrist, and Hand

Essential Anatomy

The Anatomy of Forearm Rotation

Like the anatomy of the proximal ends of the radius and ulna, so are the distal ends accommodated to each other to allow rotation of the forearm; and like the proximal radio-ulnar joint, which by its inclusion within the capsule and synovial lining of the elbow joint is thus a synovial joint, so too the distal radio-ulnar joint, by its inclusion within the capsule and synovial lining of the radiocarpal joint, is a synovial joint. Normal function of both the proximal and distal radio-ulnar joints, as well as of the radiohumeral joint are necessary for rotation of the forearm to be full, brisk, and painless. The proximal joint has been described in a previous chapter. The distal joint is the articulation between a semilunar-shaped facet on the ulnar side of the epiphysis of the radius, and the disciform surface of the radial side of the epiphysis of the ulna. (See Figure 6–1.) During rotation at the distal radio-ulnar joint, the radius glides around the arc of the ulna, while at the proximal radio-ulnar joint, the disc of the radius rotates within the radial

groove of the ulna. While the proximal end of the radius and ulna are firmly apposed by the annular ligament, the distal ends of the radius and ulna are granted somewhat more play by the pliant capsule of the distal joint. This play is critical. Because the curve of the disciform medial surface of the epiphysis of the ulna is eccentric, the ulna angulates away from the center line of the forearm 8–9° as the arm rotates from full supination to full pronation. (See Figure 6–2.) Any process which causes the capsule of the distal joint to become less pliant, thus decreasing the play of the joint, will limit forearm rotation and/or cause it to be painful.

Rotation of the forearm is effected by four muscles. (See Figure 6–3.) Two effect supination, and two effect pronation. Supination is effected by:

1. The *supinator muscle* which angulates distally over the dorsum of the proximal third of the forearm from its broad origin upon the lateral epicondyle of the humerus, the radial collateral and annular ligaments, and the proximal end of the ulna, to its insertion on the anterolateral surface of the proximal one-third of the radius. It is innervated by the radial nerve.

2. The *biceps muscle* which inserts upon the radial tuberosity on the ulnar surface of the radius, just distal to the annular ligament. It is innervated by a branch of the musculocutaneous nerve.

Pronation is effected by:

1. The *pronator teres* which angulates distally from its bicapital origin upon the medial epicondyle of the humerus and coronoid process of the ulna, to insert on the anterolateral surface of the middle one-third of the radius. It is innervated by a branch of the median nerve.

2. The *pronator quadratus* which passes transversely across the distal one-third of the forearm from its origin upon the anterior surface of the ulna to its insertion upon the anterior surface of the radius. It too is innervated by a branch of the median nerve.

It should be apparent from the discussion above that the alignment of the shafts of the radius and ulna, the independence of their mobility, the correct apposition of their two articulations, and the play at the distal articulation determine the range and comfort of forearm rotation. The principles of treatment of forearm fractures derive from a respect for these relationships.

The Anatomy of the Wrist Joint

The movements of the wrist occur at four joints (see Figure 6-4):

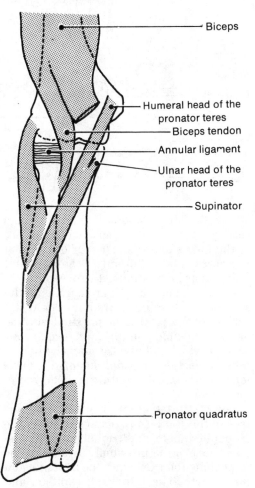

Fig. 6-3. Rotators of the forearm.

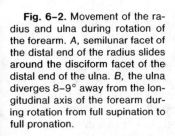

Dorsal surface

Disciform facet of the ulna

Semilunar facet of the radius

Volar surface

Fig. 6-1. Distal end of the radioulnar joint—forearm in midrotation.

Fig. 6-2. Movement of the radius and ulna during rotation of the forearm. *A*, semilunar facet of the distal end of the radius slides around the disciform facet of the distal end of the ulna. *B*, the ulna diverges 8–9° away from the longitudinal axis of the forearm during rotation from full supination to full pronation.

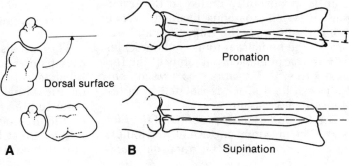

Dorsal surface

Pronation

Supination

A   B

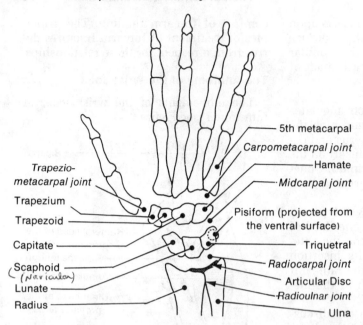

Fig. 6–4. Skeletal anatomy of the wrist—dorsal view.

The Radiocarpal Joint. The proximal surface of this joint is the articular surface of the radius and the *articular disc* which lies across the distal end of the ulna and radio-ulnar joint, attached between the ulnar styloid and the ulnar margin of the articular surface of the radius. The distal surface of this joint is the proximal surface of the *scaphoid, lunate,* and *triquetrum,* each of which is united to its neighbor by *interosseous intercarpal ligaments.* This joint communicates with the distal radioulnar joint.

The Midcarpal Joint. The proximal surface of this joint is the distal surface of the scaphoid, lunate, and triquetrum. The distal surface is the proximal surfaces of the trapezium, the trapezoid, the capitate, and the hamate. The trapezoid, capitate, and hamate are united to each other by interosseous intercarpal ligaments. The trapezium is inconstantly united to the trapezoid by an interosseous ligament. When no ligament unites the trapezium and trapezoid, the midcarpal joint communicates with the carpometacarpal joints of the fingers. When this ligament is present, the midcarpal joint space is isolated from the other three wrist joints.

The Carpometacarpal Joints of the Fingers. The proximal surface of this joint is the distal surfaces of the trapezoid, capi-

tate, and hamate. The distal surface is the proximal end of the 2nd through 5th metacarpal bones.

The Trapeziometacarpal Joint. The proximal surface of this joint is the lateral surface of the trapezium. The distal surface of the joint is the proximal surface of the 1st metacarpal. This joint space never communicates with the other joint spaces.

The radiocarpal joint allows for most of the ulnar deviation and the midcarpal joint allows for most of the radial deviation, while both joints together allow for full palmar and dorsal flexion. The carpometacarpal joints of the fingers allow for those small movements of the metacarpals which accommodate the hand to opposition and to the grasping of objects of various shapes and sizes. The trapeziometacarpal joint allows for abduction, adduction, and opposition by the thumb.

Carpal Tunnel

The carpals as a whole present a concave palmar surface which is deepened by tubercles of the scaphoid and trapezium on the radial side, and by the pisiform bone and the hamulus of the hamate bone on the ulnar side. This flume is converted into a tunnel by the tough *flexor retinaculum* which stretches between the tubercle of the scaphoid and the ulnar styloid. The eight flexors of the fingers, the long flexor of the thumb, and the median nerve share the space of this tunnel. The palmaris longus, the ulnar artery, and the palmar branch of the ulnar nerve lie on the flexor retinaculum outside the tunnel. This tunnel may be narrowed by bony deformities which result from fractures, by the bony spurs of osteoarthritis, by swelling of the synovium of the tendons, and by thickening of the flexor retinaculum. Variations in extracellular fluid volume may cause variations in the compressive symptoms resulting from a narrowing of the carpal tunnel.

The Palmar Tendons of the Wrist and Hand

While several variations will be encountered, the purposes of this text will be adequately served by a description of the usual anatomy.

Three tendons are superficial to the flexor retinaculum (see Figure 6–5):

1. The flexor carpi ulnaris which lies in the extreme ulnar palmar corner of the wrist until it inserts on the pisiform bone, which articulates with the palmar surface of the triquetrum. Its muscle is innervated by the ulnar nerve.

2. The palmaris longus, which is visible just ulnar to the midline of the wrist until it expands into the palmar aponeurosis as it enters the palm. Its muscle is innervated by the median nerve.

3. The flexor carpi radialis which is visible just radial to the midline of the wrist until it passes into a tunnel of its own, created by a splitting of the radial border of the flexor retinaculum, just before the tendon inserts on the base of the 2nd metacarpal. Its muscle is innervated by the median nerve.

The ulnar nerve lies just deep to the flexor carpi ulnaris on the outer side of the flexor retinaculum and passes on the radial side of the pisiform bone. The median nerve lies deep to the palmaris longus on the inner side of the flexor retinaculum.

Nine tendons are deep to the flexor retinaculum. (1–8) The flexor digitorum sublimis and profundus course through the middle of the wrist. The four flexor sublimis tendons lie superficial to the two fused flexor profundus tendons. About the midpalm, the two fused profundus tendons split into four. At the base of each proximal phalanx, each sublimis tendon splits, and the associated profundus tendon surfaces through the division to course superficially along the proximal and middle phalanges, to its insertion upon the base of the terminal phalanx. The divided sublimis tendon courses around the profundus tendon, comes together again dorsal to it, and separates again to insert on either side of the palmar surface of the base of the middle phalanx. The muscle of the sublimis tendons and the radial half of the muscle of the profundus tendons are innervated by the median nerve. The ulnar half of the muscle of the profundus tendons is innervated by the ulnar nerve.

(9) The flexor pollicis longus courses immediately to the radial side of the flexor tendons of the fingers. As it emerges from the carpal tunnel, it passes deep to the muscles of the thenar eminence along the palmar surface of the thumb, to insert upon the base of the terminal phalanx. Its muscle is innervated by the median nerve.

The Surgical Spaces of the Hand

As these spaces are essentially palmar spaces, they are most logically discussed at this point. Synovial and fascial planes separate the deep contents of the hand into four or five spaces. (See Figure 6–6.) Before the advent of antibiotics, knowledge of these spaces was fundamental to the accepted surgical treatment of hand infections, as hand infections tend to spread and be confined within these spaces. Today knowledge of these spaces, while less fundamental to treatment, still can lead a physician to a correct analysis of the initial extent and eventual course of a hand infection.

1. The common synovial tendon sheath of the flexor muscles. The eight flexor tendons are enclosed within this sheath in the carpal tunnel and proximal half of the palm. In the midpalm, the six tendons to the index, middle, and ring finger pass out of the common sheath and continue to their respective fingers as unsheathed tendons, while the two tendons to the fifth

finger continue within the common sheath to a point a few millimeters proximal to the attachment of the profundus tendon of the fifth finger to the base of its terminal phalanx. The six unsheathed tendons pass into individual digital tendon sheaths just proximal to each metacarpophalangeal (MP) joint and continue within these

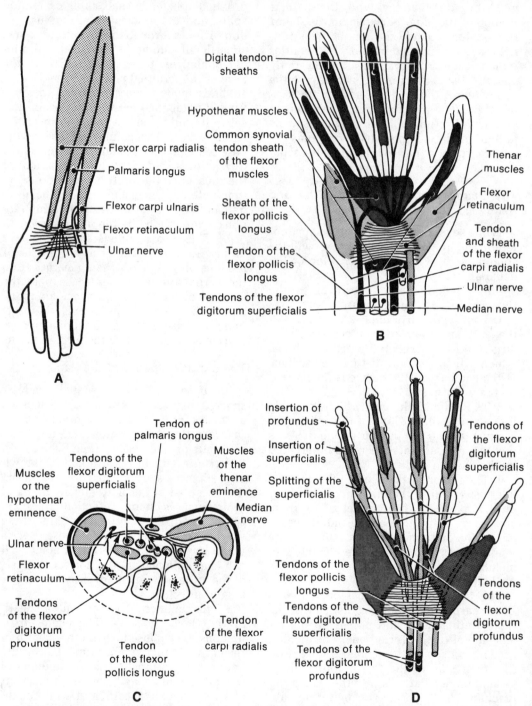

Fig. 6–5. Palmar tendons of the wrist and hand. *A*, superficial tendons. *B*, nerves and tendons deep to the palmaris longus. *C*, transverse section of the carpal tunnel. *D*, relationships of the flexor digitorum in the hand.

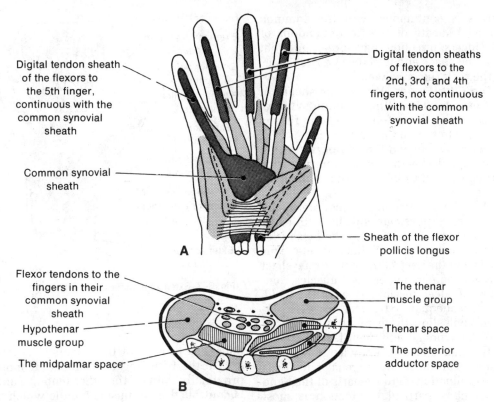

Fig. 6-6. Surgical spaces of the hand. *A,* tendon sheaths of the palm. *B,* deep palmar spaces of the hand—cross section through the palm.

sheaths to a point a few millimeters proximal to the attachments of each profundus tendon to its terminal phalanx.

2. The tendon sheath of the flexor pollicus longus. The flexor pollicus longus tendon is usually sheathed independently from the other tendons of the hand as it passes through the carpal tunnel and the palm. The tendon continues within its sheath to a point a few millimeters proximal to its attachment to the terminal phalanx of the thumb. Occasionally, the synovial space of the thumb communicates with the common synovial space of the flexor tendon to the fingers.

3-5. The deep fascial spaces of the palm. Deep to the flexor tendons and the lumbrical muscles in the palm, and overlying the metacarpals and the interosseous muscles, and the adductor muscle of the thumb, is a layer of loose connective tissue through which fluids and microorganisms can readily percolate. This layer of loose connective tissue is securely separated into

three spaces by the *midpalmar septum* and the adductor muscle of the thumb.

The *midpalmar space* lies deep to the flexor tendons of the index, middle, and ring fingers and merges with the deep fascia surrounding the proximal borders of the individual digital tendon sheaths. The *thenar space* lies between the muscles of the thenar eminence and the adductor muscle of the thumb. The posterior *adductor space* lies between the adductor muscle of the thumb and the first interosseous muscle.

Infections in the hand tend to be confined to one of the five spaces and usually do not violate the boundary of those spaces until tissue autolysis is advanced. The infection of wounds on the palmar surfaces of the fingers will spread, if at all, as follows:

The Thumb. Within the sheath of the flexor pollicus longus, and/or into the thenar and/or posterior adductor spaces. When the sheath of the flexor pollicus longus is continuous with the common synovial sheath of the flexor tendons of the fingers, infection may spread into that synovial space and into the synovial space of the fifth finger as well.

The Fifth Finger. Within the sheath of its flexor tendon to the common synovial space of the flexor tendons to the fingers and/or into the midpalmar space.

Index, Middle and Ring Fingers. Within their digital sheaths and, after rupturing through the sheaths, into the midpalmar space.

Most hand infections encountered by the primary physician still lie within the subcutaneous fascia and in the loose connective tissue between the subcutaneous fascia and the deep connective tissue sheet that surrounds the bones, muscles, tendons, and deep fascial spaces of the hand. When inadequately treated, however, autolysis will allow these infections to spread into the synovial and deep fascial spaces of the hand. Hence, knowledge of these spaces will allow the physician to focus his examination on those parts of the hand to which a particular infection is most likely to spread. Of course, wounds can directly enter those spaces and allow deep space infection at the outset.

The Dorsal Tendons of the Wrist and Hand

These are the extensor tendons to the wrist and fingers. (See Figure 6-7).

Extensors of the Wrist. The tendons which control wrist motion alone create the four corners of the wrist. The flexor tendons have been described in an earlier section. The extensors are the following:

1. Extensor carpi radialis longus and brevis together form the dorsal radial angle of the wrist and insert upon the base of the 2nd and 3rd metacarpals respectively. They are both innervated by the radial nerve.

2. Extensor carpi ulnaris forms the dorsal ulnar corner of the wrist and inserts upon the base of the 5th metacarpal. Its muscle is innervated by the radial nerve.

Extensors of the Fingers. Two muscle groups control these tendons, the extensor digitorum and the extensor indicis. The extensor digitorum splits into four ten-

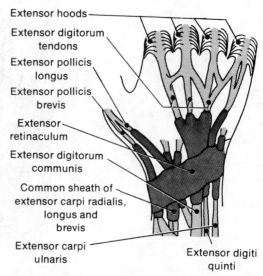

Extensor hoods
Extensor digitorum tendons
Extensor pollicis longus
Extensor pollicis brevis
Extensor retinaculum
Extensor digitorum communis
Common sheath of extensor carpi radialis, longus and brevis
Extensor carpi ulnaris
Extensor digiti quinti

Fig. 6-7. Extensor tendons of the wrist and fingers.

dons, one to each of the fingers. The tendon to the fifth finger separates off more proximally than do the other tendons, and is controlled by a muscle bundle which is rather distinct from the bulk of the extensor digitorum. Hence, this tendon and its controlling muscle bundle have been named independently the extensor digiti minimi. The extensor indicis is a shorter muscle than the extensor digitorum, entirely separate from it, which controls a tendon to the index finger which merges with the branch of the extensor digitorum to the index finger just proximal to the MP joint. Intertendinous slips cross between each of the tendons. All the tendons cross the wrist under the extensor retinaculum.

At each MP joint, each extensor tendon expands to form an *extensor hood* which tends to cover the sides of the joint as well as its dorsum and which more distally receives attachments from the lumbrical and interosseous muscles. At each proximal interphalangeal joint, each extensor hood separates into two lateral bands, and one central band. The central band inserts upon the base of the middle phalanx while the lateral bands cross the joint on either side and come together over the dorsum of the middle phalanx, to continue as a single band to an insertion upon the base of the terminal phalanx.

The Radial Tendons of the Hand

Three tendons bound what is known as the anatomic snuffbox over the radial aspect of the wrist (see Figure 6-8):

1. The extensor pollicis longus forms the dorsal boundary of the anatomic snuffbox, and continues distally to insert upon the base of the terminal phalanx. The muscle of this tendon is innervated by the radial nerve.

2-3. The extensor pollicis brevis and abductor pollicis longus form the palmar boundary of the anatomic snuffbox. The extensor pollicis brevis continues directly distally to insert upon the dorsal surface of the base of the proximal phalanx of the thumb, and the abductor pollicis longus spirals distally around the wrist to insert upon the radial surface of the base of the 1st metacarpal. The muscles of these tendons are innervated by the radial nerve.

The Intrinsic Muscles of the Hand

These muscles lie in three groups, each of which controls one of the three fundamental parts of the hand.

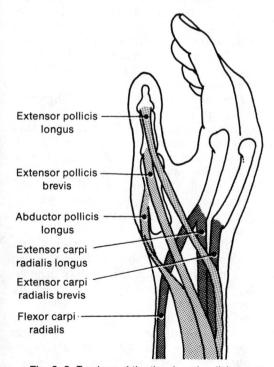

Extensor pollicis longus

Extensor pollicis brevis

Abductor pollicis longus

Extensor carpi radialis longus

Extensor carpi radialis brevis

Flexor carpi radialis

Fig. 6-8. Tendons of the thumb and radial aspect of the wrist.

The Short Muscles of the Thumb. (See Figure 6-9.) The muscles of the thenar eminence are the abductor pollicis brevis centrally, the flexor pollicus brevis on its palmar distal side, and the opponens on its radial proximal side. All three originate from the flexor retinaculum and trapezium. The abductor pollicis brevis inserts upon the base of the radial surface of the proximal phalanx, the flexor pollicis brevis inserts upon the base of the palmar surface of the proximal phalanx, and the opponens inserts on the radial side of the body of the 1st metacarpal. These muscles are chiefly innervated by the median nerve.

Deep to the thenar eminence on the floor of the thenar fascial space lies the adductor pollicis. As a palmar muscle and an adductor, it is homologous to the palmar interosseous muscles to the fingers. It arises from the bases of the 1st and 2nd metacarpal, the floor of the carpal tunnel, and the shaft of the 3rd metacarpal, and inserts upon the ulnar sesamoid and the ulnar surface of the base of the proximal phalanx. It is chiefly innervated by the ulnar nerve.

Muscles of the Central Compartment. (See Figure 6-10.) The *lumbrical muscles* are four in number and lie between the flexor tendons to the fingers. They arise from the profundus tendons and attach to the radial side of the extensor hoods. They extend the interphalangeal (IP) joints while flexing the MP joints. They are variably innervated, the radial two tending to be innervated by branches from the median nerve, and the ulnar two tending to be innervated by branches from the ulnar nerve.

The interosseous muscles lie between the metacarpals in two layers—a palmar layer and a dorsal layer. The palmar layer effects adduction of the fingers, and the dorsal layer abduction of the fingers. The palmar muscles attach to the adductor surface of each extensor hood. The dorsal muscles attach to the abductor surface of the base of each proximal phalanx. They are generally innervated by branches of the ulnar nerve, but on occasion the 1st dorsal interosseous muscle is innervated by a branch of the median nerve.

Hypothenar Muscles. (See Figure 6-11.)

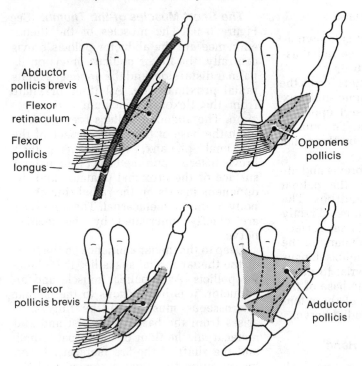

Abductor
pollicis brevis

Flexor
retinaculum

Flexor
pollicis
longus —

Opponens
pollicis

Flexor
pollicis brevis

Adductor
pollicis

Fig. 6–9. Short muscles of the thumb.

The most superficial muscle, the palmaris brevis, works with the palmaris longus from which it originates, to harden the palm. It inserts into the skin of the ulnar border of the palm.

The three deeper muscles control some of the movements and postures of the fifth finger. The abductor digiti minimi originates upon the pisiform bone and inserts into the ulnar side of the base of the proximal phalanx of the fifth finger. The flexor digiti minimi brevis arises from the hamulus and the flexor retinaculum and inserts with the abductor digiti minimi upon the ulnar side of the base of the proximal phalanx. The opponens digiti minimi lies largely deep to these muscles. It arises from the flexor retinaculum and the hamulus of the hamate, and inserts upon the ulnar palmar surface of the 5th metacarpal. All these muscles are innervated by branches of the ulnar nerve.

Fractures of the Forearm

General Principles for Treatment of Forearm Fractures

Evaluation and treatment of all forearm fractures are founded upon 15 principles.

1. When only one of two parallel bones is fractured, the fracture cannot be displaced unless one of the articulations between the two bones has been disrupted. Therefore, the displaced fracture of one bone implies a dislocation, either of the radiohumeral joint, and with it the proximal radial ulnar joint, or of the distal radial ulnar joint. (See Figure 6–12.)

2. As both supinators attach to the proximal third of the radius, and both pronators attach distal to the proximal third, the proximal fragment of any fracture through the proximal third of the radius will be rotated into supination. Therefore, fractures through the proximal third of the forearm must be immobilized with the forearm in full supination. (See Figure 6–13.)

3. As the pronator teres attaches just proximal to the midpoint of the radius, the proximal fragment of the fracture through the middle third will generally be held by the supinators and the pronator teres in neutral rotation. Therefore, fractures through the middle third of the forearm must be immobilized in neutral rotation (thumb up). (See Figure 6–14.)

4. As the pronator quadratus attaches to

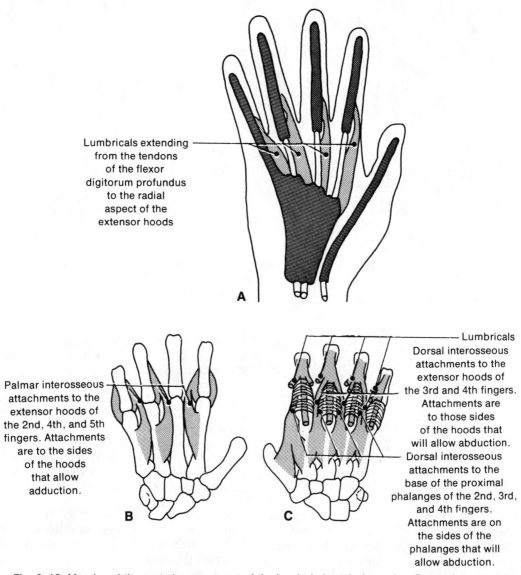

Lumbricals extending from the tendons of the flexor digitorum profundus to the radial aspect of the extensor hoods

A

Palmar interosseous attachments to the extensor hoods of the 2nd, 4th, and 5th fingers. Attachments are to the sides of the hoods that allow adduction.

B

Lumbricals

Dorsal interosseous attachments to the extensor hoods of the 3rd and 4th fingers. Attachments are to those sides of the hoods that will allow abduction.

Dorsal interosseous attachments to the base of the proximal phalanges of the 2nd, 3rd, and 4th fingers. Attachments are on the sides of the phalanges that will allow abduction.

C

Fig. 6–10. Muscles of the central compartment of the hand. *A,* lumbrical muscles. *B,* attachments of the palmar interossei. *C,* attachments of the dorsal interossei.

the volar surface of most of the distal third of the radius and ulna, fragments of fractures through the distal third are unlikely to become displaced in rotation. Therefore, experts with plaster can often hold a reduction of a distal third fracture with a forearm cast alone, allowing the patient freedom of forearm rotation and elbow motion throughout the healing period. However, to be so effective, the forearm cast must be skin tight, swelling at the time of casting should be minimal, and venous drainage must remain optimal if further swelling and the resultant ischemia are to be avoided. A somewhat looser cast can hold the reduction if the forearm is immobilized in full rotation: pronation when the distal fragment has been—and so may tend after reduction to become—dorsally angulated, supination when the distal fragment has been—and so may tend after reduction to become—ventrally angulated. (See Figure 6–15.) Note that some orthopaedists disagree with the value of prona-

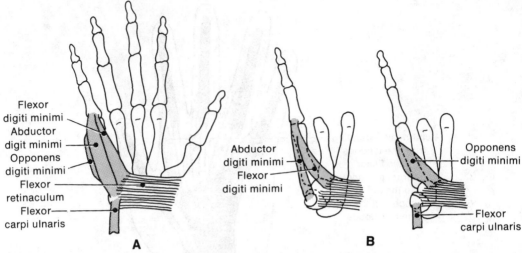

Flexor digiti minimi
Abductor digit minimi
Opponens digiti minimi
Flexor retinaculum
Flexor carpi ulnaris

A

Abductor digiti minimi
Flexor digiti minimi

Opponens digiti minimi

Flexor carpi ulnaris

B

Fig. 6–11. Muscles of the hypothenar eminence. *A,* composite view. *B,* dissected view.

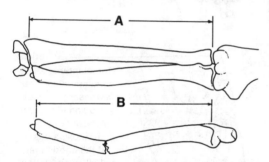

Fig. 6–12. First principle of treatment of forearm fractures. Radio-ulnar or radiohumeral joint or both must dislocate if the bone is to be free to angulate, as *B* will be shorter than *A.*

tion for immobilization of fractures of the distal third of the forearm and point out that the consequent increased stiffness far outweighs any theoretical advantage. Some of these physicians will even immobilize a Colles' fracture in supination and slight dorsiflexion. Unlike them, we have not yet abandoned the classic position for distal one-third fractures. The classic positions are justified by two presumptions:

a. When on stretch, as they would be with the forearm in full supination, the pronator teres and pronator quadratus muscles may create a ventrally directed force upon the fracture line, thereby resisting ventral angulation (apex pointing dorsally), and facilitating dorsal angulation (apex pointing ventrally).

b. A cast which holds the forearm in full

rotation will apply its rotating force upon the head of the radius, thereby tending to prevent dorsal angulation of the distal fragment when holding pronation, and ventral angulation of the distal fragment when holding supination.

5. Rotational forces may fracture both bones at different levels. These fractures should be immobilized with the forearm in that position of rotation dictated by the level of the radial fracture.

6. Fractures of the shafts of both bones of the forearm in normal adults usually require open reduction and internal fixation.

7. In contrast, fractures of both bones of the forearm in children usually can be reduced and held by closed reduction and external fixation.

8. Bone growth in children allows for a degree of remodelling that will correct greater displacements and angulations than can the remodelling available to adult bones. Hence, reductions unacceptable for adults may be quite acceptable for children, and much preferable to the risks of open reduction and internal fixation. Three rules govern the application of this principle:

a. The younger the child, the greater the correction possible.

b. The closer the fracture to an epiphyseal plate, the greater the correction possible.

c. Angulation opposite the physiologic

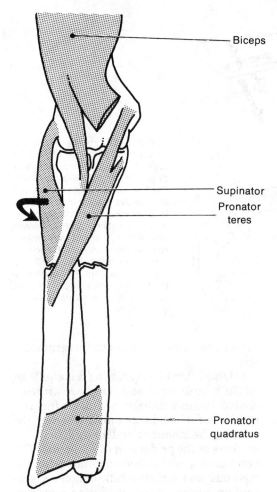

apposition and alignment, and immobilized in plaster.

10. Difficult reductions of complete fractures are often simplified by placing the arm in hanging traction with as much weight as necessary to make the bone free for manipulation.

11. When strong traction and appropriate manipulations fail to restore apposition and acceptable angulation of a fracture, muscle may be impaled between the fragments. Such fractures may require open reduction and must be referred to an orthopaedist.

12. The duration of immobilization and whether in full or forearm plaster depend

Fig. 6–13. Second principle of treatment of forearm fractures. Proximal fragment of the radius supinates following fractures through the proximal third of the forearm, as the action of the supinator is unopposed.

curve of a bone is more likely to correct than an equal angulation beyond the physiologic curve of a bone. (See Figure 6–16.)

9. Incomplete fractures that are angulated are more likely to increase their angulation after immobilization or to re-angulate after reduction and immobilization than are complete fractures. Therefore, when incomplete fractures are angulated, they should be fractured through by a quick force in the direction opposite to the initial angulation. This maneuver is conveniently executed over the operator's knee by a quick short movement identical to that used to break a stick for the fire. The fragments are then moved into proper

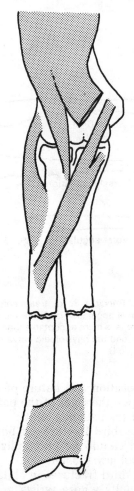

Fig. 6–14. Third principle of treatment of fractures of the forearm. Proximal half of the radius remains in neutral rotation following fractures through the middle third of the forearm, as the action of the pronator teres balances the action of the supinators.

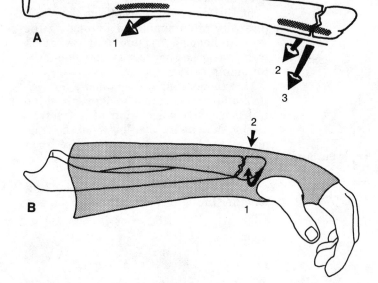

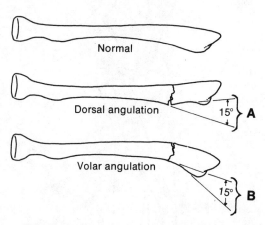

Fig. 6–15. Fourth principle of treatment of fractures of the forearm. *A, 1* and *2* are vectors of pronators when on stretch with the forearm in full supination. *3* is the resultant vector at the fracture line resisting volar displacement and angulation, and facilitating dorsal displacement and angulation. In full pronation, these vectors are eliminated. *B,* recoil vector of the forearm (*1*) is neutralized by the resistance of the rigid cast (*2*), thus opposing dorsal angulation.

Fig. 6–16. Principle 8c of treatment of forearm fractures. Dorsal angulation opposite the physiologic curve of the bone is more acceptable than equal volar angulation beyond the physiologic curve of the bone. Angle A = angle B.

upon the location and nature of the fracture and upon the vigor of the patient and the state of the patient's joints:

a. Middle third fractures of both bones in children should be immobilized for 8 weeks in full-arm plaster.

b. Distal third fractures in children and vigorous adults whose wrists and hands are not arthritic, and whose fractures are not comminuted, and are holding a near-anatomic reduction, should be immobilized for 4 weeks in full-arm plaster, and for an additional 4 weeks in forearm plaster.

c. Distal third fractures in frail adults or adults whose wrist and hand are arthritic should be immobilized in full or forearm plaster for 4 weeks at most, whether the fracture be comminuted or not, and regardless of the perfection of reduction. The additional 4 weeks recommended for the vigorous non-arthritic folk is more a precaution against re-injury during a vulnerable time than a primary necessity to prevent malunion. The frail and arthritic stand a greater chance of permanent wrist dysfunction from overlong immobilization than from refracture during an incautious moment in the vulnerable second 4 weeks.

13. Particularly in the frail and arthritic, the structure of the cast is as important to optimal rehabilitation as is the perfection of reduction. Rehabilitation begins with active finger and shoulder exercises as soon as the cast is applied. For active finger exercise to be possible, volar flexion (though a necessary position of immobilization for those fractures which were dorsally angulated by the injury) cannot be extreme, and the application of the cast to the hand must not block the MP joints. The proper cast will extend to the heads of the metacarpals dorsally, but only to the necks of the metacarpals ventrally. The

necks of the metacarpals lie deep to the distal palmar crease; that line is taken as the distal limit of the palmar surface of the cast. The entire thumb, including the 1st metacarpal and thenar eminence should be left free, such that the trapeziometacarpal joint can maintain its range of motion as well as the MP and IP joints. Where the cast passes over the thenar web, it must be kept as thin as possible, and its margins must be smoothly padded to prevent abrasions at the base of the thumb. When active finger motion is restricted by improper casting, the ensuing stiffness—which will be dramatically evident when the cast is removed—may never yield to the most persistent, tactful rehabilitation.

14. The first few days after the cast is applied, particular effort must be made to keep the hand above the level of the heart, and to keep the fingers moving, and thus the muscle pump working. If these active precautions are not taken, swelling will lead to ischemia, the cast will have to be loosened, and an optimal reduction may be lost.

15. As mentioned above, rehabilitation begins at once with finger and shoulder motion. As soon as a full-arm cast is shortened into a forearm cast, elbow motion is added to the regimen. As soon as the forearm cast is removed, wrist motion in all four directions and forearm rotation are added to the regimen. Particularly for the frail and elderly, a physical therapist's services are advisable. The duration of remobilization will last at least as long as the duration of immobilization.

Applying these principles, the primary practitioner should treat all undisplaced fractures and most displaced fractures in adults and children and should splint and refer all displaced fractures at the midshaft of both bones in adults, and all fractures that resist acceptable reduction.

Two examples of forearm fractures deserve specific discussion:

The Monteggia Fracture (See Figure 6–17)

This fracture is a classic example of the first principle stated above. This injury combines the anatomically necessary dis-

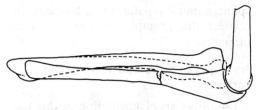

Fig. 6–17. Monteggia fracture. The distal radio-ulnar joint remains intact. Thus, the proximal radio-ulnar and radiohumeral joints must dislocate if the ulna is to angulate. The *dotted* lines indicate the position in which the radius must remain if the radio-ulnar and radiohumeral joints are to remain intact.

location of the radiohumeral and proximal radio-ulnar joints with a markedly angulated fracture through the upper third of the ulna. When the first principle has been unknown or ignored, practitioners have missed the dislocation and treated only the ulnar fracture, and the patient has developed a permanent elbow dysfunction. While the theory of the first principle implies that the ulnar fracture could displace in association with a dislocation of the distal radio-ulnar joint, the forces that produce the Monteggia fracture disrupt the proximal articulations invariably. In England, the injury occurs most typically to motorists who drive along narrow, walled or hedged lanes, with an arm resting elbow-out on the window frame until the proximal ulna impacts a rigid protrusion. The fractured ulna is typically angulated posteriorly, that is, the apex is directed toward the volar surface. When such a fracture of the proximal ulna is encountered, adequate x-rays of the elbow joint must be obtained. When the angulation is marked, x-rays will almost invariably confirm an anterior dislocation of the radial head from its articulation with the humerus and ulna. When the angulation is slight, x-rays may demonstrate a fracture of the head or neck of the radius, instead of the dislocation.

Closed manipulation under anesthesia sometimes produces a satisfactory reduction, which remains stable in plaster, but too often reduction cannot be achieved or held except by open methods of reduction and internal fixation. The primary practitioner should make the diagnosis, document the evidence for radial nerve function, immobilize the arm in a posterior splint, admit the patient to a hospital, and request the prompt services of an orthopedist.

Fractures of the Distal Third of the Forearm

We direct special attention to this fracture for these reasons:

1. In our opinion, these fractures are encountered by the primary practitioner more commonly than any other long-bone fracture except perhaps for tibial fractures during ski season.

2. Also, these are among the fractures which usually should be treated definitively by the primary practitioner.

3. Finally, one of the methods used to reduce these fractures is applicable to reductions of fractures of both forearm bones at any level.

Four distinct fractures occur at this level. All result from a fall onto the outstretched arm—two with the wrist dorsiflexed and two with the wrist volar flexed.

Colles' Fracture. This fracture is the most common of the three. It typically occurs in adults—elderly adults more commonly than in young adults. By definition, the fracture occurs within 2.5 cm (1″) of the carpal articular surface of the radius; the distal fragment is angulated dorsally and may be dorsally and radially displaced as well; the distal end of the ulna may or may not be similarly fractured. These displacements produce what has been termed the "silver fork deformity." (See Figure 6–18.) The more osteoporotic the bones, the more likely are the distal fragment and the end of the proximal fragment to be severely comminuted or impacted as well. In the face of comminution or impaction, anatomic reduction is often impossible, and when achieved, can rarely be held by external fixation. While methods of open reduction and internal fixation have been used for these comminuted or impacted fractures, we do not recommend them. The comminuted and impacted fractures are typically fractures of the elderly. When applied to the elderly, open treatment and the prolonged immobilization it imposes, too often yield permanently painful stiff wrists, much less useful than the wrists of those whose fractures were "badly set" by

closed methods. Unfortunately, however deft and appropriate the reduction and immobilization, and however tactful the rehabilitation, healing of the comminuted or impacted Colles' fracture rarely permits full restoration of wrist motion, and often leads to degenerative arthritis of the radiocarpal and distal radio-ulnar joints.

Smith's Fracture. This fracture is the least common of the three. It may be considered a reverse Colles' fracture. It occurs when an individual falls upon the outstretched arm with the wrist in volar flexion. (See Figure 6–19.) Like the Colles' fracture, it is a fracture of adults; it is more likely to be comminuted when bones are osteoporotic; and the permanent complications of its comminution are limited range of motion and degenerative arthritis of the wrist.

Barton's Fracture. The forces which usually produce Smith's fracture may produce an oblique fracture through the articular surface of the distal end of the radius. A fragment is thus separated away from the volar surface of the distal end of the radius. (See Figure 6–20.) As the articular surface is crossed by the fracture line, the reduction must be anatomic. Such a result can rarely be achieved without open reduction and internal fixation. When the

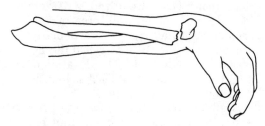

Fig. 6–18. Colles' fracture.

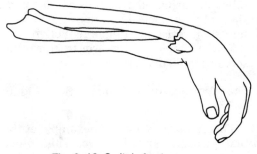

Fig. 6–19. Smith's fracture.

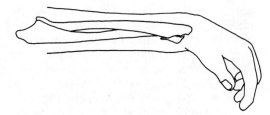

Fig. 6–20. Barton's fracture.

primary clinician encounters this fracture, he or she should splint the wrist and refer the patient promptly to an orthopaedist.

Fracture Separation of the Distal Radial Epiphysis. (See Figure 6–21.) This fracture is sustained by schoolchildren less often than the clavicle fracture and more often than the supra- and intercondylar humerus fractures. It is more likely to be displaced like a Colles' fracture than a Smith's fracture. Anatomic reduction is usually easily attained, and any irreducible deformity is usually so slight as to correct completely with continued growth of the radius. Epiphyseal injury capable of stopping growth of the radius is very unusual following this injury. That tragic complication results from axially compressed comminuted fractures, which occur very rarely in children. See the more general discussion of epiphyseal injuries in Chapter 19.

Treatment.

1. The goals of treatment of the fractures of the distal third of the forearm are: apposition of the fragments and restoration of the radio-ulnar articulation and the normal volar angulation of the radiocarpal articulation. The radio-ulnar articulation can be presumed to be restored if the distal ends of the radius and ulna lie in the same frontal plane, and the angle made by the long axis of the forearm with a line drawn through the radial and ulnar styloids is no greater than 75° in the radiodistal quadrant. Normally, the angle between the long axis of the forearm and the surface of the radiocarpal articulation is about 60° in the dorsodistal quadrant. (See Figure 6–22.)

2. The choice of anesthesia depends somewhat upon the method of reduction chosen (see the two methods described below) and somewhat upon the anxiety of the patient. The hematoma block is simple, quick, and quite effective when using the continuous traction method of reduction. While it will also allow reduction by the classic and quicker manual method, particularly if the patient is placid and lightly muscled, it usually yields incomplete pain relief, and the reactive increase in muscle tone which will accompany the pain of reduction will be too strong to allow reduction of more displaced fractures, particularly when the patient is apprehensive and heavily muscled. While the effects of the hematoma block can be potentiated by narcotics and sedatives, the narcotized patient deserves observation until independently awake and aware, which requires a bed and a knowledgeable person—usually expensive commodities. Even though successful, we feel less artful if not somewhat abashed if we reduce a fracture painfully when it might have been done painlessly. Therefore, we have come to prefer the

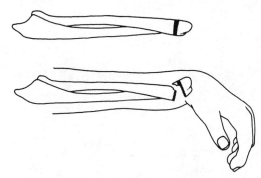

Fig. 6–21. Fracture separation of the distal radial epiphysis.

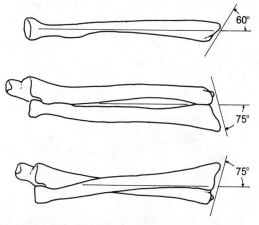

Fig. 6–22. Goals of treatment of fractures of the distal third of the forearm.

regional intravenous block (Beer block). By following the recommended protocol exactly, we have found the regional intravenous block safe, cheap, and very effective for the reduction of forearm fractures. (See Chapter 16.)

3. Once the arm is anesthetized, the reduction can be accomplished by one of two methods:

a. Manipulation alone. (See Figure 6–23.) Manual traction is applied from the hand for at least 1 minute. Particularly when deprived of blood flow, as is the arm anesthetized by regional intravenous block, the forearm muscles are fatigued by this maneuver, and any impaction of the fragments begins to loosen. When muscle tone decreases, the reduction can proceed. Further disimpaction is accomplished by gently increasing the deformity. Traction is then applied to the angulated distal frag-

ment, and the reduction is concluded by applying force with the traction hand such as will correct the angulation, while at the same time pushing the thumb of the other on the trailing surface of the distal fragment. (The trailing surface of the Colles' fracture is the dorsal surface, and the trailing surface of the Smith's fracture is the volar surface.)

b. Manipulation following traction. (See Figure 6–24.) This method can effect a reduction even without anesthesia, but as it is not painless, we precede the method with the hematoma block. The patient is instructed to lie supine on a bed or treatment table with the shoulder of the affected arm just inside its edge, and abducted to 90°. In this position, nearly all of the patient's arm will extend out from the bed. With the elbow at 90° and the forearm pointing to the ceiling, the weight of the arm is suspended from Chinese finger traps. Adhesive tapes can be used if the wire traps are unavailable. Traction applied through the thumb and index finger will reduce the radius; traction applied through the ring and fifth fingers will reduce the ulna. When both bones require reduction, we apply the traction through the thumb, index, and fifth fingers. Heavy weights are then applied to a sling which

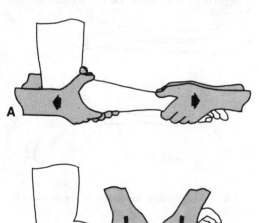

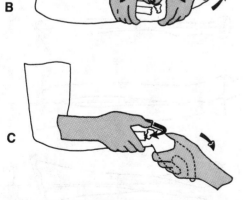

Fig. 6–23. Reduction of distal third of forearm fracture by manipulation alone. *A,* apply traction. *B,* increased angulation. *C,* correct angulation and position.

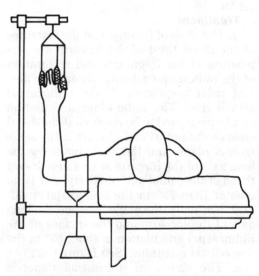

Fig. 6–24. Reduction of distal third of forearm fracture while in weighted traction. The hand is suspended from Chinese finger traps to the thumb, index, and fifth fingers. Weights as necessary are applied to distract the fracture fragments.

has been draped over the upper arm. As much as 60–80 pounds may be required. Often after 5 or more minutes in this form of traction, the fracture is nearly reduced, and gentle angular manipulation of the distal fragment will easily complete the reduction. Once the fracture is reduced, the weight is decreased to 10–15 pounds.

If the fracture is stable, it will not lose position upon decreasing the force of the traction. With the arm thus in traction, padding and plaster of Paris are applied from the hand to the elbow. When the plaster has set, the traction is removed, the forearm is placed in the appropriate rotation (see above, principles 2 through 5 un-

Table 6–1
Summary of Movements of the Forearm, Wrist, and Hand, and Their Chief Controllers

Movement	Muscles	Nerves
Pronation of the forearm	Pronator teres	Median nerve
	Pronator quadratus	Median nerve
Supination of the forearm	Supinator	Radial nerve
	Biceps	Musculocutaneous nerve
Wrist flexion	Flexor carpi radialis	Median nerve
	Flexor carpi ulnaris	Ulnar nerve
	Palmaris longus	Median nerve
Wrist extension	Extensor carpi radialis longus	Radial nerve
	Extensor carpi radialis brevis	Radial nerve
	Extensor carpis ulnaris	Radial nerve
Radial deviation of the wrist	Abductor pollicis longus	Radial nerve
	Extensor pollicis brevis	Radial nerve
	Extensor carpi radialis longus and brevis	Radial nerve
Ulnar deviation of the wrist	Extensor carpi ulnaris	Radial nerve
	Flexor carpi ulnaris	Ulnar nerve
Flexors of the thumb		
Interphalangeal joint	Flexor pollicis longus	Median nerve
Metacarpophalangeal joint	Flexor pollicis brevis	Median nerve
Abduction of the thumb	Abductor pollicis longus	Radial nerve
	Abductor pollicis brevis	Median nerve
Opposition of the thumb	Opponens pollicis	Median nerve
Adduction of the thumb	Adductor policis	Ulnar nerve
Extension of the thumb		
Interphalangeal joint	Extensor pollicis longus	Radial nerve
Metacarpophalangeal joint	Extensor pollicis brevis	Radial nerve
Flexion of the fingers		
Distal Interphalangeal joints	Flexor digitorum profundus	Medium nerve and ulnar nerve
Proximal Interphalangeal joints	Flexor digitorum sublimis	Medium nerve
Metacarpophalangeal joints	Interosseous muscles	Ulnar nerve
	Lumbricals 1 and 2	Median nerve
	Lumbricals 3 and 4	Ulnar nerve
	Flexor digiti minimi	Ulnar nerve
Abduction of the fingers	Dorsal interosseous muscles	Ulnar nerve
	Abductor digiti minimi	Ulnar nerve
Adduction of the fingers	Palmar interosseous muscles	Ulnar nerve
Opposition of the 5th finger	Opponens digiti minimi	Ulnar nerve
Extension of the fingers	Extensor digitorum	Radial nerve
	Extensor indicus	Radial nerve
	Extensor digiti minimi	Radial nerve
Extension of interphalangeal joint while metacarpophalangeal joint is flexed	Lumbricals and palmar interosseous muscles	Median and ulnar nerves

der "General Principles for Treatment of Forearm Fractures"), and the padding and plaster are carried above the elbow.

4. The duration of immobilization and the schedule of rehabilitation are as described above in paragraphs 12–15 under "General Principles for Treatment of Forearm Fractures."

Fractures and Dislocations of the Carpus

These injuries typically are sustained by adolescents and young adults during a fall onto the outstretched arm with the wrist dorsiflexed. Three of these injuries occur sufficiently often and yield to closed methods of treatment sufficiently readily as to stand among those injuries which should be definitively treated by the primary practitioner. These injuries will be discussed in some detail shortly. However, any carpal bone can be fractured or dislocated, and the painfully injured wrist can be very difficult to diagnose. Often little deformity is visible other than that fullness of the carpal space produced by blood or transudate; x-rays within the first few days of an injury may fail to show a fracture line, and practitioners unused to studying carpal films may miss a dislocation. Further danger of misdiagnosis attends the fact that fractures or subluxations of the bases of the 4th or 5th metacarpal, and subluxations of the distal radio-ulnar joint present very much as do carpal injuries. (See below under . . .) By careful palpation around the carpus, the radioulnar joint, and the bases of the metacarpals, and by careful comparison of anteroposterior, lateral, and oblique x-rays of the injured wrist, with comparable x-rays of a normal wrist (preferably the patient's other wrist), the practitioner will often identify the injury. If an undisplaced fracture is identified, the practitioner should treat it definitively as recommended below for the scaphoid fracture. If a displaced fracture or dislocation is recognized and cannot be reduced, the wrist should be splinted and the patient referred to an orthopedist. If median or ulnar nerve dysfunction are evident, the referral should occur on the day of injury. If median and ulnar nerve function are normal, the referral can be delayed for as long as, but no longer than 1 week. When clinical evidence of carpal injury cannot be explained by x-ray findings, the practitioner should be very wary of diagnosing a sprain; for injuries in this region, it is wiser to err on the side of over-referral.

The following are the three specific injuries for which primary practitioners should accept definitive responsibility:

Scaphoid Fracture

This fracture is by far the most common of the carpal injuries, occurring as it does only somewhat less frequently than do fractures of the distal third of the forearm. The scaphoid may be fractured at any of three points: the tuberosity, the waist, and the proximal pole. (See Figure 6–25.) The clinical characteristics of all scaphoid fractures are the following:

1. The patient will report a fall upon the extended arm, wrist dorsiflexed, and will complain of pain in the wrist, particularly toward the radial side.

2. Any movement of the wrist, active or passive, will produce pain.

3. In patients with lean arms, a fullness of the carpal space will be evident when the two wrists are compared.

4. While the entire carpus may appear somewhat tender, the anatomic snuffbox will be uniquely so.

When this clinical picture is encountered, anteroposterior (AP), lateral, and oblique x-rays of the carpus must be obtained. The oblique view may show a fracture line not visible on AP and lateral views. However, some fractures will not be visible during the first few days following injury. Therefore, when this clinical picture is encountered and x-rays fail to confirm the fracture, the fracture should be immobilized for 3 weeks as if the scaphoid were fractured. After 3 weeks, bone resorption at the fracture line will allow x-rays to reveal the fracture, if it exists. If a fracture does not exist, much less has been lost by 3 weeks' immobilization than can be lost if a fractured scaphoid is subject to movement during the first 3 weeks. While both poles of the scaphoid may be independently vascularized, one often is not, and depends upon the flow

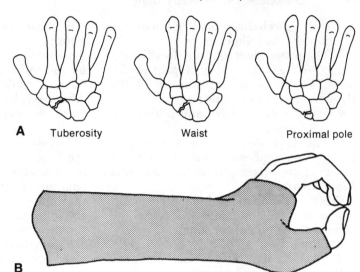

A   Tuberosity   Waist   Proximal pole

" Navicular "

Fig. 6–25. Scaphoid fractures. *A,* three varieties of scaphoid fracture. *B,* immobilization of scaphoid fractures.

B

through the bone for its nourishment. If the original injury has not interrupted such intramedullary flow, continued movement at the fracture line is very likely to do so.

The uncomplicated fracture of the scaphoid will usually unite within 10 weeks. However, because circulation to one of the poles can be decreased or interrupted, delayed union, non-union, or avascular necrosis of one of the poles may occur. Whether or not the fracture has been immobilized from the outset may be a critical determinant of the outcome.

Treatment.

1. The wrist should be immobilized in a forearm cast with the wrist in slight dorsiflexion, and the thumb in a position of opposition. Plaster should extend to the interphalangeal joint of the thumb. (See Figure 6–25.) We apply the cast while the patient holds the thumb in a position that will allow easy opposition between the thumb and the index finger. The cast must be firmly molded to prevent rotation of the forearm. If this intention cannot be realized by molding, the cast must be extended above the elbow. The forearm is immobilized in neutral rotation.

2. If after 2 months x-ray union is not nearly complete, the patient should probably be referred to an orthopaedist. Some orthopaedists prefer to do surgery at that point. Unless obvious necrosis or non-union has occurred, in our clinic it has been the practice to continue the closed method

of treatment, changing the cast at 6-week intervals, as long as some progress toward union is evident. If after 4–6 months, progress toward union appears arrested, bone graft surgery is considered.

3. Rehabilitation must begin at once in the cast with finger, elbow, and shoulder exercise. Once union has been achieved and the cast has been removed, active wrist and thumb motion must be added to the regimen. A physical therapist's services may be advisable from the outset. The duration of remobilization may last at least as long as the duration of immobilization.

Dislocation of the Lunate (See Figure 6–26)

Much less common than the scaphoid fracture is the dislocation of the lunate. The injuring force of dorsiflexion will usually displace the lunate into the volar aspect of the wrist, where it will at least severely crowd the contents of the carpal tunnel and thereby interfere with the blood supply to that segment of the median nerve. When the dislocation occurs with great force, the median nerve may be contused or even lacerated. While this injury usually occurs alone, it may be accompanied by a fracture of the scaphoid. When this combined injury occurs, the proximal fragment of the scaphoid usually dislocates with the lunate.

The clinical characteristics of lunate dislocation are the following:

1. The patient will report a dorsiflexion injury and will complain of pain in the wrist, and often of paresthesias of the thumb, index, and middle fingers.

2. Pain is induced by any attempt to move the wrist.

3. The dislocated lunate is usually palpable as an abnormal knob on the volar aspect of the wrist at the level of the distal flexor crease.

Careful examination of anteroposterior, lateral, and oblique x-rays will reveal the abnormal position of the lunate.

Treatment.

1. Anesthesia. Intravenous analgesia with meperidine and promethazine are often comforting and relaxing enough to allow a humane and successful reduction. When analgesia does not allow a reasonably tolerable manipulation, we resort to the regional intravenous block.

2. More often than not, especially if seen early, this dislocation can be reduced by closed maneuvers, and the primary practitioner should attempt the reduction. The wrist is held in a position of dorsiflexion to its maximum extent, while continuous heavy traction is applied to the hand. With the thumb of his other hand, the operator pushes distally then dorsally and finally proximally on the lunate by a rolling motion of his thumb. (See Figure 6–26.) Once the lunate feels as though engaged in its space, the operator gradually flexes the dorsiflexed wrist while continuing thumb pressure on the lunate. The reduction often occurs with a snap quite evident to the operator. Even in the face of median nerve dysfunction, the primary practitioner should attempt this reduction.

3. Once the lunate is reduced, the practitioner must re-evaluate median nerve function. If function does not return within an hour, the wrist should be splinted, and the patient should be referred immediately to an orthopedist.

4. When the dislocated lunate is accompanied by the displaced proximal fragment of a scaphoid fracture, the reduction should be attempted by the same maneuver. Reduction of this injury is often easier than reduction of the lunate alone.

5. Once the dislocation is reduced and return of median nerve function has been demonstrated, the wrist should be immobilized for 3 weeks in forearm plaster in neutral position, or in slight volar flexion. After 3 weeks, the cast is removed, and the wrist recast in slight dorsiflexion for another 3 weeks. If the scaphoid has been fractured as well, the cast must extend to the IP joint of the thumb with the thumb in opposition, and immobilization must continue for at least 10 weeks, after which the injury must be managed as advised above in paragraph 2 under "Treatment" for "Scaphoid Fracture."

6. Rehabilitation is identical to that advised above in Paragraph 3 under "Treatment" for "Scaphoid Fracture."

Perilunate Dislocation (See Figure 6–27)

Rather than force the lunate into the volar aspect of the wrist, dorsiflexion injury may force the rest of the carpus dorsally out of articulation with the radius and ulna, leaving the lunate in normal articulation with the radius. The effects on the median nerve may be identical to the effects of lunate dislocation.

The clinical characteristics of perilunate dislocation are the following:

1. The patient will report dorsiflexion injury and complain of pain in the wrist, and often paresthesias of the thumb, index, and middle fingers.

2. Pain is induced by any attempt to move the wrist.

3. Dorsal displacement of the carpus will be visible somewhat like a shallow "silver fork" deformity, and the lunate can be palpated in its position just distal to the ulnar half of the carpal articular surface of the radius.

4. Careful examination of AP, lateral, and oblique x-rays will demonstrate the lunate in articulation with the radius and the rest of the carpus dorsally displaced.

Treatment.

1. Anesthesia. We employ the same methods as described above under "Treatment" for "Dislocation of the Lunate."

2. A perilunate dislocation can be reduced by closed methods about as readily as can a lunate dislocation. (See Figure

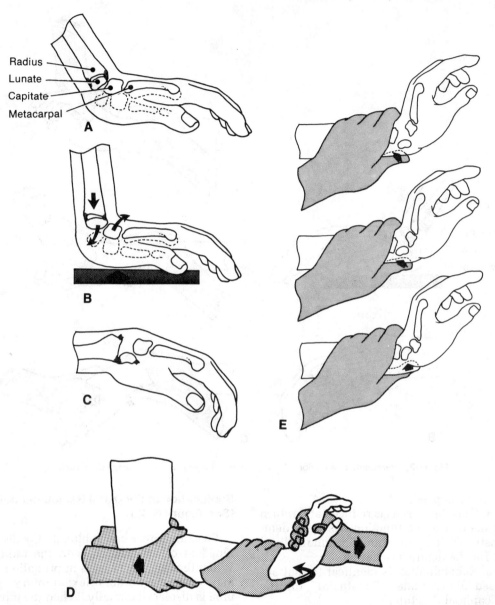

Fig. 6–26. Dislocation of the lunate. *A*, normal wrist. *B*, mechanism of injury. *C*, dislocation. *D*, reduction. *E*, detail of the manipulation of the lunate.

6–27.) The primary practitioner should attempt the reduction. The wrist is held in a position of slight dorsiflexion while continuous heavy traction is applied to the hand. With the thumb of his other hand pressing on the volar surface of the lunate to hold it in position, the wrist is gradually flexed to bring the rest of the carpus volarwise into proper articulation with the lunate, radius, and ulna. This reduction is

not rewarded by so dramatic a snap as rewards the reduction of the lunate dislocation. This reduction should be attempted even in the face of median nerve dysfunction.

3. Once the carpus is reduced, the practitioner must re-evaluate median nerve function. If function does not return within an hour, the wrist should be splinted, and the patient should be referred immediately

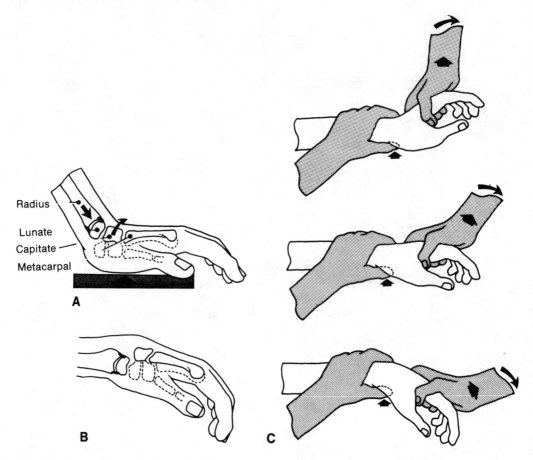

Fig. 6–27. Perilunate dislocation. *A*, mechanism of injury. *B*, dislocation. *C*, reduction.

to an orthopaedist.

4. Once the carpus is reduced and return of median nerve function has been demonstrated, the wrist should be immobilized as for the lunate dislocation.

5. Rehabilitation is identical to that advised above under "Treatment" for the "Scaphoid Fracture."

Forearm and Hand Injuries Easily Mistaken for Carpal Injuries

As suggested in the introduction to carpal injuries, it is clinically more logical to consider one forearm injury and a specific variety of hand injuries at this point, rather than in their regional sections. These are: the distal radio-ulnar subluxation and the fractures of the bases of metacarpals 2 through 5, and/or the subluxation of their articulations with the carpus.

Subluxation of the Distal Radioulnar Joint (See Figure 6–28)

Twisting forces can subluxate the distal ulna out of articulation with the radius. When the injuring twist is in pronation as may accompany a dorsiflexion injury, the ulna is displaced dorsally. When the injuring twist is in supination, as may accompany volar flexion of the wrist, the ulna is usually displaced ventrally. This injury may be more common than generally reported, as the subluxation may well relocate spontaneously. The persistent subluxation, however, is rare. It must be mentioned, as it may present clinically as a carpal injury, and unless it is specifically looked for, it may be missed, and a permanent disorder of forearm rotation may result.

The clinical characteristics of the sub-

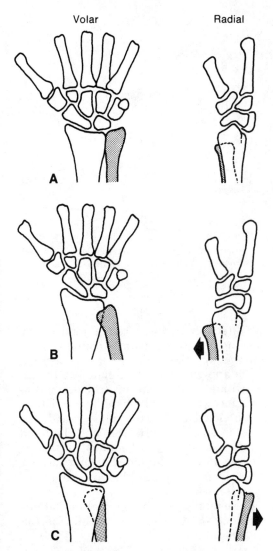

Volar   Radial

Fig. 6–28. Dislocations of the distal end of the ulna. *A,* normal relationship, *B,* volar displacement of the ulna. *C,* dorsal displacement of the ulna.

luxation of the distal radio-ulnar joint are the following:

1. The patient will report a twisting injury and will complain of pain in the wrist.

2. Any attempt to move the wrist or rotate the forearm will produce pain.

3. When both wrists are carefully compared by inspection and palpation, the displacement of the ulna—whether dorsal or volar—will usually be appreciated.

Careful comparison of AP, lateral, and oblique x-rays of the injured wrist with comparable x-rays of the normal wrist will usually demonstrate the subluxation of the radio-ulnar joint.

Treatment.

1. Anesthesia. We employ the same methods as for the lunate dislocation.

2. Reduction is accomplished by the opposite twist to that which produced the dislocation: extreme supination will reduce the dorsally subluxed ulna, and extreme pronation will reduce the ventrally subluxed ulna.

3. The position of reduction usually must be held for 4 weeks in a full-arm plaster: full supination after reduction of the dorsally subluxed ulna, and full pronation after reduction of the ventrally subluxed ulna. The wrist should be in a neutral position.

4. Rehabilitation is identical to that advised for the fracture of the distal third of the forearm.

Fractures of the Bases of Metacarpals 2 through 5, and/or Subluxation of Their Articulations with the Carpus (See Figure 6–29)

A direct blow can fracture the base of a metacarpal, and a twisting dorsiflexion force to the hand and wrist can either fracture the bases of the 4th and 5th metacarpal, or subluxate their articulation with the capitate and hamate. All of these injuries occur about as often as do the scaphoid fracture. Subluxation of the articulatims of metacarpals 2 and 3 with the trapezoid and capitate, however, are very rare. On first presentation, all these injuries can suggest a carpal injury and, unless specifically looked for, they are likely to be missed and a permanently painful limitation in hand and wrist function may result.

The clinical characteristics of these injuries are the following:

1. The patient may report either a blow to the dorsum of the wrist or hand, or a dorsiflexion injury to the hand and wrist, and will complain of pain in the wrist and hand at about the location of the injured metacarpal.

2. Any attempt to move the wrist or to make a fist will provoke pain.

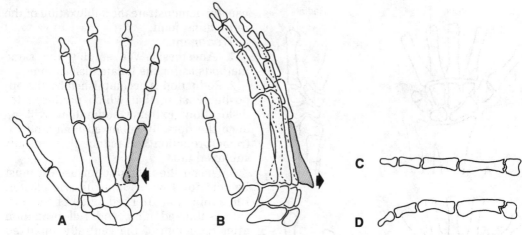

Fig. 6–29. Dislocation and fracture of the metacarpals. *A,* dislocation of the 5th metacarpal, dorsal view. *B,* dislocation of the 5th metacarpal, radial view. *C,* fracture of the base of a metacarpal, dorsal view. *D,* fracture of the base of a metacarpal, lateral view.

3. The point of the injury will be uniquely tender, and manipulation of the affected metacarpal will produce pain.

AP, lateral, and oblique views of the wrist and hand will demonstrate the fracture or subluxation.

Treatment.

1. Anesthesia. When reduction is necessary, adequate anesthesia is obtained by injection of 4–5 cc. 1% lidocaine into the hematoma of fractures or around a subluxated joint. Occasionally, a very tense individual will require intravenous meperidine and promethazine prior to the block.

2. Undisplaced fractures should be immobilized in forearm plaster with the wrist in slight dorsiflexion, and the hand firmly fixed between the dorsal surface of the cast and a well-molded palmar surface.

3. Displaced fractures are rare but are easily reduced and held in forearm plaster with the wrist in slight dorsiflexion and the hand firmly fixed between the dorsal surface of the cast and a well-molded palmar surface.

The reduction is accomplished by straight traction on the articulating finger and force applied to the displaced fragment in a direction appropriate to re-establish apposition and alignment.

4. Subluxations of the metacarpals from their articulation with the trapezoid, capitate, and hamane generally occur in a dor-

sal direction and are easily reduced by pushing toward the palm directly over the dorsum of the subluxated metacarpal while applying straight traction to the affected metacarpal and its articulating finger. Once reduced, the hand and wrist are immobilized in forearm plaster with the wrist in slight dorsiflexion, and the hand firmly fixed between the dorsal surface of the cast and a well-molded palmar surface.

5. All these injuries should be immobilized for 4–6 weeks.

6. Rehabilitation is identical to that advised above under "Treatment" for the "Scaphoid Fracture."

Fractures and Dislocations of the Hand

Injuries at the Base of the First Metacarpal

Hyperabduction and hyperflexion of the thumb may produce one of three injuries at the base of the first metacarpal: The *transverse fracture* and the *Bennett fracture,* both of which occur about as often as the scaphoid fracture, and the *trapeziometacarpal subluxation* or *dislocation* which occurs somewhat less often than the scaphoid fracture. While the patient may complain initially of pain in the radial aspect of the wrist, a fairly obvious disability and somewhat less obvious mala-

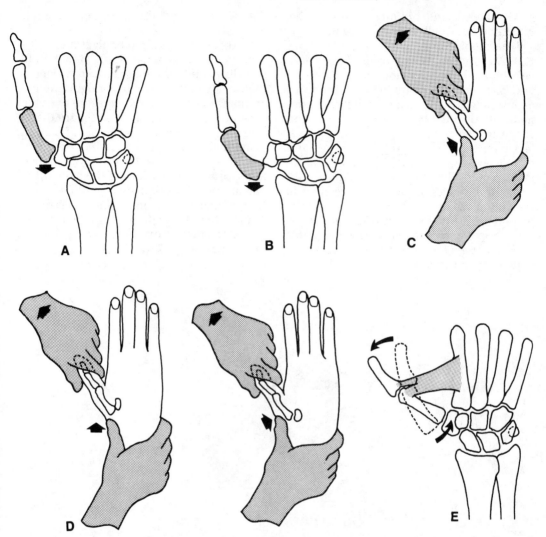

Fig. 6–30. Injury to the trapeziometacarpal joint. *A*, trapeziometacarpal subluxation. *B*, trapeziometacarpal dislocation. *C*, reduction of trapeziometacarpal subluxation. *D*, reduction of trapeziometacarpal dislocation. *E*, immobilization of trapeziometacarpal dislocations—resistance of the adductor pollicis acts as a fulcrum over which abduction force to the thumb acts to resist redislocation.

lignment of the thumb are more likely to direct the attention of the practitioner to the injured metacarpal than to the carpus—unlike the injuries at the bases of the other metacarpals. However, the complaint of pain in the radial aspect of the wrist should call to mind as a differential group these three injuries as well as the scaphoid fracture.

The clinical presentation of all three of these injuries is identical:

1. The patient may report an abduction or flexion injury to the thumb, or a fall onto the radial aspect of the hand, and will complain of pain over the radial aspect of the wrist and hand.

2. Any attempt to move the wrist or the thumb will intensify the pain.

3. Comparative inspection of the two hands will usually demonstrate an abnormal angulation and/or shortening of the 1st metacarpal and a fullness or frank knob over the radial or palmar base of the 1st metacarpal.

4. Palpation at the base of the 1st metacarpal and manipulation of the 1st metacarpal will elicit pain, and when the injury is a fracture, may elicit crepitation.

AP, lateral, and oblique x-rays of the wrist and hand will reveal the injury.

Treatment.

1. Anesthesia. Adequate anesthesia may be obtained by injection of 4–5 cc. 1% lidocaine into the hematoma of fractures or into and around a dislocated trapeziometacarpal joint. However a subluxation can often be reduced quite quickly with less pain than that of the anesthetic, and full dislocation or the Bennett fracture may require lengthy manipulation, and successful reduction will require muscle relaxation which local anesthesia and the patient's efforts to cooperate cannot always provide. Hence, we occasionally employ the regional intravenous block for reduction and immobilization of the Ben-

nett fracture and the trapeziometacarpal dislocation.

2. Reduction and Immobilization.

a. A trapeziometacarpal subluxation and dislocation are diagrammed in Figure 6–30. They are reduced by straight traction on the thumb and direct pressure over the base of the metacarpal. (See Figure 6–30.) The sooner after injury the manipulation is applied, the easier the reduction. Pressure to reduce the subluxation is applied to the protruding surface of the base of the metacarpal and is directed parallel to the trapeziometacarpal joint line. Pressure to reduce the dislocation is applied to the articular surface of the metacarpal at its protruding angle, and is directed at first distally (as the metacarpal is always prox-

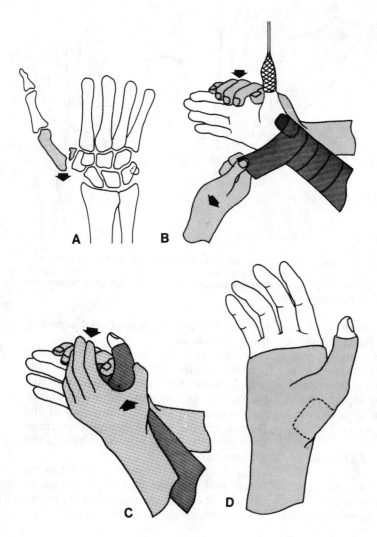

Fig. 6–31 Bennett's fracture-dislocation. *A*, the injury. *B*, reduction and immobilization. *C*, molding the cast to maintain reductive forces. *D*, appearance of the completed cast.

imally displaced) and gradually in an arc toward the direction of the joint line as the metacarpal begins to slip into re-articulation with the trapezium. Both injuries should be immobilized in a scaphoid cast for 4 weeks.

b. Transverse fractures of the base of the 1st metacarpal. These fractures are variably angulated, usually in abduction. Strong straight traction on the thumb, coupled with gentle efforts to increase the angulation, will usually free the impaction and allow the distal fragment to be moved back into fairly stable alignment. Once reduced, the orientation of the thumb must be noted, and any rotation of the distal fragment must be corrected to set the thumb in the normal position of opposition. When satisfactorily aligned and rotated, the injury is immobilized in a scaphoid cast for about 4 weeks.

c. Bennett fracture dislocation. This injury is an oblique fracture through the midpoint of the trapeziometacarpal joint. (See Figure 6–31.) The distal fragment has almost invariably been dislocated from the joint while the short proximal fragment remains in perfect articulation. If the fracture is not perfectly reduced, irregularity of the joint line may lead to a disabling degenerative arthritis of the trapeziometacarpal joint. While the reduction is simple, the immobilization is usually difficult. The same manipulation used for reduction of the trapeziometacarpal dislocation is used for the reduction of this fracture. However, the reduction is far from stable. The distal fragment will usually redislocate the moment the operator lets go of the hand. Nonetheless, the primary practitioner should attempt to immobilize the fracture in plaster as this closed method is sometimes successful, if the following details are adhered to:

(1) Traction and full abduction are maintained while the plaster is applied. These ends are most easily attained by suspension and weights as diagrammed in Figure 6–31.

(2) A felt pad is placed over the radiopalmar aspect of the base of the 1st metacarpal and plaster is applied over that. (See Figure 6–31.)

(3) Firm pressure is applied to the radiopalmar aspect of the base of the 1st me-

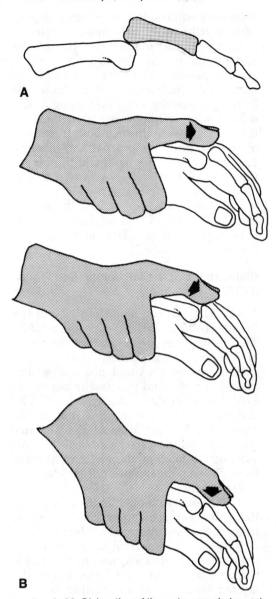

Fig. 6–32. Dislocation of the metacarpophalangeal joint. *A,* the injury. *B,* reduction.

tacarpal while the plaster is setting. The plaster is thus applied in a manner which will maintain full abduction of the 1st metacarpal and firm pressure over the radiopalmar aspect of its base. If postimmobilization x-rays show the reduction to have held, the cast is retained, and the fracture is re-x-rayed in 5 days. If the reduction is still maintained, the cast is retained for about 6 weeks. Since this fracture involves the joint surface, the reduction must be anatomic. Even 1–2 mm. separation of the fragments will result in an eventual degenerative arthritis. Hence, unless anatomic reduction is maintained by the closed method, the patient should be referred to an orthopaedist. We prefer in our clinic to immobilize the fractures which cannot be held by a cast by a method using a Kirschner wire. Without any skin incision, the wire is passed through both fragments of the fractured metacarpal and into the 2nd metacarpal. The hand and thumb are then immobilized for 4 weeks in a scaphoid cast.

3. Rehabilitation for each of these injuries is identical to that advised above in paragraph 3 under "Treatment" for the "Scaphoid Fracture."

Dislocations of the MP Joints (See Figure 6–32)

Any MP joint can be dislocated, but the thumb seems to be the most vulnerable. The dislocations are invariably the result of hyperpextension forces. The articular surface of the proximal phalanx is displaced dorsally and proximally out of articulation with the metacarpal head. The dislocation occurs through a rent in the capsule: Either the base of the phalanx tears through the dorsal aspect of the capsule, or the head of the metacarpal tears through the palmar aspect of the capsule.

Treatment.

1. If seen very soon after the injury, and the patient is placid, often no anesthesia is needed. If a first attempt at reduction fails, or if the injury be several hours old, or the patient visibly anxious, we prefer a metacarpal block about 2 cm. proximal to the injured joint. We avoid creating any further swelling about the joint itself.

2. Whichever surface of the capsule is torn, a method of reduction using absolutely no traction is most likely to succeed. We recommend the following method: Grasp the hand in such a way that your flexed thumb lies upon the dorsum of the metacarpal, up against the base of the dislocated phalanx. Then push with the thumb, gradually increasing force, so as to move the base of the dislocated phalanx distally, toward the articular surface of the metacarpal head. As the leading margin of the base of the phalanx is felt to engage

the articular surface of the metacarpal head, the force of the thumb is gradually redirected to sweep the base of the phalanx into articulation and flexion at once. When successful, this last maneuver is accompanied by a definite sense of smooth giving-way (See Figure 6–32.)

Once reduced, active flexion exercises should begin. Immobiliztion is not necessary. At most, we recommend a dorsal guard, fixed to the hand, but not to the finger, to prevent hyperextension for 2 weeks.

4. When unable to reduce the dislocation, the primary clinician must refer the patient to an orthopaedist. Open reduction is sometimes necessary.

Fractures of the Shaft of a Metacarpal

These fractures may be transverse, oblique, or spiral. (See Figure 6–33.) The transverse fractures usually result from violence to the dorsum of the hand. The oblique or spiral fractures usually result from a fall onto the palmar or dorsal surface of the metacarpal heads, or from punching with the closed fist in a manner which takes the force on the volar aspect of the knuckle. (See Figure 6–34.) Punching straight with the wrist slightly dorsiflexed, or hooking with the arm supinated, will often impact with the volar aspect of the knuckles.

The clinical characteristics of the shaft fracture are the following:

1. The patient may report a fall onto the hand, a punching mishap, or direct violence to the back of the hand, and will

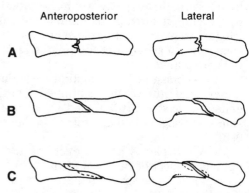

Fig. 6–33. Fractures of the shaft of a metacarpal. *A,* transverse. *B,* oblique. *C,* spiral.

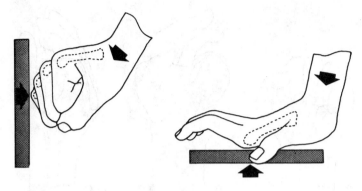

Fig. 6-34. Force tending to produce oblique and spiral fractures of the metacarpal.

complain of pain in the hand.

2. The dorsum of the hand will appear variably swollen.

3. Any effort to make a fist will increase the pain.

4. Passive manipulation of the affected metacarpal will increase the pain and may produce crepitation.

5. The articulating finger may be malrotated.

Treatment. *Anesthesia.* When reduction is necessary, adequate anesthesia is obtained by injection of 4–5 cc. 1% lidocaine into the fracture hematoma.

Reduction and Immobilization.

1. Undisplaced, unangulated transverse fractures need no immobilization, but the patient may appreciate the protection of a dorsal plaster splint extending to the knuckles. It is most important from the outset that the fingers be used for light activity and be purposely exercised in a full range of flexion and extension. The plaster can be removed within 3–4 weeks.

2. Transverse fractures which are angulated and displaced so as to distort the contour of the hand should be reduced. The reduction is effected by straight traction on the articulating finger, and direct pressure upon, or angular force at the fracture site, as appropriate to move the fragments into apposition and alignment. Once the fracture is reduced, a short arm cast is applied with the wrist in neutral position or slightly dorsiflexed, with the hand firmly held between the dorsum of the cast and a well-molded palmar surface, and with a palmar splint extending to the end of the articulating finger molded to hold the finger in position of function. Immobilization should continue for about 4 weeks.

3. Spiral or oblique fractures tend to over-ride their fragments and rotate the distal fragment. Unless the over-riding is extreme, causing a cosmetically or functionally unacceptable recession of the knuckle, it is best ignored. Reduction of over-riding can rarely be helped by any method short of traction on a Kirschner wire passed vertically through the metacarpal head or transversely through the distal phalanx of the articulating finger. In our opinion, the longer convalescence necessitated by the immobilization of the digit and the slight danger of infection along the wire are not justified by the inclination to restore the normal prominence of a minimally recessed MP joint. When knuckle recession is unacceptable, the patient might best be referred to an orthopaedist. On the other hand, rotation cannot be ignored as it will, of course, change the orientation of the articulating digit and thereby distort the grip. Various closed methods for holding normal rotation have been devised. We recommend two methods (see Figure 6–35.):

a. The articulating finger is caused to curl around a padded roll of plaster attached to the palmar aspect of the cast, and is fixed securely to the roll in the position of correct rotation with tape or padded plaster. The palmar roll is of a size that will support the finger with the MP and proximal IP joints each flexed about 75° and the distal IP joint flexed about 30° (At those angles, the distal phalanx will lie parallel to the dorsum of the hand.)

b. Palmar plaster is carried to the proximal edge of the proximal IP joint of the articulating finger, and dorsal plaster is

Fig. 6–35. Immobilization of spiral and oblique fractures of the metacarpal. *A*, when normally aligned, fingers point to a common center on the palm. *B*, first method of immobilization—the finger of the fractured metacarpal is rigidly immobilized over a gauze roll under plaster. *C*, the second method of immobilization—the finger of the fractured metacarpal is immobilized in a dorsal plaster trough, allowing for some motion of the interphalangeal joints in flexion.

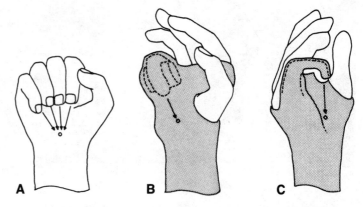

carried to its tip. The plaster is molded to prevent the MP and proximal IP joints from extending beyond about 75° flexion. The dorsal plaster is carried down the sides of the finger toward the palm. This method allows a fair degree of active flexion of the MP and IP joints during the period of immobilization. Exercise of those joints through the period of immobilization shortens the ultimate duration of convalescence. Plaster at the base of the finger must be kept as thin as possible and padded inside and out to protect the interdigital web from abrasion and possible infection. Whatever method is used, the immobilization should continue for about 4 weeks.

Rehabilitation. When the cast is finally removed, exercises are begun to restore wrist motion and the motion of the MP and IP joints of the articulating finger. The timid, the frail, and the arthritic should be referred to a physical therapist for supervision of a restorative exercise regimen.

Fractures of the Neck of the Metacarpal (See Figure 6–36)

This fracture results from punching with a closed fist in a manner which takes the force on the dorsal aspect of the knuckle: Punching straight with the wrist in slight volar flexion will often impact with the dorsal aspect of the knuckles. The knuckle is displaced toward the palm with the apex of angulation directed dorsally. The fragments are usually firmly impacted.

The clinical characteristics of this fracture are the following:

1. The patient usually reports a punching injury.

2. The affected knuckle is often recessed.

3. The neck of the affected metacarpal is tender to palpation.

AP and lateral x-rays will confirm a fracture of the neck of the metacarpal.

Treatment.

1. A hematoma block with 3–4 cc. 1% lidocaine usually provides good anesthesia. The hematoma is readily entered from the dorsal surface.

2. The impaction of the fragments is loosened by flexing the MP joint to 90° and wiggling the proximal phalanx like a lever to rotate the distal fragment back and forth. (See Figure 6–36.)

3. Once the impaction is loosened, the MP joint is straightened, and the fracture is reduced by applying direct pressure with the thumb in a distal-dorsal direction on the palmar surface of the knuckle while the fingers of the same hand grip the dorsum of the shaft of the fractured metacarpal. (See Figure 6–36.) Unless the operator has an uncommonly strong grip, this maneuver will not succeed unless the previous maneuver has fully disimpacted the fragments. A modification of the thenar grip prescribed for reduction of fractures of the distal third of the forearm is an alternative means for directing reducing force upon this fracture. (See Figure 6–36.) We do not advise the classic maneuver that applies reducing force through the flexed proximal phalanx, as this maneuver can dislocate the MP joint. Nor do we advise the classic method of immobilization which binds the MP and IP joints of the articulating finger in 90° flexion, as the stiffness which necessarily results can be most relentless.

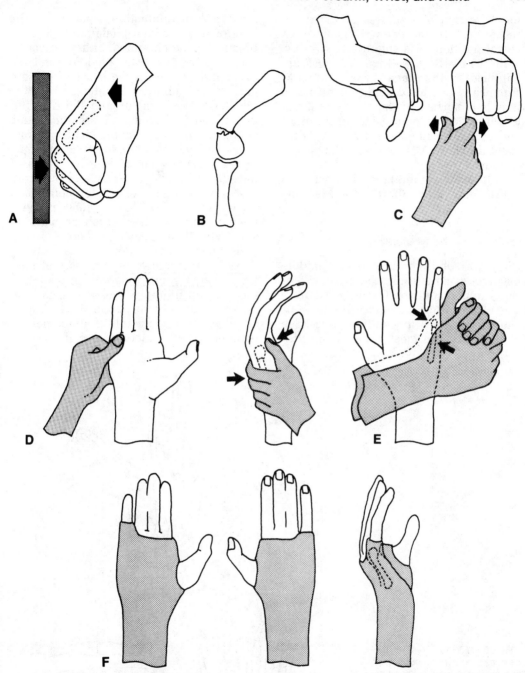

Fig. 6–36. Fracture of the neck of the metacarpal. *A,* force tending to produce the fracture. *B,* illustration of the fracture. *C,* disimpaction of the fracture with rotation forces. *D,* first method of reduction—relocation of the fragments by thumb finger pressure. *E,* second method of reduction—relocation of the fragments by the thenar grip. *F,* immobilization—volar, dorsal, and ulnar views. *Dotted lines* on the ulnar views show molding to maintain reductive forces.

4. Once reduced, the fracture is immobilized by forearm plaster which extends on the palmar surface beyond the fractured knuckle to the proximal interphalan-geal joint of the articulating finger, and which extends on the dorsal surface to the dorsum of the affected knuckle. The other MP joints are left free, as described for

immobilization of fractures of the distal third of the forearm. The wrist is placed in neutral position or is slightly dorsiflexed. While the plaster is setting, firm pressure is applied by the thenar grip: the thenar eminence of one hand applies pressure to the palmar surface of the fractured knuckle, while the thenar eminence of the other hand applies counterpressure to the dorsum of the shaft. After 4 weeks, the plaster is removed.

5. The same rehabilitation is advised as for Fractures of the Shaft of the Metacarpal (see above).

Fractures of the Phalanges

Fractures of the proximal and middle phalanges usually result from hyperextension or hyperabduction forces, while fractures of the distal phalanx usually result from crushing or heavy cutting forces (See Figure 6–37.) The most common injuries are the hyperabduction fracture of the base of the proximal phalanx of the fifth finger, the comminuted and transection fractures of any distal phalanx, and the avulsion fractures at the bases of phalanges. School children usually sustain the hyperabduction fractures of the fifth finger, school children and athletic young adults usually sustain the avulsion fractures, and preschool children and manual workers usually sustain the fractures of the distal phalanx. Preschool children crush or partially amputate their distal phalanges in doors, or in their parents' lawnmowers; workers crush or partially amputate their distal phalanges under their hammers, or in power tools.

Avulsion fractures at the bases of phalanges can accompany severe spraining of the MP and IP joints. The separated fragments are usually the points of attachment of ligaments or the points of attachment of tendons. These fractures are dealt with

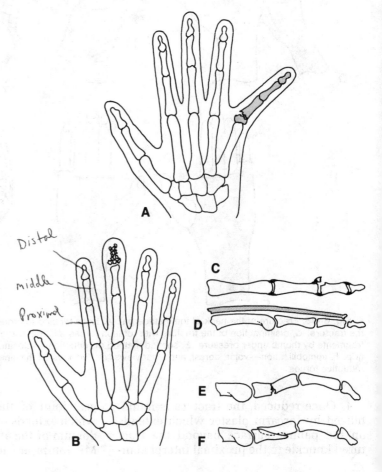

Fig. 6–37. Fractures of the phalanges. *A,* hyperabduction of the base of the proximal phalanx of the fifth finger. *B,* comminuted fracture of the distal phalanx. *C,* avulsion fracture of the base of the phalanx—collateral ligament avulsion. *D,* avulsion fracture of the base of the phalanx—tendon avulsion. *E,* transverse fracture of the shaft of the proximal or intermediate phalanx. *F,* spiral fracture of the shaft of the proximal or intermediate phalanx.

below under Ligamentous and Tendinous Injuries of the Hand.

Though encountered quite regularly, transverse or spiral fractures of the shafts of the proximal and middle phalanges are the least common of the finger fractures and are typically sustained by vigorous adults and school children during sports or rough play. These fractures are nearly all angulated.

The clinical characteristics of all these fractures are the following:

1. Undisplaced and avulsion fractures present swelling, tenderness, and occasional palpable crepitation over the fractured phalanx or sprained joint.

2. Displaced fractures and crush or partial amputation injuries to distal phalanges are visibly unmistakable.

3. AP and lateral x-rays of injured finger demonstrate the fracture.

Treatment.

1. Anesthesia. When reduction is necessary, adequate anesthsia can be obtained by a metacarpal block.

2. Reduction and Immobilization.

a. Undisplaced transverse fractures. We recommend that these be held with gauze wrapping to a dorsal plaster splint which has been incorporated into a forearm cast with the wrist in neutral position or slight dorsiflexion. The finger is immobilized in the *position of function*: the MP joint at 80° flexion, the proximal interphalangeal (PIP) joint at 30–50° flexion, and the distal interphalangeal (DIP) joint straight. The position of the PIP joint of the index finger is closer to 30°, that of the fifth finger closer to 50°, and that of each intervening finger is proportionately between those angles. (See Figure 6–38.) This position should be held for no more than 3 weeks.

b. Angulated transverse fractures of the base of the proximal phalanx. This fracture is often impacted. If so, the impaction is loosened by firm traction, followed by a gentle increase in the angulation. Once disimpacted, the angulation is corrected by levering the finger in an opposite direction from that of the deformation over a fulcrum placed against the interdigital web. One of the operator's fingers usually makes a fine fulcrum. Once reduced, a similar method of immobilization as described for undisplaced fractures is ap-

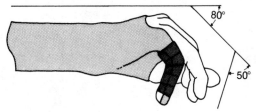

Fig. 6–38. Immobilization of the undisplaced transverse fracture of the base of the proximal phalanx of the fifth finger.

plied. The splint, however, also extends along the side of the finger toward which it has been displaced. (See Figure 6–39.) This position should be held for no more than 3 weeks.

c. Crush injuries of or near-amputations through the distal phalanx are essentially soft tissue injuries. Their treatment is discussed in the section dealing with lacerations of the hand.

d. Angulated transverse fractures of the shaft of the proximal or middle phalanx. (see Figure 6–40.) Initially, traction is applied distal to the fracture while the angulation is increased. By this maneuver, the margins on the side toward which the distal fragment is directed will be engaged. Once these margins are engaged, the distal fragment is moved to reduce the angulation. Fractures which have angulated the distal fragment dorsally, which are by far the most common, are immobilized with the finger in flexion (the MP joint 80°, the PIP joint at 30–50°, and the DIP joint straight), and fractures which have angulated the distal fragment toward the palm are immobilized in extension. Fingers mobilized in flexion are held with gauze against dorsal plaster splints, and fingers immobilized in extension are held with gauze on straight palmar plaster splints. Tips of distal phalanges are left open to allow the examiner to monitor circulation. The splints are incorporated into a forearm cast. These positions are held for 3 weeks.

e. Spiral and oblique fractures of the proximal or middle phalanx usually override as well as angulate their fragments. Strong traction accomplishes the reduction, but the reduction is invariably lost once the traction is released. Hence these fractures must nearly all be immobilized by intramedullary wire or by continuous traction. Most primary practioners can

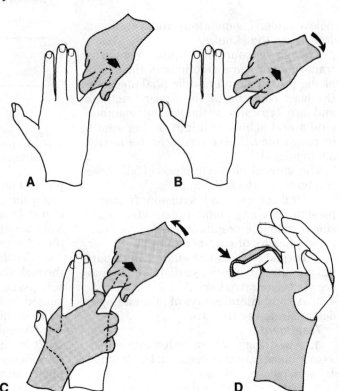

Fig. 6–39. Reduction and immobilization of angulated transverse fracture at the base of the proximal phalanx of the fifth finger. *A*, disimpaction by traction. *B*, angulation to engage the lateral cortex. *C*, realignment using the examiner's finger as a fulcrum. *D*, immobilization with metacarpophalangeal joint at 80° and the proximal interphalangeal joint at 50°.

learn a traction method. We recommend the following (see Figure 6–41):

(1) A forearm cast is applied with the wrist in neutral position or slight dorsiflexion and carried dorsally to the metacarpal heads and ventrally to the distal palmar crease, and to the neck of the first metacarpal.

(2) A coathanger wire is bent into a "U" shape, then bent again to parallel a slightly flexed finger, and adhesive strips are slung between the wires to create a hammock for the finger. This structure is then incorporated into the palmar aspect of the cast at a point which will allow the fractured finger to rest upon it. The length of the wire loop must be great enough for it to extend about 1–1½" beyond the end of the finger when in traction.

(3) The finger is scrubbed with pHisoHex for 5 minutes, then Wescodyne or Betadine solution is applied for 1 minute, and then the finger is dried with a sterile gauze. A Kirschner wire is then passed transversely through the distal phalanx about 1 cm. distal to the distal IP

joint. The wire is bent into a ring around the tip of the finger, and a short, sturdy rubber band is incorporated between the Kirschner wire ring and the coathanger loop.

(4) Traction is applied to the finger by twisting the rubber band with the wooden stick of a cotton applicator which has been shortened to a length ¼" greater than the distance across the wire loop. Once reduction is realized, the traction is maintained by jamming the twisted stick across the wire loop, and taping it securely in place. (See Figure 6–41.)

(5) If it is deemed necessary to protect the traction apparatus, padded plaster can be extended from the cast around the splint and finger as far as the DIP joint.

(6) Before accepting reduction and immobilization, the operator must assure himself that the finger lies in normal rotation; it is too easy to create or overlook a malrotation.

(7) This traction immobilization must be maintained for 3 weeks.

3. Rehabilitation of fractures of the

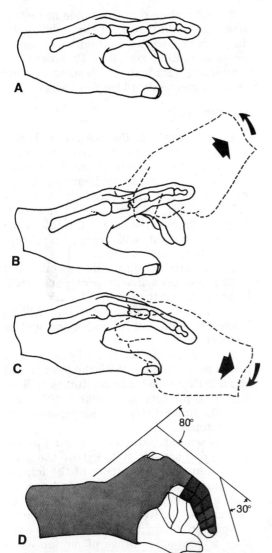

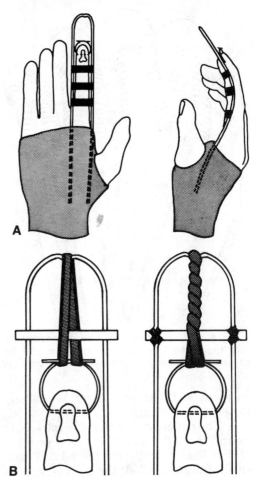

Fig. 6–41. Immobilization of spiral and oblique fractures of the proximal or intermediate phalanx by traction. *A,* incorporation of a wire hammock into the cast and placement of a Kirschner wire through the distal phalanx. *B,* application of traction.

Fig. 6–40. Reduction and immobilization of angulated transverse fracture of the shaft of the proximal phalanx. *A,* dorsally angulated fracture of the index finger. *B,* traction with increased angulation to engage the dorsal margins. *C,* realignment. *D,* immobilization with the metacarpophalangeal joint at 80° and the proximal interphalangeal joint at 30°. The tip of the distal phalanx is exposed to allow the clinician to monitor circulation to the finger.

proximal and middle phalanges is identical to that described for the fractures of the shafts of the metacarpals.

Ligamentous and Tendinous Injuries of the Hand

MP Joints—The Extensor Hood Injury

Any dislocation or hyperflexion strain of the MP joint may tear the extensor hood on one side, allowing the tendon to displace into the web space on the opposite side of the joint as the joint flexes. (See Figure 6–42.)

Clinical characteristics of this injury are the following:

1. The patient may report a hyperflexion strain, or the examiner may have just reduced an MP dislocation, or the patient may present several days after injury complaining of difficulty actively extending the MP joint from a point of full flexion and of his perception that something seems to slip when he flexes the joint.

2. The tendon may be observed to slip off the dorsum of the joint into one of the

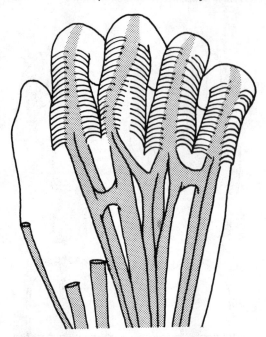

Fig. 6–42. Lateral tear of the extensor hood of the third finger. The illustration shows the tear and the consequent displacement of the extensor tendon.

adjacent webs as the finger is actively flexed.

3. The patient may be unable actively to extend the MP joint fully from a position of full flexion, but once the joint is passively fully extended, the patient will be able to hold the joint strongly in full extension.

Treatment.

1. If the finger be splinted in full extension for 3 weeks, the rent in the extensor hood may heal and function thereafter be satisfactory. Unfortunately, this closed method of treatment does not yield a good result with enough regularity to be relied upon as the treatment of choice. We recommend an open surgical repair and advise that the closed method of treatment be applied only when surgery is refused or unavailable. Therefore, the primary practitioner should splint the finger in full extension and refer the patient to an orthopaedist for open surgical repair at the earliest opportunity.

2. Whichever method is used, the joint is splinted in full extension on a plaster splint, which extends from the palmar surface of a forearm cast. Immobilization is maintained for 3 weeks.

3. Restoration of a full range of motion after discontinuance of immobilization may require weeks to months of active range of motion exercises. Progress is intentionally gradual as healing is not strongly consolidated for 6–8 weeks.

The PIP Joint

✳ ***Stable Sprain of the PIP Joint.*** Forces which laterally angulate, hyperextend, or hyperflex the joint will injure the capsule and its ligamentous thickenings. When these structures are injured short of rupture, the injury is termed a stable sprain. Clinical characteristics are the following:

1. The patient will report an abrupt painful force on the finger.

2. The affected joint will be swollen and tender, and occasionally ecchymoses will be seen around the joint.

3. Range of motion of the joint will be limited by pain, but full extension will be possible.

4. Stress to the collateral ligament will reveal no instability: With the joint flexed about 20°, modest angular forces will be unable to produce more than a 10° angulation in either direction. (See Figure 6–43.)

Treatment.

1. When the examiner is certain that the patient can actively fully extend the joint, and when the volar aspect of the joint is not uniquely tender or passive hyperextension greater than that which can be produced in the twin finger, the finger may be splinted in slight flexion for a few days after which active range of motion exercises may begin.

2. Ice during the first 48 hours may limit swelling, and ultimately either ice or heat prior to active range of motion exercise may create an analgesic effect that will facilitate the performance of the exercises.

Tear or Avulsion of the Collateral Ligament. When forces are great enough to rupture a portion of the capsule and its included ligament, the injury is termed an unstable sprain. Clinical characteristics are the same as for the stable sprain, except that stress to the joint by the method described above will produce greater than 10° angulation in one or both lateral directions. (See Figure 6–43.) Any doubt can usually be dispelled by comparison with the range of angulation possible in the

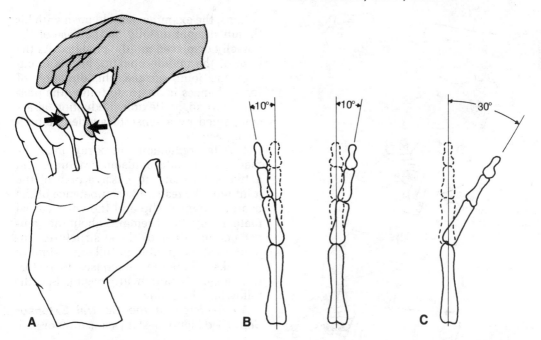

Fig. 6–43. Manipulative examination of the proximal interphalangeal joint. *A*, the manipulation illustrated. (The joint is flexed 20° during the manipula tion.) *B*, limits of normal lateral angulation. *C*, angulation possible after a tear or avulsion of a collateral ligament.

normal twin of the opposite hand.

The avulsion may or may not carry with it a fragment of bone from the ligament's point of attachment to the base of the middle phalanx. Hence, an x-ray may or may not reveal an avulsion fracture at that point.

Treatment.

1. If instability is slight, and if an attendant avulsion fracture shows little displacement, and if the examiner is certain that the patient can fully extend the joint and that the volar aspect of the joint is not uniquely tender or that passive hyperextension is not greater than that possible in the twin finger, we still believe the treatment of choice to be splintage with the injured joint in 15–20° flexion, and the MP joint in 70° flexion. However, some orthopaedists believe that any degree of instability warrants open repair.

2. The splint is a plaster extension from the dorsal surface of a forearm cast.

3. After 3 weeks' immobilization, the splint is removed and rehabilitation is begun. A restoration of full range of motion may take weeks to months of active range of motion exercises.

Dislocation of the PIP Joint. Dislocations of this joint are almost invariably the result of hyperextension injury. The base of the middle phalanx is usually displaced dorsally and proximally out of articulation with the head of the proximal phalanx. (See Figure 6–44.)

The deformity is obvious and usually quite distinct from that of an angulated fracture of the shaft of either phalanx. When in doubt, an x-ray should be made before attempting reduction.

Treatment.

1. If seen within minutes of the injury, the reduction can be effected quickly with less pain than that of a local anesthetic. When a longer period has elapsed, and the difficulty of reduction thus somewhat increased, we recommend a metacarpal block before carrying out the reductive maneuver.

2. The reduction is so easy and the manipulation so safe that it seems a shame to subject the patient to the added misery and risk of a more difficult reduction attendant on the inevitable delay which insistence on an x-ray before treatment will create—unless the examiner is patheti-

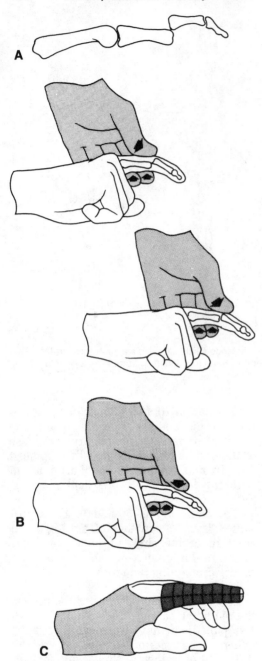

cations, the examiner should push with his thumb straight distally on the base of the dorsally displaced middle phalanx. As the base of the middle phalanx begins to engage the joint surface, the direction of force changes in an arc to follow the phalanx into slight flexion. Reduction is accompanied by a sense of sudden smooth giving way.

4. After reduction, an x-ray must be made to exclude avulsion fractures and active extension and passive play of the joint must be tested for competence of the central extensor slip and the volar carpal plate. If any doubt remains about the competence of either of those structures, the joint must be splinted in full extension for 3 weeks. Thereafter, exercises to restore full range of motion are begun. See the following discussion.

An Avulsion of the Central Extensor Slip. (See Figure 6–45.) Dislocation or sud-

Fig. 6–44. Dislocation of an interphalangeal joint. *A,* dorsal dislocation. *B,* reduction. *C,* immobilization in a forearm cast with a volar splint. The joint is in full extension.

cally in doubt as to whether the injury be a shaft fracture or a dislocation.

3. The reduction is best effected by pushing rather than pulling. (See Figure 6–44.) As recommended for the MP dislo-

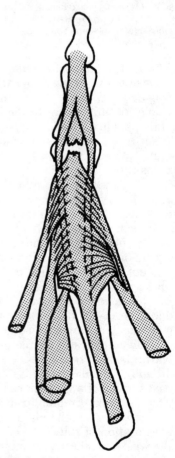

Fig. 6–45. Avulsion of the central extensor tendon slip.

den passive flexion against the patient's resistance may avulse the central extensor slip from its attachment to the dorsum of the base of the middle phalanx. Many textbooks have described this injury to present as a boutonnière deformity with the proximal IP joint in fixed flexion, herniated as it has become between the two lateral slips of the distal extensor tendon. In our experience, the fresh injury does not present with this deformity, and primary practitioners taught to look for the deformity miss the early diagnosis, mistreat the injury, and at their next encounter with the patient face an individual who cannot extend his PIP joint. Perhaps it was the relative stoicism of past generations which caused patients with avulsed central extensor slips to pay their initial visit to the authors of so many textbooks only after the boutonnière deformity had developed. We wish to warn the primary practitioner: An injury which has avulsed the central extensor slip is rarely initially deformed; it can be diagnosed by other signs; and so diagnosed, it can be treated in a manner which will prevent the boutonnière deformity.

The clinical characteristics are the following:

1. The patient may report a sudden impact which painfully forced the PIP joint into flexion, or the practitioner may have just reduced a dislocation of the PIP joint.

2. The joint is quite swollen soon after injury.

3. The patient is unable actively fully to extend the PIP joint. Occasionally the degree of swelling will prevent the practitioner from reliably assessing the degree of active extension.

Treatment.

1. When the PIP joint has been injured, and the practitioner is unable to assess the degree to which the joint can be actively extended, whatever other damage is manifest, avulsion of the central extensor slip must be assumed and the joint splinted in full extension.

2. Within a few days, when the swelling will have diminished, the finger should be re-examined. If at that time full active extension is accomplished, the central extensor slip can be presumed to be intact, and the other manifest damage may be treated in whatever position has been advised.

3. If, however, it is clear at any point that the joint cannot be fully actively extended, an avulsion of the central extensor slip must be presumed, and the finger must remain in full extension for 3 weeks before beginning rehabilitation.

4. Restoration of full motion to the joint may take weeks to months of active range of motion exercises.

Avulsion of the Volar Carpal Plate. (See Figure 6–46.) This avulsion may result from an hyperextension injury short of, or to the point of, frank dislocation of the PIP joint. When most ligament injuries are treated by closed methods, efforts are made to bring the two points of the detachment closer together. The avulsion of the volar carpal plate may be the one exception. If an avulsed volar carpal plate is treated in accordance with the general principle, bringing the points of attachment closer together by immobilizing the joint in flexion, the avulsed volar carpal plate will shorten with healing and create a flexion contracture of the joint which will resemble the boutonnière deformity.

The clinical characteristics of this injury are the following:

1. The patient may report a hyperextension injury, or the examiner may have just reduced a dislocation of the PIP joint.

2. The joint is quite swollen soon after injury.

3. Any efforts to flex or extend the joint increase the pain.

4. The palmar surface may be uniquely tender.

5. It may be possible to hyperextend the

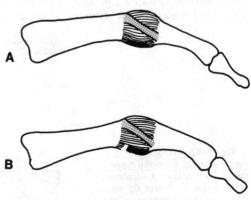

Fig. 6–46. Avulsion of the volar carpal plate. *A,* the normal joint. *B,* the carpal plate is avulsed.

joint beyond the point to which the joint of the twin finger can be hyperextended.

Treatment.

1. When the PIP joint has been injured and is quite swollen, and the palmar surface of the joint is tender and/or the joint can be passively extended to an abnormal degree, an avulsion of the volar carpal plate must be presumed, and whatever other damage is manifest, the joint must be splinted in full extension for 3 weeks before beginning rehabilitation.

2. Restoration of full motion to the joint may take weeks to months of active range of motion exercises.

The DIP Joint.

Avulsion of the Extensor Tendon (the Mallet Finger). Sudden resisted flexion of the DIP joint can avulse the extensor tendon from its attachment to the dorsal surface of the base of the terminal phalanx. (See Figure 6–47.) As late as the 1940's, baseball players—particularly catchers—were notorious for their chronic mallet fingers, called "baseball fingers" in the trade. A foul tip deflecting the ball just off the glove into an extended finger of the ungloved throwing hand was one of the risks of the catcher's position. When they remembered to do it, catchers kept the PIP and DIP joints of the throwing hand flexed while awaiting the pitch. Of course, anyone can sustain a mallet finger injury: A clumsy catch or return by basketball players or volleyball players, a thrust of a swimmer's hand against the end of a pool, a fall onto a slightly flexed and reflexly stiffened finger can all produce the injury. Fewer chronic mallet fingers should be

seen in the world today, as we known how to treat them simply and very cheaply.

The clinical characteristics of the injury are the following:

1. The patient may report a "jamming" injury.

2. Swelling and tenderness are usually evident over the dorsum of the base of the terminal phalanx.

3. When the fingers are held out stiffly, the injured DIP joint remains in slight flexion and its further passive flexion cannot be resisted.

The avulsion may or may not carry with it a fragment of the bone from the tendon's point of attachment to the base of the distal phalanx. Hence, an x-ray may or may not reveal an avulsion fracture at that point.

Treatment.

1. Whether the tendon alone is torn, or whether a piece of its attachment to the distal phalanx has been avulsed makes no difference in treatment. All these injuries must be immobilized in hyperextension for 6 weeks.

2. Because it is simple and unencumbering, and because it allows trustworthy patients to monitor and correct their immobilization themselves, we effect the immobilization with a 1″ conventional metal finger splint.

3. These splints are made bent at about a 110° angle. We widen this angle to about 150°, pad the splint with adhesive foam or Elastoplast, and apply the splint to the injured finger with the apex of the splint at the palmar surface of the dorsal IP joint. The splint is held to the finger with clear tape or standard adhesive tape. A gauze bandage may be applied over all to protect the tapes. (See Figure 6–47.)

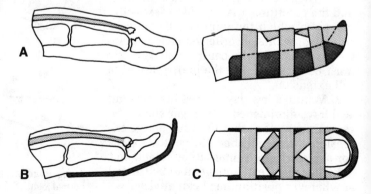

Fig. 6–47. Avulsion of the extensor tendon from the base of the distal phalanx. *A,* illustration of the avulsion. *B* and *C,* reduction and immobilization with a metal finger splint.

4. The splint must be examined weekly to insure that the positon of hyperextension is being maintained. Trustworthy patients may be trained to monitor the splints themselves.

5. This closed method of treatment may be successfully applied as late as 6 weeks after the injury. However, if over 2 months have passed without treatment, open surgical repair will generally be required. Even this repair may not at that stage restore normal extension to the DIP joint.

6. After immobilization is discontinued, restoration of full flexion to the joint may take weeks to months of active range of motion exercises.

Avulsion of the Flexor Profundus Tendon. (See Figure 6–48.) Sudden resisted extension of the dorsal IP joint can avulse the flexor profundus from its attachment to the palmar surface of the base of the terminal phalanx. While avulsion is the more common injury, occasionally the body of the tendon will be ruptured instead. The injury is most prevalent among athletic school children, and occurs most commonly to the middle or ring fingers.

Clinical characteristics are the following:

1. The patient may report a "jamming" injury to the finger.

2. The palmar aspect of the middle phalanx and dorsal IP joint are usually swollen and tender.

3. The patient is unable actively to flex the terminal phalanx.

Treatment. The primary practitioner should splint the finger in a position of function and refer the patient to an orthopaedist for open surgical repair at the earliest opportunity.

Lacerations in the Hand and Wrist

It is hardly hyperbolic to assert that clumsy treatment of hand wounds can devastate the patient's dexterity: Infection in the deep spaces can autolyze tendons or immobilize them in scar tissue; missed or improperly repaired tendon and nerve injuries can prevent an optimal restoration of function; improper repair of fingertip injuries can result in disabling tenderness.

This section will review three large groups of principles with which any practitioner who treats hand injuries should

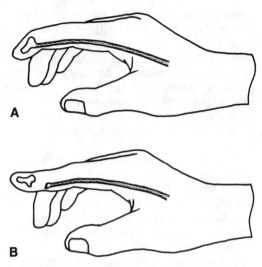

A

B

Fig. 6–48. Avulsion of the flexor profundus tendon from the base of the distal phalanx. *A,* normal. *B,* avulsed.

comply:

1. The general principles of wound repair that minimize unnecessary pain, infection, and avoidable deformity.

2. The nerves and tendons that lacerations are likely to injure and the principles of their repair.

3. The principles of repair of fingertip injuries.

General Principles of Wound Repair

We assume the reader is already thoughtfully acquainted with the general principles of wound care, and intend merely to list for emphasis those principles which in our opinion the occasional operator tends to overlook.

1. An assessment of motor and sensory function should be attempted prior to any manipulation of the wound.

2. When pain appears to be intense, an intravenous analgesic should be administered before proceeding further (morphine grains ⅙ to ¼, or meperidine 50–100 mg.). Patients distracted by pain may cooperate more reliably with an assessment of function after adequate analgesia.

3. The depth of the wound, the availability of skin for wound closure, and the state of the bones and joints should then be assessed by gentle manipulation, and a tentative plan of treatment devised.

4. Local or regional anesthesia should be administered before any further manip-

ulation. We recommend the choice of procedure be determined by the following:

a. Because it is quick and, if injected slowly, is painless, local anesthetic is best for simple lacerations. We use plain lidocaine in wounds of the finger, but take advantage of the hemostatic effect of the lidocaine-adrenalin mixture in most wounds of the palm and dorsum of the hand.

b. All wounds of fingers, except the simplest, uncontused, uncomplicated lacerations, should be anesthetized by a metacarpal or digital block. We prefer the metacarpal block, as it anesthetizes the entire finger and does not swell the finger. Plain 1% lidocaine is used.

c. Complicated or contused lacerations or avulsions to several fingers and extensive injuries of the body of the hand should be anesthetized by lidocaine block at or above the wrist, or the patient should be given a general anesthetic. The axillary block, which requires only one injection, is usually the block of choice. (See Chapter 16.)

5. Adequate exploration of the wound and repair of tendons and nerves usually cannot be accomplished in a bloody field. A digital or brachial tourniquet, applied after draining the venous blood by elevation, should be used when bleeding obscures the operative field. However, *tourniquets should be avoided if at all possible, when repairing a partial amputation of a digit, or a partial amputation of the pad of the fingertip,* as hemostasis encourages the formation of thrombi in small vessels which may obstruct the few remaining vessels to the distal part.

6. There is no "golden period" of safe primary closure. Whether any laceration should be closed primarily or not will depend on the circumstances of that particular laceration. For example, if a clean instrument has lacerated a clean hand, and the wound has been kept clean and shows no evidence of infection, when first seen, the wound may be closed whenever it is first seen. Most contaminated wounds which can be debrided and thoroughly irrigated can probably be closed safely within 10 hours of the injury. On the other hand, bites should almost never be closed primarily.

7. All wounds must be thoroughly irrigated with saline, whether they are to be left open or closed. The word "thoroughly" is a relative word. The greater the presumed contamination, the greater the volume of irrigant used. We may irrigate some wounds with 1000 cc. of saline, and others with only 3-5 cc. of lidocaine remaining in the anesthesia syringe. We conclude the irrigation of the more contaminated wounds with 50 cc. or less of a solution of penicillin in normal saline (20,000 units/cc.), or if the patient be allergic to penicillin, with a solution of neomycin in normal saline (1 mg./cc.).

8. All visible debris must be removed from the wound unless the tissue debridement necessary to achieve that end threatens to be too extensive. For example, dirt stain which may be ground into ligaments and bones may be removed only by removing the ligament or part of the bone. We are content to leave this dirt stain in the hands of the body's defenses.

9. To avoid injury to digital nerves, and to preserve skin for wound closure, debridement must be performed very cautiously. Only obviously avascular tissue should be removed. Contusion alone is no reason for debridement.

10. Skin sutures may be removed from hand and wrist injuries after 10-12 days.

The Injuries Deep to the Skin

1. *Lacerations of the radial aspect of the wrist and hand* may transect one or more of five tendons and the digital branches of the superficial radial nerve (see figures 6-7 and 6-8.) In the wrist, the *extensor pollicis longus* crosses over the *extensor carpi radialis longus* and *brevis* at the dorsal border of the anatomic snuffbox, and the *extensor pollicis brevis* lies just dorsal to the *abductor pollicis longus* at the volar border of the anatomic snuffbox. The digital branches of the radial nerve ramify superifical to these tendons. In the hand, the extensor pollicis longus and brevis angle toward one another from the borders of the anatomic snuffbox to the insertion of the extensor pollicis brevis at the first MP joint. Lacerations into the dorsal border of the anatomic snuffbox may transect the extensor pollicis longus and the extensor

carpi radialis longus and brevis. If all three tendons are lacerated, extension of the DIP joint of the thumb will be lost, and radial bending of the wrist may be weakened. Lacerations into the volar border of the anatomic snuffbox may transect the extensor pollicis brevis, and the abductor pollicis longus. If both tendons are transected, abduction of the thumb and radial bending of the wrist will be distinctly weakened. Laceration into the radial aspect of the hand over the 1st metacarpal may transect the extensor pollicis longus and brevis. Transection of the brevis tendon alone may not produce a visible dysfunction, whereas transection of the longus tendon will prevent extension of the DIP joint of the thumb. Variable dysesthesias to the thumb, index, and/or middle fingers will result from transection of the digital branches of the superficial radial nerve. Lacerations into the volar radial border of the wrist are also likely to enter the dorsal and/or palmar branches of the radial artery. Most orthopaedists will always repair the extensor pollicis longus, abductor pollicis longus, and one of the extensor carpi tendons. Some will repair both extensor carpi tendons and will be prepared to re-open the wound at a later date to lyse the adhesions that almost inevitably will form.

2. *Lacerations into the dorsum of the wrist and hand* may transect an extensor tendon to the fingers. The patient with such an injury is unable to extend the MP joint controlled by that tendon, but is able to extend the PIP joint, and the distal IP joints. The reader will remember that extension of those joints is partially controlled by the intrinsic muscles of the hand through their insertion into the extensor hood distal to the MP joint. These tendons should be repaired on the day of injury.

3. *Lacerations into the ulnar aspect of the wrist* can transect the flexor carpi ulnaris and/or extensor carpi ulnaris. (See Figures 6–5 and 6–7.) Only a little more force than that necessary to transect the flexor carpi ulnaris will carry the injuring instrument into and through the ulnar nerve. Transection of both flexor and extensor tendons will prevent active ulnar deviation of the wrist, but transection of only one or the other may not result in any visible dysfunction. Transection of the ul-

nar nerve will paralyze the intrinsic muscles of the hand, except those of the thenar eminence, thus preventing flexion of the MP joints of the fingers during extension of the PIP and DIP joints, and will prevent abduction and adduction of the fingers. If both tendons are transected, at least the extensor tendon should be repaired. If the ulnar nerve is transected, it is best repaired primarily. If the only available physician seriously doubts his ability to repair it, he should leave the nerve untouched and close the wound. That patient should be referred after 6 weeks to an orthopaedist or neurosurgeon for secondary repair.

4. *Lacerations into the volar aspect of the wrist* are quite likely to transect the palmaris longus and the flexor carpi radialis tendons, and are slightly less likely to pass through the transverse carpal ligament (flexor retinaculum) to transect the median nerve. Those lacerations that injure the flexor carpi radialis are likely to also lacerate the palmar branch of the radial artery. Deeper injuries transect the flexors to the fingers, as well as the more superficial tendons, and are much less commonly encountered. The dysfunction characteristic of transection of the flexors to the fingers and thumb, and of the median nerve, are summarized in paragraphs 5 and 6 immediately following. When all flexor tendons have been transected, most surgeons will repair the flexor profundus tendons and the flexor pollicis longus and leave the rest, on the grounds that the minimal procedure is less likely to result in adhesive scarring than would repair of all the flexors at once. When the flexor sublimis tendons have been transected and the flexor profundus tendons spared, many surgeons will repair the flexor sublimis tendons. Transection of the palmaris longus and the flexor carpi radialis tendon need not be repaired, but when both ends of the tendons are readily accessible, their repair is not contraindicated, and should restore to the wrist a more normal appearance.

If it can be done well, a transected median nerve should be primarily repaired. Should the primary practitioner seriously doubt his ability to repair the nerve and no other surgeon be available, he should leave the nerve alone and close the wound. That patient should be referred after 6 weeks to an orthopaedist or neurosurgeon for secondary repair. At the wrist level, the median nerve and the flexor tendons have been mistaken for one another, and the tendon has been sutured to nerve. This costly if not tragic error can be avoided if one keeps the possibility of the error and the different appearance of nerve from tendon in mind. The nerve is softer than tendon, does not share a tendon's glistening white appearance, but is rather a dull yellow, and is often accompanied by a thin blood vessel which courses on its surface.

5. *Lacerations into the thenar eminence* may transect the motor branch of the median nerve, paralyzing the muscles of the thenar eminence and may transect the flexor pollicis longus tendon. The function of the nerve is tested by instructing the patient to make an "O" with the thumb and the fifth finger. The nerve can be presumed to be intact only if the thenar muscles become palpably firm during this effort, and if the examiner experiences moderate resistance when attempting to pull one of his own fingers through the ring of the "O" while the patient resists. The function of the tendon is tested by instructing the patient to flex the IP joint of the thumb while keeping the MP joint in extension. An inability to do so implies transection of the tendon. Most surgeons prefer to repair these injuries primarily.

6. *Lacerations into the palm* may transect the flexor tendons to the fingers and/or the digital nerves. Perception of light touch and pinprick are tested on each side of the tips of each finger, and flexor tendon function is tested as follows:

Flexor profundus. The MP and PIP joints of one finger are held in extension by the examiner while the patient is instructed to flex the DIP joint of that finger. Inability to do so implies a transection of its deep flexor. Each finger is tested in turn.

Flexor sublimis. The DIP and PIP joints of the fingers adjacent to the finger to be tested are fully extended by the examiner while the patient is instructed to flex the PIP joint of the test finger. Because the flexor profundus tendons are fused at the wrist level, passive extension of PIP and DIP joints of the neighboring fingers pre-

vents any application of muscle force to the flexor profundus of the test finger. Any flexion of the PIP joint under those circumstances must thus be attributed to the sublimis tendon alone. Inability to flex the PIP joint during this testing maneuver implies a transection of the superficial flexor to that finger. Each finger is tested in turn.

Most surgeons prefer to repair these injuries primarily.

7. *Lacerations into the palmar aspect of the proximal phalanx of a finger* may lacerate both the flexor sublimis and flexor profundus tendons. Transection of both tendons in this region prevents flexion of the PIP and DIP joints, but does not prevent flexion of the MP joints. When the patient is instructed to flex the finger, the MP joint will flex while the PIP and DIP joints will remain in extension. This area has been called "no man's land," in deference to the classic opinion that tendon injuries in this area should not be primarily repaired. This opinion is based on the observation that adhesions are more likely to form between the tendons and their common sheaths when healing in the depths of an accidental injury, than they are at a later date when healing in the depths of a clean, neat, surgical wound. However, we have been tending more to suture these tendons primarily, provided the laceration is clean and the tissues are not contused. After repair, the injured fingers are splinted in a position of function.

8. *Lacerations into the palmar aspect of the middle phalanx or DIP joint* may transect the flexor profundus tendon. When the patient with such an injury is instructed to flex the finger, the MP and PIP joints will flex while the DIP joint will remain extended. Many surgeons prefer to repair this injury primarily.

9. *Laceration into the dorsum of a MP joint* can variously disrupt the extensor hood. Axial lacerations, like tears of the extensor hood, can so split the hood as to make the lie of the tendon over the apex of the joint unstable. During full flexion, the tendon will slip off into the trough of the interdigital web. Lacerations to either side of the apex will allow the tendon to slip to the opposite side, and lacerations through the apex will allow the tendon to split half into each groove. With the ten-

don thus displaced, active extension of the MP joint from a position of full flexion becomes impossible. Transverse lacerations will transect the tendon and the adjacent portions of the hood, making full extension of the MP joint impossible. All of these lacerations, except perhaps the deepest and widest transverse lacerations, leave at least one attachment of the intrinsic muscles undisturbed; thus like tears of the extensor hood, these lacerations do not prevent full extension of the PIP and DIP joints, but only of the MP joint. These injuries should be primarily repaired.

10. *Lacerations over the dorsum of a proximal phalanx* may transect the extensor tendon at that level, preventing extension of the PIP and DIP joints. These injuries should be primarily repaired.

11. *Lacerations over the dorsum of the PIP joint* can variously disrupt the three slips of the extensor tendon. Axial lacerations through the apex of the joint may split the central slip, allowing the joint to herniate between the two halves during full flexion, and the transverse lacerations through the apex of the joint can transect the central slip, allowing the joint to herniate between the lateral slips during full flexion. Both of these injuries, like the avulsion of the central slip, will result in a boutonnière deformity. More laterally placed transverse lacerations may transect the underlying lateral slip of the extensor tendon. This injury may not result in any visible dysfunction, or it may—by changing the direction of the tendon's force—prevent full extension of the DIP joint. The widest transverse laceration may transect all three slips, preventing the extension of the DIP as well as the PIP joint. Many surgeons prefer not to repair these extensor slip lacerations primarily, but rather to splint them in full extension and attempt a secondary repair after 6 weeks' healing, if function is not normal at that time. If the wound is clean and not contused, we prefer primary repair.

12. *Lacerations into the dorsum of the middle phalanx and DIP joint* may transect the terminal portion of the extensor tendon, preventing extension of the DIP joint. This injury should be primarily repaired.

13. *Lacerations into the lateral aspect of the fingers* may transect the digital nerves, yielding various dysesthesias, and if over the PIP or DIP joints, may transect the capsule and its ligamentous thickening, yielding an unstable joint. The ligamentous injury should be primarily repaired. If at all possible, the digital nerves should be primarily repaired. When the only available physician cannot repair the nerves, the nerves should be left alone and the wound closed. The patient should be referred after 6 weeks to an orthopaedist or neurosurgeon for consideration of secondary repair.

Repair of Tendons, Ligaments, and Nerves

We recommend the Bunnell stitch and the near-and-far stitch for repair of hand and wrist tendons, and a simple running stitch for repair of lacerations of the extensor hood and of ligaments. The near-and-far stitch is particularly useful for repairing the flat, fairly narrow extensor tendons in the fingers. The near-and-far stitch can often be placed through a small laceration which would have to be extended, were one to place the Bunnell stitch. But the greater security of the Bunnell stitch recommends it for the larger tendons,

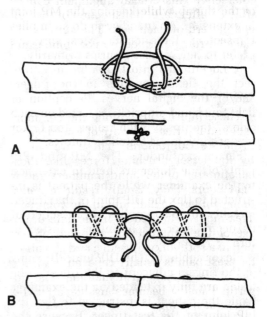

Fig. 6–49. Tendon repair. *A,* near and far stitch. *B,* Bunnell stitch. The near and far stitch leaves the knot exposed, while the Bunnell stitch buries the knot between the tendon fragments.

whether at hand or wrist levels (see Figure 6–49). 4-0 or 5-0 monofilament nylon, Prolene, or wire are the suture materials of choice for tendon repair. The following is a summary of those tendon injuries which we feel can be satisfactorily repaired in an outpatient setting:

1. Lacerations of the extensor hood.
2. Extensor tendons on the wrist, hand, and phalanges including the isolated injury of the extensor pollicis longus tendon. However, we do not recommend outpatient repair of transections about the PIP joint beyond that point where the tendon is split into three slips, unless the outpatient surgery is quite clean and the outpatient surgeon very adept.

3 and 4. Palmaris longus and flexor carpi radialis tendons, when both ends are clearly accessible, and the transection neat and clean.

5. Flexor digitorum profundus when lacerated at the level of the middle phalanx, the laceration is neat and clean, and the tendon ends are readily retrieved.

The ends of severed nerves are approximated with interrupted 8–10 ϕ nonabsorbable suture. The fascicles or nerve bundles of each end must line up with those of the other end. This crucial alignment can be affected after careful inspection of the mosaic pattern of each end. The sutures are placed through perineurium or epineurium not through nerve bundles.

Fingertip Injuries

These injuries are among the commonest hand injuries. They are of four degrees:

Simple Contusions. These are caused by the lesser crushing forces like those encountered under hand hammers and in light doors. They usually result in hematomas under the nail, and in the volar pad. Treatment is limited to immediate drainage of the subungual hematoma, protection in a soft bulky dressing, and elevation. Severest pain is usually relieved by drainage of the subungual hematoma. The fingertip usually becomes usable after 1–2 weeks of healing.

Complicated Contusions. These are caused by the moderate crushing forces. The nail plate may be avulsed, and the nail bed disrupted, the volar pad may be burst. the distal phalanx may be fractured, and/or the insertion of the flexor or extensor tendons avulsed.

Treatment. Open wounds are thoroughly irrigated and debrided, then treated as follows: The architecture of the nail bed should be restored as accurately as possible. Wound margins must be held in close approximation by suture or adhesive strips ("Steri-Strips"), and any avulsed nail bed should be replaced by split thickness grafts from the volar forearm. The avulsed nail plate should be trimmed to fit exactly over the nail bed and fixed in place with sutures or adhesive strips. It should be left on the nail bed for 2–3 weeks, after which the nail bed will have healed and toughened sufficiently to withstand exposure. The margins of the wound of the burst volar pad should be closely approximated by percutaneous sutures. Fractures of the distal phalanx should be molded manually to proper shape and splinted in a soft bulky dressing. The patient must be instructed to flex and extend the DIP joint actively. An inability to do either will often correlate with x-ray evidence of an avulsion fracture of the base of the phalanx. These avulsions are treated as described above under "The DIP Joint."

Volar Pad Avulsions. Slicing or heavy crushing forces may remove the volar pad from the fingertip. We are accustomed to covering avulsed surfaces greater than 1 sq. cm. in area with a split thickness graft or a rotation flap. Avulsions less than 1 sq. cm. in area we leave to heal by secondary intention. Recent publications and the experience of some of our emergency physicians suggest that the final outcome can be expected to be just as satisfactory whether an avulsion be grafted or left to heal by secondary intention regardless of size. In either case, the wound is thoroughly cleaned by irrigation, scrubbing, and debridement as necessary. When ground-in grease or dirt cannot be removed, the wound is best left open for 1–2 weeks before attempting a graft procedure.

Basic Principles of Skin Graft. (See Figure 6–50.) The split thickness graft is most likely to take, but the full thickness graft entirely separated from subcutaneous fascia provides a thicker and thus tougher volar pad. Indeed, if the avulsed volar pad is available and has not been contused, it can be converted by sharp scraping into a

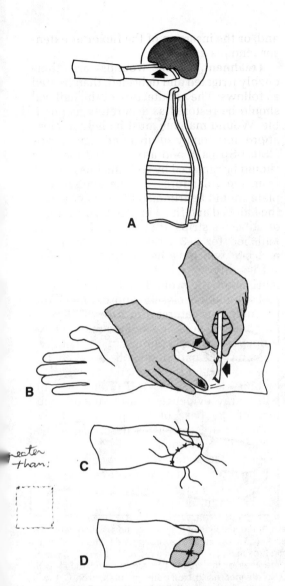

greater
than:

Fig. 6–50. Preparation of split thickness skin graft. *A*, conversion of an avulsed volar pad to a split thickness graft—viewed from the deep surface. *B*, creation of a split thickness graft from skin of the volar forearm. *C*, the split thickness graft attached with interrupted sutures, four of which are cut long. *D*, pressure pad tied in place by the long sutures.

thick split thickness graft which often takes, is tough, and is cosmetically most satisfactory. (See Figure 6–50.) Grafts taken from the volar forearm are obtained as diagrammed in Figure 6–50. Split thickness grafts are taken by a tangential cut in the center of a field previously anesthetized by 1% lidocaine. We find a No. 10 blade quite adequate for the size of graft we generally need. The proper thickness carries no fat and leaves punctate bleeding

at the graft site. The graft is fitted to the margins of the wound, and sutured in place of interrupted 4-0 suture. The graft is kept in close apposition to the wound with a gauze or Telfa pad which has been tied firmly over the graft by long threads of four of the interrupted marginal sutures. (See Figure 6–50.) A soft bulky dressing is applied over the graft pad and the finger. After 4 days, the bulky dressing and graft pad are removed, and the graft is inspected for fluctuance. Any fluctuance implies the accumulation of blood or serum between the wound surface and graft, or between the epidermis and the dermis of the graft. To distinguish where this fluid is is difficult. It must be drained off, and another pressure pad applied, and held in place with adhesive strips. Bulky soft dressing is reapplied over all, and the wound is ignored for another 6 days. On the 10th day after injury, the pressure dressing and marginal sutures are removed. Most grafts, especially full thickness grafts, will appear blistered at this time, if not earlier, causing the novice to fear for the graft. But within the following 1–2 weeks, it often becomes clear that the dermis has taken and that only the epidermis has sloughed, and a new epidermis has begun to regenerate. Indeed, if properly prepared and carefully applied after this fashion, nearly all split thickness grafts and most full thickness grafts will take. The patient is instructed to bathe the wound in warm soapy water twice daily, rinsing thoroughly afterward, and to protect the wound with Band-Aids to the pad of which has been applied an antibiotic ointment, until the graft has been fully re-epithelialized. When the wound fully matures, the size of the grafted site will be somewhat smaller than the original wound. The cutaneous sensation in these fingertips will always remain impaired, but they rarely remain painfully sensitive beyond 8 weeks. On the other hand, wounds left alone to heal entirely by secondary intention may remain painfully sensitive for a somewhat longer time and they also fail to regain normal cutaneous sensation.

The Rotation Flap. Skin defects in inelastic areas like fingertips can sometimes be closed by rotation flaps which transfer the defect to an elastic area where, after adequate undermining, skin will stretch

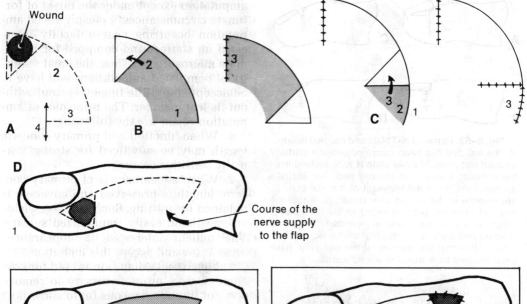

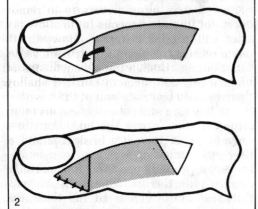

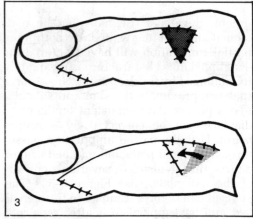

Fig. 6–51. Principles and application of the rotation flap. *A,* modification of the wound and creation of the flap. The wound is converted to a wedge (*1*). A curvilinear incision (*2*) is extended in a circular arc to the chosen area of elastic skin. The direction of the circular arc in the elastic area must be such that a radial incision (*3*) will cross perpendicular to the axis of greatest elasticity (*4*). As the lines of the wedge (*1*) are oriented radial to the curvilinear incision, the direction of the wedge must be so planned as to cause the radial incision (*3*) to be oriented perpendicular to the axis of greatest elasticity (*4*). *B,* undermining (*1*), rotation of the flap (*2*), and closure of the original defect (*3*). *C,* extension of the curvilinear incision (*1*) and undermining (*2*) to allow closure of the created defect (*3*) by stretched skin. *D,* application of the rotation flap for closure of a finger wound. *1,* conversion of the wound to a wedge, and creation of a flap. Note the incisions avoid crossing the nerve supply to the flap. *2,* undermining and rotation of the flap and closure of the original defect. *3,* the new defect can be closed by extension of the incision, undermining and stretch, or by split thickness graft, depending on the size of the new defect relative to the elasticity of the surrounding skin.

sufficiently to bridge the defect. When thick skin and normal sensation seem advisable, as over the pinching surfaces of the thumb and index finger, we prefer closure by rotation flap to closure by split thickness graft or secondary intention healing. When a defect is too large for closure by a rotation flap alone, we sometimes combine the two methods, thus grafting over a smaller area than would have been necessary by grafting alone.

Figure 6–51 diagrams the principles of the rotation flap and illustrates two uses for the method in repair of finger wounds.

Partial and Complete Amputations. Slicing and heavy crushing forces may completely or partially sever part or all of the distal phalanx. A partially amputated portion may be reattached if the distal fragment remains well perfused as evidenced by bleeding, pink color, and capillary return. If in doubt, or if the patient is

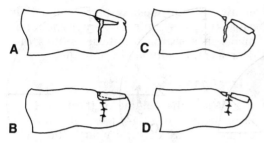

Fig. 6–52. Repair of nail plate and nail bed injuries. A, the nail bed has been lacerated under a partially avulsed nail plate. The nail plate is fully avulsed from the proximal fragment of the nail bed, and partially avulsed from the distal fragment of the nail bed. B, appearance of the wound after repair. Note that the nail plate has not been replaced under the epionychium. C, the nail bed has been lacerated through the severed nail plate. D, illustration of the wound after repair. Note that the margins of the nail plate have been trimmed back from the wound margin.

urgent, the distal fragment can be reattached and its fate awaited. By definition, partial amputation will have fractured the distal phalanx. This fracture is adequately immobilized by the deep soft tissue sutures that reapproximate the skin and subcutaneous planes. Any persistent tendency to displace can be corrected by a proper splint. Usually, partial amputation passes through the nail plate and nail bed or nail matrix, thus *avulsing* or *severing* a portion of the nail plate. (See Figure 6–52.) The *avulsed* nail plate is trimmed to fit the nail bed and is reapplied to it after repairing the injury to the nail bed. The two portions of the *severed* nail plate may be left attached as they are to the proximal and distal protions of the nail bed, and allowed thus to come into reapproximation, along with the two portions of fingertip. However, occasionally the nail bed at the wound margins is prevented from close approximation by the nail plate. If so, when all else seems to be healing well, granulations will form in the nail bed wound and emerge between the two portions of the nail plate. While repeated cautery will eventually lead to healing, the resultant scar in the nail bed will distort the new nail. This complication cannot be predicted. We prefer to prevent its occasional occurrence by clipping back the two portions of nail plate 2–3 mm. from the wound margin, to allow precise and confirmed approximation of the margins of the nail bed.

One cannot hope to restore a completed amputation except under the rarest of fortunate circumstances: a cleanly sliced amputation occurring near a facility interested in, staffed, and equipped for immediate microsurgery. Thus, the great majority of completed amputations will have to be accepted and the finger repaired without its lost member. The principles of amputation repair are the following:

1. When function is of primary concern, length may be sacrificed for strong, normally sensitive coverage.

2. When appearance is of primary concern, length is preserved and coverage is obtained by grafting. Such coverage yields an anesthetic easily traumatized surface. The patient interested in appearances must know and accept this limitation.

3. When remaining skin is used for coverage, it may prove necessary to remove some of its subcutaneous fat to allow neat but still padded coverage. However, the skin receives its blood supply from vessels that course through the subcutaneous fat, hence this debridement must be shallow, particularly centrally and at the base.

4. The skin and its subcutaneous fat are applied snugly over the end, but not so snugly as to prevent a brisk capillary return.

5. Length with good function can sometimes be preserved when available volar skin allows coverage to the volar two-thirds of the tip. The remaining dorsal defect can be covered by a split or full thickness graft.

Amputation wounds are variously oriented and include various excess or deficiency of well-perfused volar skin. Thus, every repair requires some creative planning. By strict adherence to the above five principles, the primary practitioner who is comfortable with that kind of mechanical creativity can and should repair fingertip amputations. The only instrument he will need, in addition to those on the standard laceration set-up, is the rongeur.

Soft Tissue Syndromes of the Wrist and Hand

The primary practitioner commonly encounters each of nine syndromes:

Carpal Tunnel Syndrome

The anatomy of the carpal tunnel was reviewed above under "Carpal Tunnel."

The volume of the tunnel is only slightly greater than the volume of its soft tissue contents. Any process which decreases the volume of the tunnel or increases the volume of its contents will so crowd the median nerve as to interfere with its blood supply and cause it to malfunction. Early malfunction presents as a dysesthesia; late malfunction presents as thenar atrophy and weakness of abduction and opposition of the thumb. The volume of the tunnel may be decreased by the deformity of a Colles' or a carpal fracture, by arthritic spurs, or by a tumor or by a thickening of the flexor retinaculum. The volume of the contents can be increased by simple fluid retention, by fat deposition, by carpal synovitis, and by tenosynovitis.

Characteristic clinical features are the following:

1. Patients will complain of paresthesias and hypesthesias in the hand. Initially, many patients will insist that the entire hand becomes numb, and only after careful questioning and not until a second visit are they able to acknowledge the median nerve distribution of this numbness—thumb, index, middle and radial aspect of the ring finger. Often patients will complain of one finger more than the others, which finger will vary from patient to patient.

2. Many but not all patients will complain of pain in the wrist.

3. Symptoms tend to emerge during sleeping hours and during sustained manual activity, like driving and knitting.

4. While both hands may be symptomatic, one hand is usually more severely so than the other.

5. Particularly in the face of carpal synovitis and tenosynovitis, the wrist may appear unusually full and be unusually tender, and wrist motion may be restricted by pain.

6. Extreme palmar flexion may aggravate the dysesthesias, and extreme dorsiflexion is somewhat less likely to do so. *Phalen's*

7. Tapping over the volar aspect of the wrist at the level of the distal crease may produce painful paresthesias in the median nerve distribution. This phenomenon is called Tinel's sign.

Diagnosis is made when most of these characteristics are evident and when an examination of the neck, shoulder, and elbow fails to detect a more compatible cause for the symptoms. X-rays should be made, in a search for those entities that decrease the volume of the tunnel.

Treatment.

1. When the volume of the tunnel has been decreased by a persistent Colles' or carpal fracture deformity, arthritic spurs, or tumor, or when thenar wasting is evident, the patient should be promptly referred to an orthopedist for consideration of surgical decompression of the tunnel. Otherwise, the following conservative measures should be employed.

2. When history and examination suggest recent weight gain and/or fluid retention, diuretics and a diet for salt restriction or weight loss should be prescribed.

3. When fullness, tenderness, and painful motion suggest carpal synovitis or tenosynovitis, the cause for the inflammation should be sought. (See Chapter 18) If the cause is degenerative, oral anti-inflammatory agents may be employed. (See Chapter 18) Alternatively, a corticosteroid may be injected—0.5 cc. of any intra-articular corticosteroid is injected just distal to the distal carpal crease, to one side or the other of the palmaris longus tendon. We use a No. 25 needle and introduce it perpendicular to the surface to a depth of about 1 cm. (See Figure 6–53.) Should the needle provoke median nerve paresthesias, it

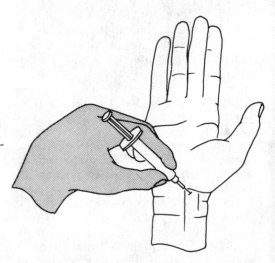

Fig. 6–53. Injection of the carpal tunnel. The needle enters just distal to the distal carpal crease, to one side or the other of the palmaris longus tendon.

must be withdrawn and repositioned to a point that does not provoke the paresthesias. A corticosteroid should be injected into the free space, not into any structure, and its instillation should be painless. Should the inflammation appear to stem from other causes (rheumatoid, gout, pseudogout, gonococcal), treatment should follow the regimen recommended for those diseases. (See Chapter 18) Degeneration is far and away the most common cause of these carpal synovial and tenosynovial inflammations, as it is for all synovial tenosynovial inflammations.

4. Ice should be applied in the face of acute inflammatory signs.

5. The patient must be instructed to avoid extreme wrist movements and repetitive gripping activities. A removable dorsal splint may be used as a reminder through the day, but is particularly beneficial during sleeping hours. The wrist is held in neutral position.

6. When 6–8 weeks of conservative measures fail, it may be quite appropriate to refer the patient to an orthopaedist. However, the appearance of thenar weakness or atrophy at any point is an indication for immediate referral.

DeQuervain's Syndrome

This syndrome is less common than the carpal tunnel syndrome. The tendons of the abductor pollicis longus and extensor pollicis brevis share a common tendon sheath as they cross the radial styloid and create the volar border of the anatomic snuffbox. This sheath may become painfully inflamed, especially in those who use their thumbs repetitively, as in knitting. The digital branches of the radial nerve which course over the tendons may become irritated as well, particularly when swelling is extreme. Characteristic clinical features are the following:

1. Patients will complain of pain in the radial aspect of the wrist and thumb, which may be intensified by wrist and thumb movement.

2. If digital branches of the radial nerve are irritated, patients may complain of pain and paresthesias in the dorsum of the thumb, index, and middle fingers. This complaint may cause the unwary to mistakenly diagnose a carpal tunnel syndrome.

3. Swelling may be palpable or visible over the tendons, just distal to the radial styloid, and tenderness may be distinguished over the course of the tendon near the radial styloid.

4. Occasionally, a creaking crepitation may be palpable over the tendons during thumb motion.

5. Active or passive adduction of the thumb across the palm increases pain.

6. Resisted abduction and extension of the thumb increases pain.

Treatment.

1. The wrist and trapeziometacarpal joint should be immobilized in a dorsoradial plaster splint.

2. Ice should be applied in the face of acute inflammatory signs. Otherwise, the patient may use either heat or cold, whichever is more comforting.

3. One-half cubic centimeter of any intra-articular corticosteroid may be injected in and around the tendon sheath. This injection may give dramatic relief and is the anti-inflammatory treatment of choice.

4. Oral anti-inflammatory agents may be employed, as for the carpal tunnel syndrome, should the patient refuse an injection.

5. If symptoms persist after 6 weeks' immobilization and a trial of the various anti-inflammatory medications, the patient may quite reasonably be referred to an orthopaedist who may consider incision or excision of the tendon sheath. That treatment usually grants dramatic relief.

Tenosynovitis of the Extensor Tendon Sheath

This syndrome is less common than is DeQuervain's syndrome. The sheath of the common extensor tendon to the fingers at the wrist may become painfully inflamed, particularly after activity requiring repetitive wrist flexion-extension, as is required in the game of badminton. Characteristic clinical features are the following:

1. The patient may complain of pain in the dorsum of the wrist and hand, worsened by wrist movement.

2. Active or passive volar flexion and resisted dorsiflexion of the wrist may augment the pain.

3. Visible or palpable swelling may be

evident over the dorsum of the wrist, and the common tendon may be tender.

4. A creaking crepitation may be palpable during wrist flexion and extension.

Treatment.

1. The wrist should be splinted in 30° of dorsiflexion.

2. Ice should be applied, in the face of acute inflammatory signs. Otherwise, the patient may use either heat or ice, whichever is more comforting.

3. Oral anti-inflammatory medications or injectable intra-articular corticosteroids may be used as prescribed for De-Quervain's syndrome. As in the De-Quervain's syndrome, an injection of corticosteroid may give dramatic relief.

Inflammation of the Ulnar Flexor Mechanism

The flexor carpi ulnaris inserts upon the pisiform bone, which is palpable just distal to the distal flexor crease of the wrist on the ulnar side. The pisiform transmits the force of the flexor carpi ulnaris through ligaments to the triquetrum. The sheath of the tendon and/or the pisiform-triquetral ligaments may become inflamed, particularly during activity requiring repetitive ulnar bending as occurs during fly casting, or prolonged ulnar friction as occurs during lengthy writing. The ulnar nerve, which lies just deep to the flexor carpi ulnaris, and just radial to the pisiform, may become irritated as well.

Characteristic clinical features are the following:

1. Patients may complain of pain over the ulnar aspect of the wrist and hand, worsened by movement, and may complain of paresthesias in the ulnar distribution (fifth finger and ulnar aspect of the ring finger).

2. Passive or active dorsiflexion and radial deviation, and resisted active volar flexion and ulnar deviation may increase the pain.

3. The volar ulnar aspect of the wrist may be visibly swollen and is usually tender.

4. When ulnar nerve irritation is advanced, intrinsic muscle weakness and wasting in ulnar distribution will become evident. The hypothenar eminence will be visibly flattened and the force of abduction and adduction of the fingers will be weakened.

Treatment.

Immobilization, ice, or heat, and anti-inflammatory medications are employed as for the DeQuervain's syndrome. Again, corticosteroid injection into and around the tendon sheath and around the pisiform bone may afford dramatic relief. Injection technique should avoid injury to the ulnar nerve. Evidence of intrinsic muscle weakness or wasting is indication for prompt referral to an orthopaedist, who may consider release of fibers which pass from the pisiform superficial to the ulnar nerve, and attach to the flexor retinaculum, which lies deep to the ulnar nerve. The ulnar nerve is held firmly in this short canal, vulnerable to pressure from the swelling of the inflamed sheath of the flexor carpi ulnaris, and the inflamed pisotriquetrous ligaments. Release of the constraining fibers frees the nerve from the pressure created upon it by these inflamed structures.

The Trigger Finger and the Clutched Thumb

A fibrous sheath crosses over each flexor tendon at each MP joint, thereby creating a pulley-like restricting canal for the tendon. These sheaths may thicken, narrowing the canals beneath them, while the underlying segments of tendon may enlarge as a nodule. (See Figure 6–54.) Tendons involved in this process are the flexor pollicis longus, the flexor digitorum profundus, or the bifurcation of the flexor digitorum sublimis. Passage of such a nodule through the narrowed restricting canal will produce a sensation of snapping. Eventually, active flexion of the joint may become very difficult, and subsequent active extension nearly impossible. The underlying cause of the trigger finger and clutched thumb is usually unknown, though benign. Occasionally, it represents the first appearance of rheumatoid tenosynovitis.

Characteristic clinical features are the following:

1. Patients will complain of a snapping when actively flexing and extending the affected finger. They will often attribute these symptoms to a locking of the PIP joint.

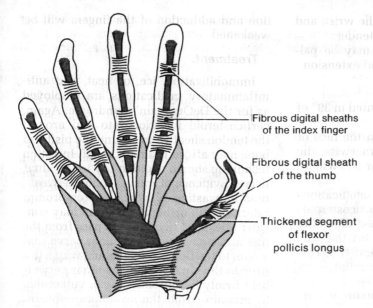

Fibrous digital sheaths
of the index finger

Fibrous digital sheath
of the thumb

Thickened segment
of flexor
pollicis longus

Fig. 6-54. Fibrous digital sheaths of all the fingers are illustrated. A thickened tendon segment of the flexor pollicis longus is trapped proximal to the fibrous digital sheath of the thumb. The extensor policis longus may not be able to overcome the resulting resistance.

2. Patients will occasionally complain of pain or of tenderness over the palmar aspect of the MP joint.

3. A nodule which moves with active flexion and extension may be palpable in the palm, just proximal to the affected MP joint.

4. From a position of extension, the finger can be passively fully flexed and subsequently fully extended actively or passively without any snapping. After the finger has been actively flexed, any effort to extend it passively will provoke a snapping through a point of resistance.

5. Snapping during active flexion is palpable over the palmar aspect of the MP joint.

Treatment. Occasionally, injection of an intra-articular corticosteroid into the restricting canal, and rest of the tendon, by immobilization of the finger in a splint will yield a remission within 1-2 weeks. Often, the fibrous sheath overlying the tendon must be longitudinally incised, fully opening the canal to free the tendon from its entrapment. Because a rheumatoid tenosynovitis may be encountered, requiring a tenosynovectomy, the procedure should be done in hospital by an orthopaedist or hand surgeon.

The Ganglion   Cyst

These are cystic masses that emerge from tendon sheaths or joint capsules. The pathogenesis of these cysts is not certainly known.

Ganglions are quite common about the wrist and hand. They are typically encountered in one of four locations:

1. On the dorsal aspect of the wrist, emerging from the sheaths of the tendons of the extensors to the fingers, or from the joint capsule of the wrist (usually the interosseous intercarpal ligaments).

2. On the radiovolar aspect of the wrist, either from tenosynovium of radially placed tendons, or from the joint capsule of the wrist. These are often intimately bound to the radial artery.

3. On the dorsal aspect of the hand, emerging from the sheaths of the extensor tendons to the fingers.

4. On the palmar aspect of fingers, usually near the MP joint. Ganglions in this location present as hard nodules, sometimes seeming to the novice to be bony projections.

Characteristic clinical features are the following:

1. Patients who consult about ganglions are nearly all troubled about their significance.

2. Some will also complain of pain, occasionally of rather intense pain, worsened by movement.

3. Patients often become aware of ganglions rather abruptly, as though they had appeared overnight.

4. The size of ganglions will vary spontaneously over time, occasionally seeming to disappear entirely, but nearly always reappearing, within weeks or months.

Treatment. We do not believe that ganglions need to be excised. Indeed, a permanent cure by excision is not easily obtained. The dissection always must be meticulous and extensive to insure removal of the entire cyst and its connection to the tendon sheath or joint capsule. Even in the most experienced hands, such a complete dissection cannot always be accomplished, and recurrences are common.

Once reassured that the unfamiliar lump is not a dangerous tumor, many patients are content with symptomatic treatment repeated whenever necessary. Prominent cysts may be drained through a No. 18 needle. Gelatinous cysts will drain only when forced by pressure over the cyst, coupled with aspiration by a syringe 10 cc. in size or larger. Following aspiration, an intra-articular corticosteroid may be instilled through the same needle. Any pain will subside with this treatment, and the occasional cyst may "never" return. When patients refuse drainage, splintage and oral anti-inflammatory drugs like phenylbutazone may relieve pain quite successfully. Some patients will report that they periodically have "cured" their own cysts by bursting them, either by strong manual pressure or by sharply striking them with a book.

Dupuytren's Contracture

The palmar fascia may undergo a nodular, hypertrophic degeneration of uncertain cause, which will in time yield the deformities known as Dupuytren's contracture. This degeneration usually begins in the distal palm as a palpable nodularity densely adherent to the overlying palmar skin. These adhesions to the skin pucker and fix it to the palmar fascia. As the degenerative process extends into the digital slips, the contraction of the degenerating fascia may pull the finger over into a fixed flexion deformity at the MP joint, and/or at the PIP joint, or both. The ulnar half of the palm and the fourth and fifth fingers are much more commonly involved

than are the rest of the palm and the other fingers. Some patients complain that the degenerating areas are tender, others do not.

Treatment.
1. Local injection of any intra-articular corticosteroid may temporarily relieve the tenderness which some complain of.
2. Probably no approved conservative measure, whether corticosteroid injection or simple passive stretching, poses a significant deterrance to the process. (Dr. Jack Leversee of the University of Washington department of Family Medicine has pointed out in a personal communication the possible efficacy of corticosteroid in a DMSO vehicle. Such a mode allows corticosteroid to be applied daily over an extended period. His personal use of the material has been encouraging. DMSO is not yet approved for general use with humans in the United States, though it is approved in Britain. Proper clinical trials may be attempted in the next few years.
3. Ultimately, surgical excision of the affected fascia is the only treatment currently available. The dissection is difficult and should be done in hospital by an orthopaedist or hand surgeon. Recurrence is common.

Mucus Cyst

Deep fascia over the dorsal aspect of a distal phalanx may undergo a mucoid degeneration of uncertain cause, creating a tense cyst that protrudes between the proximal nail fold and the attachment of the extensor tendon of the DIP joint. Such a cyst is usually a worry to the patient, and may be painful. Once present, they often do not spontaneously remit.

Treatment. Draining the cysts or unroofing the cysts and cauterizing their bases are always followed by a recurrence. We recommend that the cysts be removed with the overlying skin and surrounding deep fascia down to periosteum. The extensor tendon attachment should not and need not be disrupted. The wound may be closed by a split thickness graft taken from the volar forearm, or by a local rotation flap. (See above under "Basic Principles of Skin Graft and "The Rotation Flap.")

CHAPTER 7

Injury to the Nerves of the Upper Extremity Summarized

A collective summary may facilitate mastery of these essentially simple but often misremembered anatomic facts.

The Radial Nerve (See Figures 4-1, 4-4)

On entering the axilla, the radial nerve courses posteriorly within the spiral groove of the humerus, where it lies against the shaft of the humerus. At the lateral side of the junction of the middle and lower third of the arm, it pierces the lateral intermuscular septum, to enter the anterior compartment of the arm between the brachioradialis and the extensor carpi radialis laterally, and the brachialis medially. As it courses distally between these muscles, it lies directly against the anterior surface of the lateral epicondyle of the humerus. At the elbow, it gives rise to motor branches to the brachioradialis and extensor carpi radialis muscles, then divides into a superficial sensory branch and a deep mainly motor branch, called the posterior interosseous nerve. The posterior interosseous nerve pierces the supinator muscle, courses around the neck of the radius distal to the annular ligament, and passes distally deep in the posterior compartment of the forearm, giving off motor branches to the deep extensor muscles to the wrist and fingers.

The radial nerve thus innervates the triceps, the brachioradialis, the supinator, and the extensors to the wrist and fingers. Sensory branches of the radial nerve pass to the dorsum of the thumb and index finger, and sometimes the middle finger.

Fractures of the upper half of the humerus may injure the radial nerve in the spiral groove. Fractures of the lateral condyle may injure the radial nerve as it approaches the anterior aspect of the elbow. Fractures of the head or neck of the radius may injure the radial nerve near its division into its superficial and deep branches.

Injury to the radial nerve will result in a wrist drop and inability to extend the wrist, fingers, and thumb, and unique loss of sensation in the dorsum of the hand between the thumb and index finger.

The Median Nerve (See Figures 4-1, 6-5)

The median nerve courses along the medial aspect of the arm in its anterior compartment. It lies upon the branchialis muscle in the groove between that muscle and the biceps muscle. It is accompanied by

the brachial artery which lies posteromedial to it. As it approaches the front of
the elbow, the median nerve crosses over
the front of the brachial artery, to lie on
its medial side. The biceps tendon crosses
the elbow just lateral to the radial artery
and inserts upon the tuberosity of the radius. The median nerve enters the forearm
between the two heads of the pronator
and courses deep to the belly of the flexor
digitorum sublimis, where it gives rise to
muscle branches to the flexors of the wrist
and the superficial flexors to the fingers.
Its last motor branch, the largest, is the
anterior interosseous nerve which iner-
vates the deep flexors to the thumb, first
and second fingers. From the point of origin of the anterior interosseous nerve, the
median nerve continues distally deep to
the transverse carpal ligament in the carpal tunnel, wherein, just deep to it, lie the
tendons to the thumb and fingers—the
flexor pollicis longus on its radial side, and
the combined flexors to the fingers on its
ulnar side. As they emerge from the carpal
tunnel the sensory branches of the median
nerve pass to the palmar aspect of the
thumb, index, middle, and radial half of
the ring fingers, and the final motor branch
passes to the muscles of the thenar eminence which it innervates in company
with the ulnar nerve.

The median nerve is likely to be injured
by displaced supracondylar fractures of
the humerus, by Colles' fractures, and by
lacerations of the wrist, and lacerations at
the thenar eminence. Injury to the median
nerve at the supracondylar level will result
in an inability to flex the thumb and index
finger, to abduct the thumb across the
palm, to oppose the thumb strongly with
the index or middle finger, and to perceive
normally cutaneous stimulation to the palmar aspect of the thumb, index, and middle fingers. Injury to the median nerve at
the wrist will result in an inability to abduct the thumb across the palm, to oppose
the thumb, and to perceive normally cutaneous stimulation to the thumb, index,
and middle fingers. Injury to the motor
branch of the median nerve in the thenar
eminence will result in an inability to abduct the thumb across the palm, and to
oppose the thumb.

The Ulnar Nerve (See Figures 4-1, 6-5)

Upon entering the arm from the axilla,
the ulnar nerve courses in the anterior
compartment, parallel to the median nerve
but posterior to the brachial artery. At the
junction of the middle with the lower third
of the arm, it pierces the medial intermuscular septum and courses posteriorly behind the medial epicondyle of the humerus. Distal to the medial epicondyle, it
enters the forearm between the heads of
the flexor carpi ulnaris, and courses distally between the flexor carpi ulnaris and
the flexor digitorum profundus, where it is
accompanied by the ulnar artery. Along its
course, it gives rise to motor branches to
the flexor carpi ulnaris, and that portion
of the flexor digitorum profundus which
controls the flexion of the distal interphalangeal (DIP) joints of the fourth and fifth
fingers. It enters the hand just radial to the
flexor carpi ulnaris and the pisiform bone,
at which point it divides into the deep and
the superficial branches of the hand. The
deep branch is a motor branch which supplies all the intrinsic muscles of the hand,
except those of the thenar eminence and
the first and second lumbricals, and the
superficial branch is a sensory branch
which passes to the ulnar side of the palm
and the flexor aspect of the fourth and
fifth fingers.

The ulnar nerve is most likely to be
injured by fractures of the medial epicondyle, by lacerations or contusions posterior
to the medial epicondyle, and by sprains,
lacerations, and contusions to the ulnar
aspect of the wrist.

Ulnar nerve injury at any level results in
an inability to abduct and adduct the fingers, to flex the metacarpal joints while
the IP joints are in full extension, and to
perceive normal cutaneous stimulation to
the fourth and fifth fingers. The motor
disabilities produce what is termed the
"claw hand," the position assumed when
the patient with ulnar nerve injury tries to
produce the position of function: metacarpophalangeal joints of all the fingers are
extended while IP joints of the fourth and
fifth fingers are flexed.

CHAPTER 8
Neck, Shoulder, and Arm Pain Summarized

As a consequence of pain referral, whether by interpretive perception, segmental spread, or nerve root stimulation, soft tissue pathology in the neck, shoulder, or arm can generate pain of quite similar distribution. Particularly when the pain syndromes do not emerge from recognized injuries, this similarity of distribution creates a diagnostic riddle which frequently may be cracked only after thoughtful examination of the neck and entire forequarter with the full spectrum of neck and forequarter pathology clearly in mind. To facilitate a mastery of the analysis of the soft tissue pain syndromes, this chapter summarizes that spectrum of pathology in Table 8–1.

Table 8–1

Region and Syndrome	Pain Location	Pain Radiation	Diagnostic Features	Absent Symptoms and Signs
Cervical spine Mild cervical sprain and cervical myalgia.	Back of the neck.	Occasionally to the top of both shoulders.	Muscular tenderness. Some painful restriction of cervical spine movement.	No tenderness in the shoulders. Shoulder movement normal and painless.
Severe cervical sprain and facet syndrome.	Back of neck and occiput and interscapular region. (Interscapular pain is nearly pathognomonic of cervical facet pain.)	Occasionally to the top of both shoulders.	Tenderness over the facet column, with or without muscular tenderness. Manipulation by traction and vertebral thrust increases pain. Cervical spine movement is greatly restricted by pain, particularly the movements of extension and rotation.	No tenderness in the shoulders. Shoulder movement normal and painless.

Table 8-1—Continued

Region and Syndrome	Pain Location	Pain Radiation	Diagnostic Features	Absent Symptoms and Signs
Cervical disc and cervical spine arthritis with nerve root irritation.	Back of the neck and occiput and interscapular region.	To one shoulder, lateral aspect of the arm, radial aspect of the forearm, thumb, index, and middle finger of one or both arms.	Painful restriction of cervical spine movement, particularly in extension and rotation. Neurological changes: dysesthesias referred to the shoulder, lateral aspect of the arm, radial aspect of the forearm and thumb, index, or middle finger; diminished biceps or triceps tendon reflex.	No sensory signs or symptoms on the inner aspect of the arm, the ulnar side of the forearm, or in the ring and 5th fingers.
Thoracic outlet syndrome	Base of the neck and shoulder.	Neurosensory: aching pain in the shoulder, inner aspect of the arm, ulnar aspect of the forearm and into the 4th and 5th fingers. Vascular: burning pain in the tips of the fingers.	Tenderness in the supraclavicular region. Adson's maneuvers may reproduce the pain. Dysesthesias may be evident over the inner aspect of the arm, the ulnar aspect of the forearm and within the 4th and 5th fingers. Signs of impaired circulation.	No tenderness in the shoulder. Shoulder movement normal and painless. The radial aspect of the forearm, thumb, index and middle fingers are not affected.
Shoulder Tendinitis.	Over the top of the shoulder and over the deltoid insertion.	The outer or anterior aspect of the arm and along the extensor aspect of the forearm.	Tenderness over involved portion of the tendinous cuff or biceps tendon. Abduction and rotation of the shoulder are painfully restricted.	Normal cervical spine. No definite neurological changes.
Tendinous cuff tear.	Over the top of the shoulder and over the deltoid insertion.	The outer or anterior aspect of the arm and along the extensor aspect of the forearm.	Tenderness over involved portion of the tendinous cuff. Occasionally a palpable gap in the tendinous cuff. Active abduction is restricted and usually painful. Passive abduction beyond the range of active abduction.	Normal cervical spine. No definite neurological changes.
Subacromial bursitis.	Over the top of the shoulder and over the deltoid insertion.	Outer or anterior aspect of the arm and along the extensor aspect of the forearm.	Severe diffuse tenderness over the region of the tendinous cuff. The shoulder may be swollen and red. All movements are severely restricted.	Normal cervical spine. No definite neurological changes.
Elbow Tennis elbow.	Lateral aspect of the elbow.	Extensor aspect of the forearm. Occasionally paresthesias extend along the radial aspect of the forearm and into the thenar web.	Tenderness over the lateral epicondyle, the radiohumeral bursa and/or the annular ligament. use of the arm with the forearm in pronation is painful, while use with the forearm in supination is either less so or may not be painful at all.	Cervical spine and shoulder are normal Neurological examination is normal.

Table 8-1—Continued

Region and Syndrome	Pain Location	Pain Radiation	Diagnostic Features	Absent Symptoms and Signs
Pitcher's elbow.	Medial aspect of the elbow.	Flexor aspect of the forearm. Occasionally, paresthesias extend along the ulnar aspect of the forearm and into the 4th and 5th fingers.	Tenderness over the medial epicondyle. Use of the extremity with the forearm in supination is painful, while use with the forearm in pronation is less so, or may not be painful at all.	Cervical spine and shoulder are normal. Neurological examination is normal.
Bicipitoradiobursitis.	Flexor aspect of the upper forearm.	Anterior aspect of the arm and flexor aspect of the entire forearm.	Pain with active resisted supination and elbow flexion. Tenderness just distal to the antecubital fossa.	Cervical spine, shoulder and elbow are otherwise normal.
Olecranon bursitis.	Posterior aspect of the elbow.	Up the posterior aspect of the arm, and along the posterior aspect of the forearm.	A cystic mass is visible and palpable over the olecranon. This mass will be tender if the inflammation is acute.	Cervical spine, shoulder, and elbow are otherwise normal.
Wrist Tendinitis of the extensor aspect.	Dorsum of the wrist.	Dorsal aspect of the forearm and dorsum of the hand.	Local tenderness over the dorsum of the wrist. Movement of the wrist is painful and extension and flexion of the fingers may be painful. The dorsum of the wrist may be swollen.	Cervical spine, shoulder and elbow are normal.
Tendinitis of the flexor aspect. (Variant of the carpal tunnel syndrome.)	Flexor aspect of the wrist.	Thumb, index, middle, and radial half of ring fingers, due to median nerve neuritis.	Tenderness over the flexor aspect of the wrist. Hyperflexion increases paresthesias along the median nerve distribution. Tinel's sign is present. The thenar eminence may be weak and atrophic.	Cervical spine, shoulder, and elbow are normal.
Tendinitis of the radial aspect of the wrist (de Quervain's syndrome).	Radial aspect of the wrist and over the radial styloid.	Along the radial aspect of the forearm and thumb.	Tenderness and swelling are evident over the radial styloid. Adduction of the thumb across the palm causes pain.	Cervical spine, shoulder and elbow are normal.
Tendinitis of the ulnar aspect of the wrist. (Tenosynovitis of the flexor carpi ulnaris or a strain of the ligamentous attachments of the pisiform bone.)	Ulnar aspect of the wrist.	Ulnar aspect of the hand and forearm. Paresthesias over the ulnar aspect of the palm and into the 4th and 5th fingers.	Tenderness over the pisiform bone. Occasional swelling over the pisiform bone. Movement of the wrist may be painful.	Cervical spine, shoulder, and elbow are normal.

CHAPTER 9
The Back

Essential Anatomy

An understanding of certain structural characteristics unique to the thoracic spine and to the lumbosacral spine is fundamental to an understanding of back pain syndromes. The material will be presented in five subsections:

1. The normal structure and clinical importance of the functional units of the thoracic and lumbosacral spine.

2. The structural anomalies of the lumbosacral spine that predispose to low back pain.

3. The ligaments of the thoracic and lumbosacral spine.

4. The musculature of the spine.

5. The distribution of nerve roots L_3 through L_5 and S_1.

The Functional Units

Thoracic Vertebrae. (See Figure 9–1.) The *bodies* of the thoracic vertebrae are rather heart-shaped as viewed from above, with the "apex of the heart" pointed anteriorly. Perhaps the narrowness of this anterior apex contributes, along with the normal anteriorly concave curvature of the thoracic spine, to facilitate the gradual an-

terior wedging of osteoporotic vertebrae, and the resulting *thoracic kyphosis of the osteoporotic.*

The bodies of all vertebrae, including the thoracic vertebrae are rimmed superiorly and inferiorly by *epiphyses* of bone more dense than the cancellous bone of the greater bulk of the vertebral bodies. When the ossification of these epiphyses in the thoracic spine is disordered during midadolescence, another form of thoracic vertebral wedging occurs called *adolescent kyphosis.*

The *pedicles* of the thoracic vertebrae emerge posteriorly from the upper border of the lateral posterior angle of the vertebral bodies, thus creating a deep inferior vertebral notch and no superior vertebral notch. Each pedicle expands into four processes:

1. The superior facet.
2. The inferior facet.
3. The transverse process.
4. The lamina.

On the body of each thoracic vertebra, at the superior and inferior ends of the posterolateral angles, are joint surfaces called costal foveae. The superior fovea of one vertebra and the inferior fovea of the next superior vertebra form together the verte-

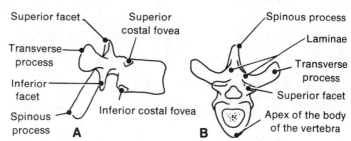

Fig. 9-1. *A* and *B*, a thoracic vertebra. Lateral and superior views.

bral acticulation for the head of the rib which takes the numerical designation of the inferior vertebra. Every rib articulates in this fashion with the bodies of the thoracic spine. These articulations are called *costovertebral* joints.

The planes of the *thoracic facets* are oriented only 10-15° from the true frontal plane. The superior facets face slightly superiorly and laterally, and the inferior facets face slightly inferiorly and medially. The articulations of the superior with the inferior facets create the facet joints, which—like all the facet joints of the spine—are true synovial joints. Normal thoracic facet joints allow for most of the rotation of the trunk. The orientation of the thoracic facets and the attachments of the thoracic spine to the rib cage prevent the thoracic spine from contributing substantially to flexion, extension, and lateral bending, though slight even imperceptible movements in these directions can be of therapeutic value. Disorders of these joints can result in thoracic, posterior flank, and abdominal pain, usually worsened by prolonged activity or prolonged inactivity, and abruptly sharpened by straining or by twisting movements.

The *transverse processes* project posterolaterally at an angle of about 45° from the frontal plane and very slightly superiorly. At the tip of each transverse process is an articular surface, the costal fovea, which articulates with the tubercle on the dorsal surface of one of the first 10 ribs. Ribs 11 and 12 usually do not articulate with any of the transverse processes. These articulations between the ribs and the transverse processes are called *costotransverse joints*. The costovertebral and costotransverse joints are both true synovial joints. Disorders of the costovertebral and costotransverse joints typically result in pleuritic

pain. A thrusting manipulation of each rib will open its costovertebral and costotransverse joints, thereby stretching their capsular ligaments. (See Figure 9-8.)

The *laminae* of each vertebra fuse at the midline to form the long spinous process the axis of which parallels the planes of the facets and overlaps the spinous process of the vertebra next inferior. The laminae lateral to the spinous process are as wide from top to bottom as the distance between the superior and inferior facets. Thus, the laminae of articulating vertebrae slightly overlap one another. A thrusting manipulation to either side of and 1 cm superior to the tip of each dorsal spinous process will apply force to the transverse processes of the inferior vertebra of that functional unit. (See Figure 9-7.) This force will rock the inferior vertebra of that functional unit so as momentarily to open the facet joints of that unit and thereby stretch their capsular ligaments.

On each side of a functional unit, bounded by the pedicles superiorly and inferiorly, the facet joints posteriorly, and the superior vertebral body and intervertebral disc anteriorly is a wide *intervertebral foramen* through which passes a thoracic nerve root. The nerve root of each functional unit is designated by the same number as is the superior vertebra of that unit. While degenerative arthritis and rheumatoid spondylitis can provoke soft tissue and bony encroachments on these foramina, symptomatic thoracic nerve root compression is relatively rare.

Lumbar Vertebrae and the Sacrum.
(See Figure 9-2.) The *lumbosacral lordosis* is one of the evolutionary adaptations which facilitate standing erect. It is this necessary lordosis that underlies the *human predisposition to low back pain.* The erect trunk posture transfers the full

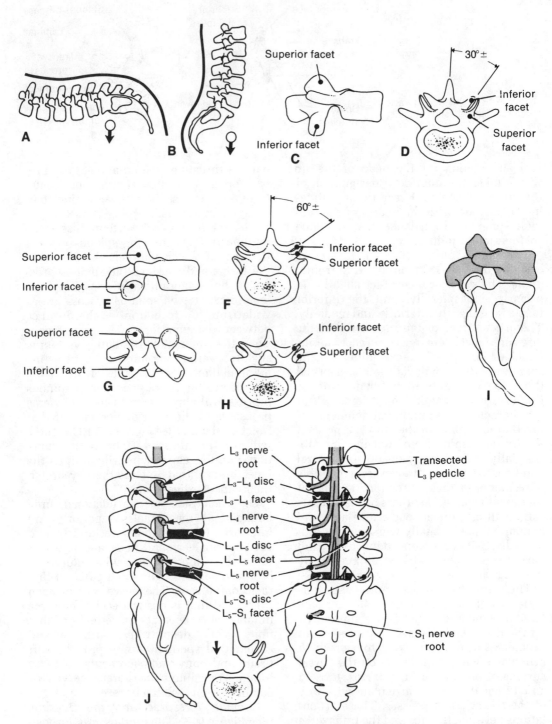

Fig. 9–2. The lumbosacral spine. *A* and *B* the lumbosacral lordosis. *C* and *D*, the 3rd lumbar vertebra. Lateral and superior views. *E* and *F*, the 5th lumbar vertebra. Lateral and superior views. *G* and *H*, the 5th lumbar vertebra. Posterior and inferior views. *I*, the 5th lumbar vertebra, in articulation with the sacrum. *J*, the relationship of nerve roots to discs and the facet joints.

weight of the upper body onto the L_4–L_5 and L_5–S_1 functional units, and the lordotic lumbosacral curve so inclines the weight-bearing surfaces of those units that the weight of the upper body applies shearing stress across them. As will be clarified later in this section, with the rest of the lumbar functional units, the L_4–L_5 and L_5–S_1 functional units afford the trunk its greatest range of motion on the fixed pelvis. During trunk movements, the entire moment arm of the upper body acts on the L_4–L_5 and L_5–S_1 functional units. These functional units are as yet poorly adapted to these static and dynamic stresses and are thus peculiarly vulnerable to injury and wear, and to the consequent pain syndrome to be outlined later in this chapter.

The *bodies* of the lumbar vertebrae are elliptically shaped as viewed from above, with the long axis in the frontal plane, and the short axis in the sagittal plane. Commensurate with the greater weight they bear, they are four to five times more massive than midcervical vertebrae, and about two times more massive than mid-dorsal vertebrae. The body of the 5th lumbar vertebra is wedge-shaped, with its anterior surface taller than its posterior.

The *pedicles* of the lumbar vertebrae emerge posteriorly from the upper half of the lateral posterior angles of the vertebral bodies. Their superior borders are near to, but not flush with, the superior border of the vertebral bodies, thus with the bodies and facets, they create a shallow superior vertebral notch and a deep inferior vertebral notch. Each pedicle expands into four processes:

1. The superior facet.
2. The inferior facet.
3. The transverse process.
4. The lamina.

The planes of the *facets* between the 1st through the 4th lumbar vertebrae are very close to the true sagittal plane, the superior facets facing laterally, and the inferior facets facing medially. However, the planes of the inferior facets of the 4th lumbar vertebra, all the facets of the 5th lumbar vertebra, and the facets of the superior articular processes of the sacrum are oriented closer to the frontal plane, the

inferior facets of the 4th and 5th lumbar vertebrae facing laterally and anteriorly, and the superior facets of the 5th lumbar vertebra and the facets of the superior articular processes of the sacrum facing medially and posteriorly. Normal facet joints of the upper lumbar spine allow for most of the flexion, extension, and lateral bending of the spine, but for nearly no rotation. The facet joints between the 4th and 5th lumbar vertebrae, and between the 5th lumbar vertebra and the sacrum allow for some rotation.

A thrusting manipulation to either side of, and 1 cm. superior to the tips of each lumbar spinous process will apply a force to the transverse process of that same vertebra. This force will rock the vertebra, so as to open the facet joints betweens its superior facets and the inferior facets of the next-higher vertebra, thereby stretching their capsular ligaments. (See Figure 9–7.)

Disorders of the lumbar and lumbosacral facet joints can result in posterior flank, inguinal, lumbosacral, and buttock pain, usually worsened by prolonged inactivity or prolonged activity, and abruptly sharpened by straining and by bending movements.

The *transverse processes* project more laterally than posteriorly, and very slightly superiorly. They are rather broad when viewed face-on, as in an anteroposterior x-ray of the spine, but thin when viewed from the top. Deep ventral muscles that help effect lumbosacral flexion and hip flexion take origin from these transverse processes. They can be fractured by blunt trauma to the posterior flanks. Forces that can fracture these processes can also contuse or lacerate a kidney.

The laminae fuse in the midline to become the *spinous process*. They are narrower from top to bottom than is the distance between the superior and inferior facets, hence the laminae and spine of one lumbar vertebra are separated from those of its articulating vertebra by a space which is covered only by the ligamentum flavum. (See below.) Lumbar puncture is performed through one of these spaces.

On each side of a functional unit, bounded by the pedicle superiorly and inferiorly, the facet joints posteriorly, and the bodies of the vertebrae and the intervertebral disc anteriorly, is a wide *intervertebral foramen* through which passes a lumbar nerve root. As each nerve root enters its foramen, it clings to the superior pedicle and thus is rarely vulnerable to protrusion of the disc which forms part of the anterior boundary of the foramen. However, as it approaches its foramen, it is held laterally in its dural sleeve over the disc next higher. Nerve roots L_4, L_5, and S_1 are most characteristically suspended in this fashion. Hence, these nerve roots are particularly vulnerable to irritation by protrusion of the disc next above the foramen: L_4 by the L_3–L_4 disc, L_5 by the L_4–L_5 disc and S_1 by the L_5–S_1 disc. Degenerative arthritis can also provoke soft tissue and bony encroachments on these foramina. These encroachments are more likely to cause irritations of the lumbar nerve roots than are similar encroachments on the dorsal nerve roots, particularly at the L_4–L_5 and L_5–S_1 units. Figure 9–2*J* illustrates the relationship of nerve roots to discs and facet joints.

Structural Anomalies of the Lumbosacral spine (See Figure 9–3)

In our opinion and in the opinion of other authors, two structural anomalies of the lumbosacral spine predispose to low back pain: malformation of the L_5–S_1 facets, and spondylolysis, usually of the 5th lumbar vertebra. Three other structural anomalies have been implicated in the literature: sacralization of the 5th lumbar vertebra, lumbarization of the 1st segment of the sacrum, and spina bifida occulta. Clear evidence of their predisposing influence is lacking in our experience and, as far as we know, in the literature as well. We discount the implication.

The plane of the facet joints changes direction, from near-sagittal at the L_1–L_2 unit, to near-frontal at the L_5–S_1 unit. The orientation of the facets determines the motions possible at a functional unit and the direction of the forces these motions apply to the articulation of a functional unit. The frontal orientation at L_5–S_1 prevents the spine from sliding forward on the inclined upper surface of the sacrum. Two kinds of *facet malformation* predis-

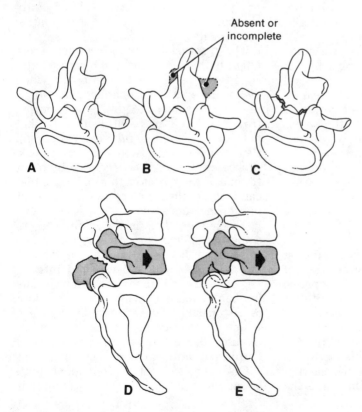

Fig. 9–3. Structural anomalies of the lumbosacral spine. *A,* normal 5th lumbar vertebra. *B,* atresia of the inferior facets of the 5th lumbar vertebra. *C,* spondylolysis. *D,* spondylolisthesis complicating spondylolysis. *E,* spondylolisthesis complicating atresia of the inferior facets of the 5th lumbar vertebra.

pose to the back pain syndrome: *asymmetric rotation* or *tropism* and *atresia*. When the facets on one side of the lumbosacral functional unit are *rotated* differently relative to the coronal plane than are the facets on the opposite side, they may so transmit the forces of movement as to apply unusual torque to the disc and they will subject themselves to unusual pressure. Thus degenerative changes may be accelerated. When the inferior facets are *atretic,* bony articulation between L_5 and S_1 will be prevented, and the full sliding weight of the spine will be transferred onto the ligaments of the L_5–S_1 functional unit. *Spondylolysis* is a disunion between two parts of a vertebra: the lamina, spinous process, and inferior facets in one part; the body, pedicles, transverse processes, and superior facets in the other part. The inferior facets keep the one part in bony articulation with the sacrum, and the superior facets keep the other part in bony articulation with the rest of the spine. The disunion between the two facets transfers the full sliding weight of the spine to the ligaments of the L_5–S_1 functional unit. Often a spondylolysis can be recognized only

on an oblique x-ray of the lumbosacral spine. On the true lateral view, the transverse process obscures the laminar defect between the facets.

These anomalies can occur unilaterally or bilaterally. When facet atresia or spondylolysis occurs bilaterally, the spine eventually may slide forward on the inclined sacrum, creating thereby a *spondylolisthesis* which will strain the posterior longitudinal ligament and which can in time do damage to the cauda equina. When they occur unilaterally, the total L_5–S_1 articulation tends to rotate around the intact facet, throwing the intact facet into malalignment. This malalignment subjects the facet to greater wear and tear, both in the form of acute sprain, and in the form of chronic friction and capsular irritation, and subjects the disc to unusual torque. Thus, these anomalies predispose abnormally to low back pain.

The Ligaments and Discs of the Thoracic (Dorsal) and Lumbosacral Spines (See Figure 9–4)

The *supraspinous and interspinous ligaments* exist as distinct entities in the dor-

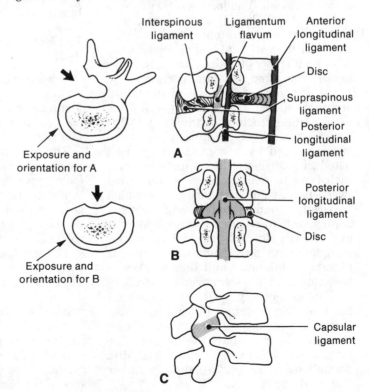

Fig. 9–4. *A–C,* ligaments and discs of the dorsolumbar spine.

sal and lumbosacral spines, while they are lost in the ligamentum nuchae of the cervical spine. Like the ligamentum nuchae, however, they are relatively weak ligaments, vulnerable to sprain, which give little support to the spine. The other ligaments of the dorsal and lumbosacral spines are a continuation of those in the neck: the *ligamenta flava* remain the segmental strong ligaments chiefly responsible for maintaining the posterior articulations of the functional units; the *capsular ligaments* remain flaccid structures which allow for the play of the facet joints necessary for normal range of motion; the *posterior longitudinal ligament* remains the multisegmental strong ligament that helps to limit flexion of the spine; the *anterior longitudinal ligament* remains the multisegmental strong ligament that helps to limit extension of the spine. All these ligaments are probably pain sensitive except perhaps the anterior longitudinal ligament.

The structure of the posterior longitudinal ligament in the dorsal and lumbosacral spines differs from its structure in the neck. In the neck, it remains a broad ligament across all functional units, while in the dorsal and lumbosacral spines, it is wide over the intervertebral discs and narrow over the vertebral bodies. (See Figure 9–4.) As it crosses the disc, its central portion is strong and its lateral portion weak.

The structure of the discs of the dorsal and lumbosacral spines is essentially the same as the structure of the discs in the neck. A central gel, the *nucleus pulposus*, is surrounded by a concentrically laminated fibrocartilage, the *annulus fibrosus*, each layer of which passes obliquely between two hyaline cartilage plates which are firmly bound to the bodies of the articulating vertebrae. The nucleus pulposus is excentrically situated, near to the posterior margin of the disc. Hence, the annulus fibrosus is thinnest—and thus weakest—posteriorly. This weak portion is strongly reinforced centrally by the strong central band of the posterior longitudinal ligament, but is weakly reinforced laterally by the weak lateral bands of the posterior longitudinal ligament. Hence, most disc herniations occur posterolaterally rather than posterocentrally.

The Sacroiliac Joint (See Figure 11–1)

Since sacroiliac sprain often presents as hip pain and as the two coxal bones that articulate with the sacrum to form the sacroiliac joint are intimately involved in the anatomy and disorders of the hip, a careful description of the anatomy of the sacroiliac joint has been deferred to Chapter 11. However, sacroiliac sprain can present as low back pain and must be considered during evaluation of patients with low back pain; and body surface landmarks adjacent to the joints are useful to the clinician when examining the low back. It is enough for this purpose to know that:

1. The sacroiliac joints are combination synovial and fibrous joints powerfully stabilized by ligaments and the locking action of the joints themselves.

2. The posterior surface of the joints are buried beneath attachments of the erector spinae and gluteus maximus muscles.

3. The posterior iliac spines are in transverse line with the postero-inferior third of the joints and are about 1 inch postero-inferior to the L_5–S_1 joints.

4. A line between the iliac crests falls barely superior to the L_4–L_5 joint.

The Musculature of the Back (See Figure 9–5)

When analyzing and treating back disorders, the clinician deals directly with members of four muscle groups: the splenius, erector spinae, segmental, and abdominal groups.

The *splenius capitis and cervicis*, which were mentioned in Chapter 1, originate from upper thoracic spines. One cause for interscapular pain is strains and cryptogenic myalgias of these muscles. These muscles help to extend, laterally bend, and rotate the neck.

The *erector spinae* are the prominent paraspinous muscles of the lumbar back. They separate into three divisions over the dorsal back, which cannot be distinguished as such through the overlying latissimus dorsi and trapezius. One cause for low back pain and interscapular pain is strains and cryptogenic myalgias of this group. These muscles are the chief extensors of the back.

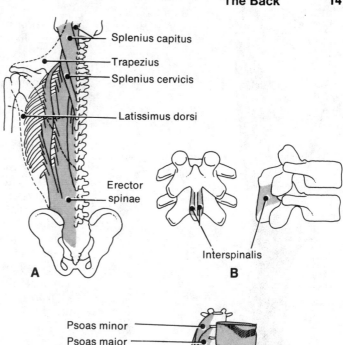

Fig. 9-5. Musculature of the back. *A,* splenius and erector spinae muscle groups. *B,* interspinalis, posterior and lateral views. *C,* flexors of the lumbosacral spine.

The *interspinales* are four pairs of muscles, which extend between the five spinous processes of the lumbar spine. They are members of the segmental group. One of the causes of low back pain is strain and cryptogenic myalgias of these muscles. They contribute to lumbar extension.

The *abdominal and iliopsoas muscles* are the chief flexors of the spine and, as such, resist lumbosacral lordosis and its consequent acute and chronic wear to discs and facet joints. Regimens intended to rehabilitate from and prevent low back disorders place primary emphasis on abdominal muscle conditioning.

Distribution of Nerve Roots L₃ through S₁ (See Figure 9-6)

Nerve roots L_3 through S_1 are the most likely of nerve roots to be injured by low back disorders. Disorders of the L_4–L_5 disc and L_5–S_1 facet joints are most likely to injure L_5 nerve roots, and disorders of the L_5–S_1 disc are most likely to injure the S_1 nerve roots. Nerve roots L_3 and L_4 are uncommonly injured, L_3 by disorders of the L_3–L_4 facet joints and L_4 by the L_3–L_4 disc or L_4–L_5 facet joints.

The cutaneous dermatomal pattern remains in some dispute, but it is generally agreed that L_3 serves cutaneous sensitivity to the anterior surface of the knee and inner aspect of the thigh, L_4 serves cutaneous sensitivity to the inner aspect of the lower leg and ankle, L_5 serves cutaneous sensitivity to the dorsum of the forefoot, and S_1 serves cutaneous sensitivity to the lateral plantar aspect of the entire foot.

All leg muscles are innervated by several segments, but L_3 and L_4 dominate control of the quadriceps and the patellar tendon

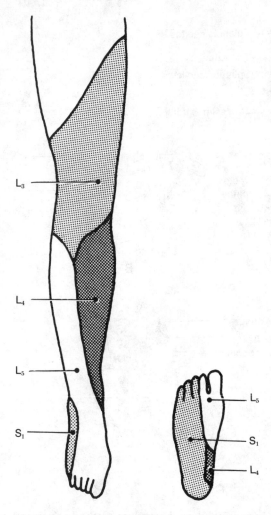

Fig. 9–6. Sensory distribution of nerve roots, L_3 through S_1.

2. Spondylitis (i.e., degenerative arthritis and rheumatoid spondylitis).

3. Costovertebral and costotransverse joint dysfunctions.

4. Costochondritis.

5. Muscle strains and myalgias.

Disruptions of the Architecture of the Vertebral Bodies

A brief review of infections, and of osteoporosis and Paget's disease of bone may be found in Chapters 19 and 20 respectively, but the pathology and treatment of neoplasms and the less common bone diseases are not reviewed in this text. It is quite enough that the primary clinician knows when to suspect and how to confirm a painful disorder of bone. The clinical findings characteristic of bone pain and the radiographic techniques used to confirm bone pathology are summarized in Chapter 20.

Scheuermann's Disease. Persistent dorsal backache in early adolescence may herald the development of Scheuermann's disease, know also as adolescent kyphosis. Classically, the disease was considered to represent an avascular necrosis of the ring-like epiphyses around the upper and lower margins of the dorsal vertebral bodies that begin to ossify in early adolescence. More recently, the pathogenesis has been viewed as a primary disorder of ossification without any underlying disorder of vascularization. Untreated, the disease leads to a permanent dorsal kyphosis of variable degree, established by the end of the adolescent growth period.

Diagnosis can be made from a lateral x-ray of the dorsal spine which will demonstrate (usually in the mid-dorsal region) wedging of one or more vertebral bodies, fragmentation of the epiphyseal rings, and concave osteolytic defects into the disc surfaces of the bodies known as Schmorl's nodes and thought to represent the herniation of disc material into weakly ossified bone.

Primary clinicians should refer children so afflicted to an orthopaedist for treatment. The child will be required to perform active dorsal extension exercise and may be required to wear a dorsolumbar brace whenever upright until growth is

reflexes, L_5 dominates control of dorsal flexion of the ankle and extension of the great toe, and S_1 dominates control of plantar flexion of the ankle and the achilles deep tendon reflex.

Thoracic Back and Trunk Pain

Among the kinds of musculoskeletal pathology that can produce pain in this part of the body, five are of particular concern to the primary clinican:

1. Disruption of the architecture of the vertebral bodies (i.e., neoplasms, infections, metabolic and vascular bone disorders).

complete. Such treatment may decrease the inevitable deformity.

Spondylitis

Pathology, diagnosis and treatment of degenerative and rheumatoid spondylitis is reviewed in Chapter 18. This section will review the characteristics of facet joint pain.

Recognition of Facet Pain. The clinical findings characteristic of facet pain are the following:

1. Steady pain is quite notable after a prolonged period of inactivity, is intensified on first resuming activity, is temporarily eased after several minutes to an hour of activity, and is again intensified after activity continues for several hours.

2. The augmentation of pain by movement is often intense but not so shockingly intense as is bone pain. Rarely, a nerve root may be impinged by the swelling of a spondylitis. Under that circumstance the augmentation of pain by movement can be shockingly intense.

3. Manipulation of the joint will provoke pain—more pain with the initial movement than with subsequent movements. The manipulations most useful for diagnosis of dorsal facet pain are rotation and anterior thrusts. (See Figure 9–7.)

4. While compression of the spine may provoke pain by flexing the dorsal spine and thus stressing the facet joints, jarring percussion over the spinous process is not likely to provoke pain unless the patient has developed considerable hyperalgesic spread of pain. Thus facet pain can usually be distinguished from bone pain.

Confirmation of Facet Pathology. Confirmation can be made by x-ray. However, x-ray evidence of facet pathology does not confirm the pain to originate from the facet. That determination can be made only from the evidence provided by a carefully taken history and carefully performed physical examination. Even then, the determination occasionally may remain rather uncertain.

Costovertebral and Costotransverse Joint Dysfunctions

Pleuritic chest pain, of course, does not necessarily imply pleuritis—indeed, in a North American primary practice, it is least likely to imply pleuritis. Much more common are costovertebral and costotransverse joint dysfunctions. We must emphasize that we refer here strictly to *pleuritic chest pain:* that is, pain which is provoked by ventilatory movements as such and which is not felt when a breath is held. Pleuritic pain must be distinguished from two other kinds of chest pain: (a) persistent chest pain which raises crucial non-orthopaedic questions with which the primary practitioner dare not procrastinate; (b) abrupt fleeting pains, unrelated to movement, usually intense and of boring or searing quality, which nearly always represent a common self-limited disorder which has been variably named, and which we prefer to designate *benign cryptogenic neuralgia.*

The pathology of costovertebral and costotransverse joint dysfunction is unknown. The disorder is defined by clinical findings alone, and these findings necessarily implicate both or either joint and do not distinguish between them.

Recognition of Costovertebral and Costotransverse Joint Dysfunction. Clinical findings characteristic of this disorder are the following:

1. Pain is by definition pleuritic.

2. The onset may be gradual, but in our experience is usually startlingly abrupt.

3. The patient's ventilatory excursions are usually quite restricted by anticipation of the pain, and may be accompanied by some grunting.

4. Active rotation of the trunk will often provoke the pain.

5. Thrusting manipulations of the affected joints will provoke the pain. Each rib is manipulated until the pain is elicited. (See Figure 9–8.)

6. Deep palpation over the costotransverse member of the affected joint pair may provoke the pain.

Treatment of Costovertebral and Costotransverse Joint Dysfunction.

1. The diagnostic manipulation may be rewarded also by distinct relief.

2. When relief is incomplete and the costotransverse joint tender, lidocaine may be injected into and around the joint. Often, substantial relief will follow and will persist even after the anesthetic effect

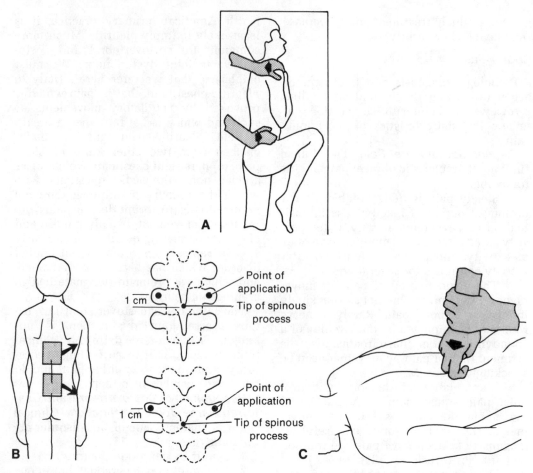

Fig. 9–7. Manipulation of dorsal and lumbar facets. *A,* rotation. *B,* points of application of anterior thrusts. *C,* the anterior thrust manipulation illustrated.

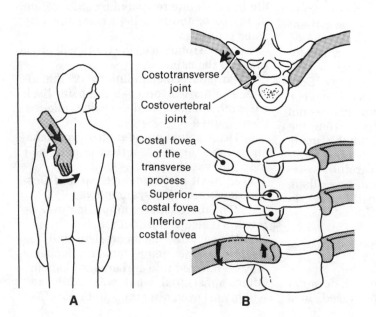

Fig. 9–8. Manipulation of costovertebral and costotransverse joints. *A,* the maneuver. *B,* the joints and the motions imparted to them by the manipulation, superior view and three-quarter view.

of the lidocane can be presumed to have worn off.

3. All patients are instructed to perform trunk rotation exercises, to further manipulate these joints. They are to perform these for 3–5 minutes at least four times daily, until a remission is complete.

4. Adult patients are instructed to take aspirin grains 10 four times a day, or its equivalent. Occasionally, stronger analgesics are added.

5. Patients may be assured of a full remission within 2–3 days. Should this prediction prove false, other causes for the pain must be searched out.

Costochondritis

This disorder presents as a persisting and usually unilateral anterior chest pain which has often alarmed the patient with thoughts of heart disease or cancer. Though the name implies an inflammation, the nature of the pathology remains unknown. Like the costovertebral-costo-transverse joint dysfunctions, it, too, is best considered to be defined by clinical findings alone.

Recognition of Costochondritis. Clinical findings characteristic of costochondritis are the following:

1. Pain is persistent, usually unilateral, and sometimes augmented by a full ventilatory excursion or full and vigorous trunk rotation.

2. Though worried, the patient looks otherwise quite well and reports no change in symptoms with exertion and only that decrease in activity which is compatible with their anxiety.

3. Examination of heart, lungs, and abdomen, which may be extended to a chest x-ray and electrocardiogram, does not demonstrate evidence of visceral disease which could account for such pain.

4. Several of the costal cartilages are very tender. The tenderness may be bilateral but is usually unilateral and directly at the site of pain referral.

Treatment of Costochondritis.

1. Effective reassurance and a minor analgesic are often all that are necessary. Patients must be warned of the duration of the problem, which can be measured in weeks rather than days.

2. When a patient asks for a definitive treatment, we suggest a trial of icing or heat as experience guides them, and sometimes we prescribe indomethacin or phenylbutazone as for myofascial periarthropathies (see Chapter 18), or if tenderness is well localized, we inject 0.5–1.0 cc. of a corticosteroid into the tender focus.

Muscle Strains and Cryptogenic Myalgias

Interscapular and chest pains seem occasionally to be most compatible with a muscle disorder. We are referring to relatively well-localized and rather intense pain syndrome, not to the generalized aching that follows unaccustomed exercise. These pains can emerge abruptly with straining efforts, and can emerge gradually without following a recognized precipitating event. Several theories of pathogenesis for the syndrome of gradual onset have been proposed, but none have been securely confirmed. The more popular theories have proposed viral inflammation of muscle, degeneration and/or congestion of intermuscular fibrous tissue, and tetanic contractions of the fibrils of a cluster of motor units. (See also the discussion of the cryptogenic periarticular pain syndromes in Chapter 18. There may be a relationship between the cryptogenic periarticular pain syndromes and the cryptogenic myalgias.) Any of the splenius muscles, any of the thoracic divisions of the erector spinae, any of the muscular shoulder girdle attachments (trapezius, rhomboid, serratus anterior, and pectorals), and any of the intercostal muscles may be involved.

While muscle strains and cryptogenic mayalgias can appear to account for high interscapular pain, they must be differentiated from the referred pain of the cervical facet syndrome. (See Chapter 1.) High interscapular pain is more likely to be referred pain. When it is referred pain, it is typically intensified by active and/or passive neck movement and/or by deep palpation over the disordered cervical facet. While these findings can distinguish the cervical facet syndrome from interscapular strains and myalgias, referred hyperalgesia and the segmental reactive increase in muscle tone which can accompany the facet syndromes can produce a confusing interscapular tenderness.

While cryptogenic myalgias can produce pain very similar in quality to the pain of costochondritis, the location of the myalgias vary more widely as the thoracic muscles girdle the thorax.

Strains generally occur during sudden contractions of near-maximum intensity. The following muscles tend to be strained by the following efforts:

1. Splenius and thoracic divisions of erector spinae. Violent sneezing, overhead lifting, "bridging" efforts while wrestling, efforts to resist sudden forward accelerations of the trunk, as often occurs in an auto accident.

2. Trapezius and rhomboids. Violent sneezing, pulling with the hands in front or above the shoulder girdle, pushing with the hands below the shoulder girdle and at the sides—retraction and depression.

3. Serratus, pectoralis major and pectoralis minor. Violent sneezing and pushing with the hands in front of the shoulder girdle (all three); pushing or lifting efforts which require elevation of the shoulder (serratus anterior), and pushing or lifting efforts which require depression of the shoulders (the pectorales)—protraction, elevation, depression.

4. Intercostals. Violent sneezing or any other Valsalva maneuver.

The cryptogenic myalgias of the splenius, the thoracic divisions of the erector spinae, the trapezius or rhomboids will produce interscapular pain. The cryptogenic myalgias of the serratus anterior, the pectorales, and the intercostals will produce anterior and/or lateral thoracic pain.

Clinical Findings Characteristic of Thoracic Muscle Strains and Myalgias.

1. The pain is usually dull, persistent, and fairly well localized, but an intercostal tetanic contraction may produce a pleuritic syndrome similar to that produced by costovertebral/costotransverse joint dysfunctions.

2. The pain usually augments with the development of fatigue, and abates somewhat with rest.

3. Movements that stretch the affected muscles usually augment the pain. Less often, movements that contract the affected muscles will also augment the pain.

4. A portion of the affected muscle is uniquely tender to palpation.

Treatment of Muscle Strains and Myalgias.

1. Exercise. Mild pain syndromes need not curtail the patient's usual activities. However, patients suffering the more severe syndromes should be encouraged to rest. At least four times daily, for 3–5 minutes at a time, the affected muscle should be stretched repetitively as follows:

a. Splenius and thoracic division of erector spinae. Rhythmic neck and back flexion, and recovery in the sitting position.

b. Trapezius and rhomboids. Rhythmic protraction of the arms and shoulders as though hugging oneself.

c. Serratus anterior and pectorales. Rhythmic retraction of the shoulders while fully inspiring.

d. Intercostals. During a full thoracic inspiration, rhythmic lateral bending away from the affected side.

2. Heat and cold. Strains should be iced the first several days, at least four times daily, before performing the stretching exercises. Either heat or cold may be applied thereafter, whichever seems more comforting. The cryptogenic myalgias may be treated from the outset with either heat or cold, as seems the most comforting. Counterirritants like methyl salicylate will augment the analgesic effect of heat.

3. Analgesics. Aspirin or its equivalent should be taken four to six times per day. (See Chapter 18.) Rarely is a stronger analgesic like codeine necessary.

4. Injection. Lidocaine injected into a discretely tender focus may yield a lasting remission.

Low Back Pain

The Variable Predisposition to Musculoskeletal Low Back Pain

As a consequence of the lumbosacral lordosis, everyone is vulnerable to low back pain, but some are more vulnerable than others. The vulnerability of some derives from an imbalance between circumstantial stresses and physical condition (by which we mean muscle strength and tone, joint mobility, and efficiently coordinated movement habits). Any circumstance, weakness or postural habit that increases the lumbosacral lordosis will magnify the vulnerability–e.g., pregnancy, abdominal obesity, high heels, and lax abdominal muscles. In the anatomic section of this chapter, we mention the importance of lumbosacral flexor tone to low back stability. Strong flexor tone decreases the lumbosacral lordosis and thus decreases the shearing stresses across the L_4, L_5, and L_5-S_1 units. In contrast, lax abdominal muscle tone allows the lordosis to increase, thus increasing the shearing stresses and the vulnerability to wear and tear.

The vulnerability of others derives from two developmental and acquired anomalies of structure that increase the instability of the L_4-L_5 and L_5-S_1 functional units: malformation of facets and spondylolysis. The nature of these anomalies was described in the anatomic section of this chapter.

Classification of Low Back Pain

A number of classifications of soft tissue musculoskeletal low back pain have been devised over the years. Some derive from a unified theory of pathogenesis that views disc degeneration as central to all soft tissue low back pain syndromes. Others, like our own, while recognizing the responsive interdependence of the various parts of the functional units of the spine, derive from a pleural theory of pathogenesis which credits four soft tissue parts with a capacity to initiate a low back pain syndrome. We believe our classification to be closer to the clinical facts and thus readily and usefully applicable to clinical problems.

As in the cervical and thoracic spine, disruptions of the architecture of the vertebral bodies can cause pain. The principles of recognition and diagnosis are as summarized in Chapter 20 for disruptions of the thoracic vertebral bodies.

Also, like cervical and thoracic pain, low back pain can represent a referral of pain from visceral disease. The following is a listing of visceral diseases most likely to present as low back pain:

Dysmenorrhea, pelvic inflammatory disease, ovarian cysts, tubal pregnancy, and abruptions of the placenta; urinary tract infections and ureteral colic; colitis and diverticulitis; dissecting aortic aneurysm.

Often, other associated symptoms or coincidences will direct the attention to the viscera. In their absence, it will be helpful to recognize that all of these disorders except pelvic inflammatory disease, tubal pregnancy, ovarian cysts, and perforated diverticulitis elicit a pain which is not affected by back movement as such. However, pelvic inflammatory disease, tubal pregnancy, ovarian cysts, and perforated diverticulitis usually produce low abdominal pain as well, and usually produce some distinct structural change which can be detected by abdominal and/or pelvic examination, either in the form of a mass, or of unique tenderness. When a patient is past 50 years of age, the clinician must actively consider a dissecting aortic aneurysm, when seeking the cause of obscure low back pain.

In the majority of instances, individuals presenting with low back pain might as well wear a sign pointing to the soft tissues of the functional units, so typical is the presentation (see below). However, while proceeding directly in such cases with the orthopaedic analysis, the clinician should remain intentionally circumspect and ready to consider bone and visceral disease, should the findings fail to fit the musculoskeletal soft tissue patterns. The following is our classification of the musculoskeletal soft tissue disorders of the low back:

Disc Degeneration. Pain does not necessarily accompany disc degeneration. It does so only when the annulus fibrosis ruptures, transferring the pressure of the extruding nucleus pulposus and fragments of annulus directly onto the posterior longitudinal ligament or through it, onto the adjacent nerve root or roots. When the posterior longitudinal ligament is strained by the pressure of the extruding disc fragments, low back pain results. When the posterior longitudinal ligament gives way and the extruding disc material impinges on nerve tissue, nerve pain and dysfunction result. Because the central band of the posterior longitudinal ligament is so much

Table 9A-1.

Low Back Pain Syndrome Summarized

Clinical Characteristics	Disc Syndrome	Acute Facet Syndrome	Chronic Facet Syndrome	Sacroiliac Sprain, Arthritis,* and Paget's Disease†	Myofascial Pain Syndrome
Location and radiation of pain.	*Posterior longitudinal ligament strain* – across the low back. *With nerve root compression* – L_4: inner aspect of calf and ankle; L_5: back of thigh and lateral calf, dorsum of foot, great toe: S_1: back of thigh and calf, lateral aspect of the heel and plantar aspect of the forefoot and 4-5 toes. *Central rupture* – bilateral generalized leg and low back pain.	*Without nerve root pain* – across the low back (may be unilateral or bilateral), into the ipsilateral buttock and thigh. *With nerve root pain* – L_3 (L_3–L_4 facet joint) knee and inner aspect of thigh; L_4 (L_4–L_5 facet joint) inner aspect of lower leg and ankle. L_5 (L_5–S_1 facet joint) back of thigh and lateral calf, and dorsum of foot and great toe.	*Without nerve root pain* – same as with the acute facet syndrome. *With segmental nerve root pain* – same as with the acute facet syndrome. *With narrow canal syndrome* – bilateral burning paresthesias.	Unilaterally over the affected sacroiliac joint, and into the ipsilateral buttock and hip.	Unilaterally over the point of muscle irritation when an erector spinal is irritated, or across the low back when an interspinous muscle is irritated. May refer into the ipsilateral buttock and hip.
Nature of onset.	Repeated episodes of low back pain which by middle age are provoked by straining and become very persistent. Nerve root symptoms may appear rapidly early or late in the course. Transient relief may be afforded by rest and by movement.	Any age, but typically in early middle age. Abrupt onset, often during an easy body movement. Any trunk movement increases the pain. Usually resolved within 2–4 weeks.	Usually over 50 years of age. Worsened by immobility, by straining, and by prolonged weightbearing. Usually preceded in youth by episodes of acute facet syndrome. Extension augments the symptoms of segmental nerve root pain and narrow canal syndrome.	Usually with a fall onto a buttock. Worsened by most pelvic movements. Axial jarring, particularly on the side of the injury, increases the pain.	When of abrupt onset, usually occurs while lifting from a forward bending position. When gradual in onset, usually is related to an excessive lordosis or scoliosis, whether primary or secondary to an unequal leg length.
Associated symptoms.	*Dysesthesias:* L_4 – inner aspect of lower leg and ankle. L_5 – back of thigh and lateral calf into the dorsum of foot and great toe. S_1 – back of thigh and calf, into the lateral plantar aspect of the foot and 4th and 5th toes. *Central rupture* – generalized dysaesthesias in the legs. *Weakness:* L_5 – Patients may complain of foot drop. S_1 – patients may compalin of weak pushoff. *Central rupture* – bilateral generalized leg weakness and	Rarely dysesthesias and weakness as follows: L_3 (L_3–L_4 facet joint) – dysaesthesias in the knee and inner aspect of thigh; may be some complaints of weakness of "knee." L_4 (L_4–L_5 facet joint) dysaesthesias in the inner aspect of lower leg and ankle; may be some complaints of weakness of the knee. L_5 (L_5–S_1 facet joint) – dysaesthesias in the back of thigh, lateral calf and the dorsum of foot; may be some foot drop.	Occasionally dysesthesias and weakness as described for the acute facet syndrome or occasionally as the Narrow Canal Syndrome – bilateral leg weakness.	None.	None.

(handwritten margin notes: "For anatomy", "p. 136 / 139", "p. 142")

Table 9A-1 – *Continued*

Clinical Characteristics	Disc Syndrome	Acute Facet Syndrome	Chronic Facet Syndrome	Sacroiliac Sprain, Arthritis,* and Paget's Disease†	Myofascial Pain Syndrome
Spinal curvature	Lumbar lordosis may be decreased or normal. A reactive scoliosis may appear convex to the affected side.	Lumbar lordosis is usually markedly decreased. A scoliosis in either direction may antedate the episode, and occasionally emerges as a reactive postural adjustment to the pain. (When reactive, the curve is usually convex to the affected side.)	An excessive lumbar lordosis or a lumbosacral scoliosis to either side may be long standing. In some cases, the lumbar lordosis is normal or slightly decreased.	Lumbosacral lordosis may be normal or decreased.	Lumbosacral lordosis is usually normal. A reactive scoliosis concave to the affected side may emerge.
Tenderness.	*Posterior longitudinal ligament strain* – no tenderness. L_5 *nerve root irritation* – deep tenderness 1" above the posterior iliac spine in the sagittal plane midway between the posterior iliac spine and the spinous process. S_1 *nerve root irritation* – deep tenderness midway between the posterior iliac spine and the spinous process. Nerve root irritation is not always accompanied by tenderness.	L_3–L_4 *facet* – deep tenderness 2" above posterior iliac spine in the sagittal plane midway between posterior iliac spine and spinous process. L_4 *and* L_5 *facet* – deep tenderness 1" above posterior iliac spine in the sagittal plane midway between the posterior iliac spine and spinous process. L_5–S_1 *facet* – deep tenderness midway between posterior iliac spine and the spinous process.	Same as for the acute facet.	Tenderness over the affected joint, inferior and medial to the posterior iliac spine.	Tenderness over the affected portion of the erector spinae muscles or between the spinous processes over an affected interspinous muscle. When erector spinae muscles are affected, the focus of irritation is usually adjacent to the iliac crest.
Forward, backward and lateral bending.	Pain usually on forward bending, relieved by recovery. Extension may produce a catching pain, but often has no effect on the pain. Lateral bending to the affected side may increase the pain of nerve root irritation.	Pain produced by forward bending and/or by recovery. Extension also produces pain. Lateral bending toward the affected side usually increases the pain, and toward the opposite side may increase the pain.	Same as acute facet syndrome. In the face of segmental nerve root and narrow canal syndromes, the radiating pain of these disorders may emerge during backward and lateral bending.	Forward bending and recovery usually do not produce pain. Extension may produce pain. Lateral bending, if done smoothly, often does not change the pain.	Forward bending and recovery may produce pain. Extension usually does not produce pain. Lateral bending away from the affected side usually produces pain.
Buttock rocking.	Shifting weight from one buttock to the other has no effect on the pain.	Shifting weight from one buttock to the other does not affect the pain if the movement is effected cautiously.	Same as acute facet syndrome.	Pain is often increased when shifting the weight to the affected side.	Shifting weight from one buttock to the other may increase erector spinae pain when weight is on the opposite buttock.

Table 9A–1—*Continued*

Clinical Characteristics	Disc Syndrome	Acute Facet Syndrome	Chronic Facet Syndrome	Sacroiliac Sprain, Arthritis,* and Paget's Disease†	Myofascial Pain Symdrome
Heel-toe walking.	*Posterior longitudinal ligament strain*—normal. L_5 *nerve root syndrome*—weak heel walking. S_1 *nerve root syndrome*—weak toe walking.	Usually normal.	Normal, unless nerve roots are irritated, then same as for the advanced disc syndrome.	Normal, although sometimes inhibited by pain.	Normal.
Straight leg raising.	*Posterior longitudinal ligament strain*—usually no effect on the pain. *With nerve root irritation*—pain increased in the affected leg, usually before the leg is elevated to 60°, or if sitting, before the knee is extended beyond 60°. At the point of leg pain, the pain can be augmented by dorsiflexion of the ankle and/or popliteal space compression. Some quadriceps weakness may be evident if L_4 nerve root is disordered.	Low back pain is increased by straight leg raising to 70° bilaterally and by abrupt recovery bilaterally. Some quadriceps weakness may be evident if L_3 or L_4 nerve roots are disordered.	Usually painless to full hamstring stretch unless nerve roots are irritated, then pain is as described for advanced disc syndrome. Some quadriceps weakness may be evident if L_3 or L_4 nerve roots are disordered.	Low back pain may be increased by straight leg raising to 70° and by abrupt recovery bilaterally.	Occasional increase in back pain by straight leg raising beyond 70° on the affected side.
Manipulation by passive anterior flexion.	No change in the pain, except perhaps some decrease.	Pain may be increased or decreased.	Pain may be increased or decreased.	If performed smoothly, pain may not be affected at all.	Full flexion may increase the pain on the affected side.
Manipulation by passive lateral bending.	No change in the pain.	Pain increased by lateral bending to either or both sides, but usually to the affected side only.	Same as with acute facet syndrome.	Pain usually not affected if the exercise is performed smoothly.	Pain may be increased by bending to the opposite side of a disordered erector spinae.
Manipulation by passive rotation.	No effect on the pain.	Pain is increased by rotation in either or both directions.	Same as acute facet syndrome.	Pain provoked by rotation in either or both directions.	No effect.
Cutaneous sensation.	*Posterior longitudinal ligament strain*—normal cutaneous sensation. *With nerve root irritation: L_4*—hypesthesia over the medial aspect of the leg &	Usually normal. If nerve roots are irritated, then: L_3—hypesthesia over anterior surface of knee and inner surface of thigh. L_4—hypesthesia	Normal, unless nerve roots are irritated; then as in acute facet syndrome.	Normal.	Normal.

Table 9A-1—Continued

Clinical Characteristics	Disc Syndrome	Acute Facet Syndrome	Chronic Facet Syndrome	Sacroiliac Sprain, Arthritis,* and Paget's Disease†	Myofascial Pain Syndrome
	ankle; L_5—hypesthesia over the dorsum of the foot. S_1—hypesthesia over the lateral aspect of the heel and plantar surface of the forefoot.	over medial aspect of lower leg and ankle. L_5—hypesthesia over dorsum of foot.			
Deep tendon reflexes.	*Posterior longitudinal ligament strain*—no change in reflexes. *With nerve root irritation:* L_4—Diminution of patellar tendon reflex. L_5—no change in patellar or achilles tendon reflexes. S_1—diminution of achilles tendon reflex.	Usually normal. If nerve roots are irritated, reflexes may be diminished: L_3 (L_3–L_4 facet joint) and/or L_4 (L_4–L_5 facet joint)—diminution of patellar tendon reflex. L_5 (L_5–S_1 facet joint)—no change in reflexes.	Normal unless nerve roots are irritated, then as acute facet syndrome.	Normal.	Normal.

* See "Psoriatic Arthritis," "Arthritis of Intestinal Disease," "Reiter's Syndrome," and "Ankylosing Spondylitis," Chapter 18.
† See "Paget's Disease," Chapter 20.

stronger than the lateral bands, a disc usually ruptures posterolaterally, rather than posterocentrally, sending its extruding contents against the single nerve root that crosses that side of the disc before entering the next lower neural foramina: L_4 when the disc of L_3–L_4 functional unit has ruptured; L_5 when the disc of the L_4–L_5 functional unit has ruptured; and S_1 when the disc of the L_5–S_1 functional unit has ruptured. The nerve root syndromes are summarized later in this chapter. Though most ruptures occur through one lateral band, somewhat more than 10% occur through both lateral bands as the so-called "dumbbell" rupture, or through the central band. The "dumbbell" rupture will produce nerve root symptoms and signs like the classic unilateral rupture, but bilaterally, and the central rupture when massive will produce a dramatically disabling neurologic dysfunction as all nerve roots below the level of rupture are crowded: both lower extremities become paresthetic and weak, and bladder and bowel control are often lost.

Facet Dysfunction and Degeneration. A low back pain associated with facet dysfunction and degeneration probably brings people to primary care offices somewhat more often than does the pain associated with posterior longitudinal ligament sprains, and nerve root injuries.

It will be recalled that facet joints are surrounded by synovial membrane and a fibrous capsule called the capsular ligament, and that this capsular ligament is lax and relatively weak. Add to these facts the additional fact that articulating facets change their relationship to one another by settling even to the point of becoming frankly subluxed when the disc of their functional unit narrows in response to degeneration, and we know enough to postulate the causes for most if not all facet joint pain.

Sudden movements in the bent position which are inadequately controlled by trunk movements may transfer forces to a facet joint which effect a sudden excessive movement in play, which may either sprain the relatively weak capsular ligament, or — on reapposition of facet surfaces— contuse a redundant fold of synovium. Either event could cause a sudden pain and reactive muscle spasm characteristic of *acute facet syndrome*. In our opinion, a unilateral spondylolysis subjects the facet joint of the intact lamina to a greater risk of this kind of injury.

As discs narrow and articulating facets change their relationship, movements of the facet joints become more wearing, both to the articular surfaces and to the capsular ligaments. These events constitute the degenerative arthritic process and produce the long-standing remitting and relapsing low backache and stiffness called the *chronic facet syndrome*. It is this relationship between discs and facets that has led some clinical theorists to their unified theory of low back pain. However, in our opinion other circumstances and relationships can lead to similar wear:

a. One severe or several lesser facet sprains.

b. An extreme lordosis or any scoliosis — abdominal obesity, pregnancy, and a weak abdominal wall all increase the normal lumbar lordosis; lower extremities of unequal length, weak hip abductors, and unknown processes that afflict some adolescents will create a scoliosis. (Adolescent scoliosis is reviewed at the end of this chapter.)

c. Unilateral spondylolysis.

d. Rotational facet malformations.

Two distinct neurologic syndromes can present with the chronic facet syndrome. Settling of facets and spur formation from the margins of facets and vertebral bodies can encroach upon neural foramina and/or the spinal canal itself. Encroachments upon neural foramina produce a *nerve root syndrome* which is usually confined to one or two segments and which may be either unilateral or bilateral. Encroachments upon the spinal canal itself may produce the narrow canal syndrome which is constituted by burning paresthesias and weakness in both legs, typically when the lumbosacral spine is held in lordotic posture as is usual when walking. The paresthesias and weakness are usually relieved by lumbosacral flexion as is usual when sitting. The narrow canal syndrome has been mistaken for claudication, emerging as it often does while walking. This complication of the chronic facet syndrome is receiving increasing attention in the literature. It probably is more prevalent than is usually appreciated. It is also called spinal stenosis, pseudoclaudication, and spondylitic caudal radiculopathy.

Sacroiliac Sprain and Arthritis. A painful disorder of the sacroiliac joint is nearly always the result of abrupt injury, usually sustained by a fall on one buttock. The sudden straining efforts probably stretch or frankly tear the sacroiliac ligaments, and conceivably lead to an irritation of the synovial lining of the joint as well. Ankylosing spondylitis, Reiter's syndrome and those forms of psoriatic arthritis and the arthritis of inflammatory intestinal disease that resemble ankylosing spondylitis, and Paget's disease may all present initially as a sacroiliac pain syndrome.

Myofascial Pain Syndrome. The erector spinae and the interspinous muscles of the lumbar back may be more vulnerable to strain and the cryptogenic myalgias than are the thoracic muscles. These problems account for the low back pain that brings people to primary care offices about as often as do the facet dysfunctions and degenerations. These muscles are commonly strained during a violent sneeze or when extending strongly against resistance as when lifting from a bent position. The strains are obviously characterized by an abrupt onset correlated with a forceful muscular act. The cryptogenic myalgias are characterized by a more gradual onset, and their pathology is unknown. (See page 145: "Muscle Strains and Cryptogenic Myalgias.") They are most likely to be located just above and below an iliac crest. They can be very persistent. Individuals with any degree of scoliosis seem to be more vulnerable to these myalgias. Scoliotics are also more vulnerable to ligamentous pain, presumably capsular ligament pain. Lordotics are vulnerable to ligamentous pain (capsular ligament and sacroiliac ligament pain).

Diagnosis of Musculoskeletal Soft Tissue Low Back Pains

Diagnostic precision requires a careful analysis of a number of subjective and objective variables, and despite thoughtful care cannot always be attained. To facilitate comparison, the variables discussed below are summarized in Table 9A-1.

History. The history of the four soft tissue disorders differs in three respects.

The Location and Radiation of Pain. Disc Syndrome. When disc degeneration has led merely to posterior longitudinal ligament sprain, pain is typically felt across the low back, but sometimes to one side or other of the midline. Persistent pain may eventually refer into the ipsilateral buttock and thigh. When disc degeneration has led to frank herniation of disc material, nerve root pain results. L_4 nerve root pain (L_3–L_4 disc) radiates into the inner aspect of the lower leg and ankle. L_5 nerve root pain (L_4–L_5 disc) radiates into the back of the thigh, the lateral aspect of the calf, the dorsum of the foot, and sometimes into the great toe. S_1 nerve root pain (L_5–S_1 disc) radiates into the back of the thigh, the back of the calf, the bottom of the heel, the plantar aspect of the foot, and sometimes the fourth and fifth toes.

Facet Syndrome. Which facet joint is disordered, whether the L_3–L_4, L_4–L_5, or L_5–S_1 makes no difference in the location and radiation of pain, unless the associated nerve root is crowded by arthritic swelling or bone spurs. The pain is typically felt across the low back, but sometimes to one side or other of the midline. Persistent pain may eventually refer into the ipsilateral buttock and thigh. Often facet joints are disordered bilaterally, in which case pain will refer into both buttocks and both thighs. When disorders of the L_3–L_4 facet joint irritate the L_3 nerve root, pain will radiate into the knee and inner aspect of the thigh. When disorders of the L_4–L_5 facet joint irritate the L_4 nerve root, pain will radiate into the inner aspect of the lower leg and ankle. When disorders of the L_5–S_1 facet joint irritate the L_5 nerve root, pain will radiate into the back of the thigh, the lateral aspect of the calf, and the dorsum of the foot. When degenerative changes have produced the narrow canal syndrome, burning causalgia-like pain will be felt in both lower extremities.

Sacroiliac Joint Sprain. Typically, pain is felt unilaterally and over the affected sacroiliac joint. When persistent, the pain may refer into the ipsilateral buttock and hip, so that patients may even present complaining of "hip pain."

Myofascial Pain. Typically, pain is felt unilaterally and over the point of muscle irritation. When persistent, the pain may refer into the ipsilateral buttock and hip.

The circumstantial and temporal nature of the onset and continuance of the pain. Disc Syndrome. A middle aged patient usually reports episodes of low back pain of one to several weeks' duration, which have occurred repeatedly since the early 30's, and which has now recurred but is lasting unusually long. While early episodes may sound like the acute facet syndrome, occurring suddenly during a body movement, more recent episodes seem to have been initiated by more vigorous exertions. The prolonged episodes of back pain may eventually remit, and though they may recur, may eventually remit and stay away indefinitely; but often these episodes progress to the stage of frank herniation and nerve root pain. Initially, nerve root pain may occur in transient episodes that follow periods of activity. Occasionally, these episodes become less severe and eventually cease to recur. Usually, the episodes become increasingly severe and persistent until eventually the pain is nearly continuous, remitting only briefly early in a period of rest, and intensifying always during even so slight a straight leg movement as a normal walking stride.

Acute Facet Syndrome. An adult of any age, but usually in the 30's, presents in severe pain which appears to hold him in a slight bent posture. The onset was abrupt and accompanied a quick body movement. Pain is less and ranges of motion greater usually by the end of 1 week, and recovery is usually complete by the end of 3 weeks. For the 1st day or two, pain is usually continuous, worsened by any low back movement and any straining. Thereafter, pain may be felt only with movement.

Chronic Facet Syndrome. An adult, usually over 50 years of age, complains of daily low back pain, worse on first rising and after prolonged sitting or standing, which may be sharply intensified by a straining effort. The patient will acknowledge episodes which sound like the acute facet syndrome in early adulthood. At this stage, the history is quite like the history of the early disc syndrome. In time, bony spurs may so crowd the neural foramina as to produce symptoms of nerve root irritation or may so crowd the spinal canal as to produce the narrow canal syndrome.

Like disc degeneration, the degeneration of facet joints typically affects the L_3–L_4, L_4–L_5 and L_5–S_1 functional units, thus causing L_3, L_4, and/or L_5 nerve root symptoms. Distinction of the chronic facet syndrome from the disc syndrome will usually be possible after physical examination alone, but in the face of nerve root pain, may require myelography. When disc herniation occurs, it tends to occur early in the course of degenerative change before x-ray signs of degeneration have become distinct. In contrast, the chronic facet syndrome occurs late in the course of degeneration when x-ray signs of degeneration are advanced. Awareness of this contrast can be diagnostically helpful.

The paresthesias and weakness of the narrow canal syndrome are typically provoked by lumbosacral extension and relieved by lumbosacral flexion. Most people walk with the lumbosacral spine somewhat extended and thus experience onset of their symptoms while walking. Most people sit with the lumbosacral spine somewhat flexed and thus experience relief of their symptoms while sitting. It is understandable why many clinicians would think of claudication when first hearing such a history. The other features of chronic facet syndrome, a normal peripheral vascular examination, and an abnormal neurologic examination, typically revealing diminished achilles tendon reflexes and diminished vibratory sensation, will suggest the correct diagnosis.

Individuals with malfunctioning facets or unilateral spondylolysis, persistent scoliosis, and excessive lordosis may develop the chronic facet syndrome in the 20's or 30's.

Sacroiliac Sprain. An individual of any age presents with low back pain, reporting a fall onto the buttocks. The pain is continuous and worsened by most low back movements, particularly those necessitated by sitting, lying, rising, and walking. Unilateral axial jars, such as would be provoked by stepping off a curb, will abruptly sharpen the pain.

Myofascial Pain. An individual of any age presents with low back pain, either of abrupt onset during a resisted extension maneuver, or of gradual onset, without obvious circumstantial correlations. Individuals with reactive lordosis or scoliosis (pregnant women, persons in walking casts, or persons adjusting to leg length differences following fractures or osteotomies) may suffer a persistent low backache, worsened by prolonged walking or standing. The scoliotic may suffer both muscular pain and ligamentous pain (presumably facet capsule pain). The lordotic probably suffers ligamentous pain (facet capsule and sacroiliac ligament pain).

Associated Symptoms. The disc syndrome and the acute and chronic facet syndrome may be associated with nerve root dysfunction other than pain: dysesthesias and weakness. These are reviewed in the discussion of the physical examination. Sacroiliac and myofascial pain are not associated with other distinguishing symptoms.

Physical Examination. The proper examination includes an orthopaedic examination and a neurologic examination. It has been our experience that young primary care clinicians tend to limit their examination to a neurologic examination. Such an examination, of course, merely gives information about nerve root involvement, but no information about the cause of the back pain.

We recommend the following examination in the following sequence:

Begin with the patient standing.

(1) Sit behind the patient and inspect the back. Reactive spasm of pelvic flexors and of erector spinae muscles will decrease or obliterate the normal lumbar lordosis and/or create a lumbosacral scoliosis. (See Figure 9-9.) Regardless of cause, severe pain tends almost invariably to be associated with the kyphotic shift away from lumbar lordosis and may be associated with lumbosacral scoliosis. Chronic moderate pain may be associated with a flat lumbosacral spine, or with accentuated lumbar lordosis, or with lumbosacral scoliosis. The presence of scoliosis and lordosis may represent the etiology of chronic myofascial pain.

(2) Palpate superficially and deeply over to either side of the midline. Superficial

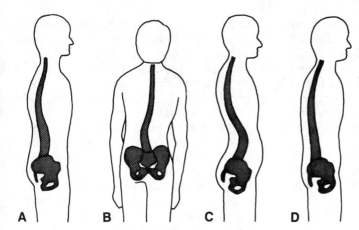

A   B   C   D

Fig. 9–9. Lumbosacral postures associated with low back pain. *A,* normal. *B,* lumbosacral scoliosis. *C,* lumbosacral lordosis. *D,* lumbosacral kyphosis.

palpation over and between the spines will elicit tenderness when the interspinous muscles are strained or otherwise painfully disordered. This tenderness is usually localized to only one or two segments. Superficial or deep palpation over an erector spinae muscle group will elicit fairly localized tenderness when that muscle group is strained or otherwise painfully disordered. Deep palpation over the facet joints and neural foramina will elicit pain when the facet joints or nerve roots are irritated. When nerve roots are irritated, the pain will often radiate into the affected dermatome.

The facet joints and neural foramina can be localized relative to the posterior iliac spines and the iliac crest (see Figure 9–10.):

a. L_5–S_1 facet joints and neural foramina—about 1 inch superior to the posterior iliac spines.

b. L_4–L_5 facet joints and neural foramina—about 2 inches superior to the posterior iliac spines at about the level of the iliac crests.

c. L_3–L_4 facet joints and neural foramina—about 3 inches superior to the posterior iliac spines and about 1 inch superior to the iliac crests.

Occasionally a nerve root irritated by a disc may be tender to palpation over the neural foramen above that through which it emerges. It is at that level that the nerve root passes over the ruptured disc.

Reactive spasm of erector spinae muscles results in superficial tenderness over the entire muscle mass. Hyperalgesic

spread results in superficial tenderness over the entire low back.

3. Watch the patient bend forward and straighten up. The movement may or may not be restricted, and it may or may not be accompanied by flexion to one side. Bending may be painful and the recovery not, or vice versa, or both may be painful. Both bending and recovery are likely to increase the pain of a muscle disorder. While bending may, it does not always increase the pain of a facet disorder, but recovery will always increase the pain of a facet disorder. Bending is likely to augment the pain of the disc syndrome (whether posterior longitudinal ligament strain or nerve root irritation), and straightening is likely to relieve that pain but will occasionally produce a catching pain. Neither bending nor straightening is as likely to affect sacroiliac joint pain.

4. Watch the patient attempt to extend the lumbosacral spine. The attempt may be free and painless, free and painful, or inhibited by pain. This movement often increases the pain of a facet disorder,

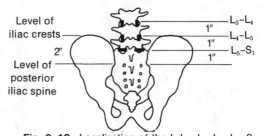

Level of iliac crests

Level of posterior iliac spine

2″

1″ — L_3–L_4

1″ — L_4–L_5

1″ — L_5–S_1

Fig. 9–10. Localization of the L_3L_4, L_4–L_5, L_5–S_1 facet joints and their neural foramina. Posterior view.

sometimes increases the pain of the sacro-iliac disorder, and usually has no influence on the pain of the other disorders.

5. Watch the patient walk on heels and toes. The L_5 nerve root dysfunction can weaken the dorsiflexors and prevent heel walking. S_1 nerve root dysfunction can weaken the gastrocnemius and soleus group and prevent toe walking.

Continue with the patient sitting, with knees flexed and legs dangling over the edge of the exam table. Sit in front and to one side of the patient.

6. Observe the patient actively extend each knee. Full extension may be possible and painless, or may be possible though painful, or may be limited by pain. The pain provoked by this movement may be felt in the low back, and/or in one or both legs. Pain felt only in the low back and posterior thigh usually represents facet pain. (The maneuver may move the facets by a slight pelvic flexion.) Pain felt in the lower leg as well usually represents nerve root pain. When dorsiflexion of the ankle at the point of pain increases the leg pain, nerve root pain is confirmed. (Dorsiflexion of the ankle places additional stretch on the sciatic nerve.) This maneuver serves the same purpose as the classic straight leg raising test, but in a way which may confuse some malingerers, and because of the effect of upright trunk weight on the discs, may be a more sensitive test for postero-lateral disc protrusion than the classic straight leg raising test. Some quadriceps weakness may be evident if L_3 and/or L_4 nerve roots have been disordered.

7. Test the patellar and achilles deep tendon reflexes. The patellar reflex will be lost when the L_3 nerve root has been disordered by an L_3–L_4 facet degeneration or when the L_4 nerve root has been disor-dered by an L_3–L_4 disc rupture or an L_4–L_5 facet degeneration. The achilles reflex will be lost when the S_1 nerve root is disordered by an L_5–S_1 disc rupture, but will not be affected when the L_5 nerve root is disor-dered by an L_4–L_5 disc rupture or L_5–S_1 facet degeneration.

8. Attempt two manipulations (see Figure 9–11): Ask the patient to rock from one buttock to the other. Sacroiliac pain will usually be increased when the patient sits on the affected side. Facet pain will usu-ally not be affected if the patient moves slowly. Posterior longitudinal ligament pain will not be affected. Erector spinae pain on the opposite side may be in-creased. As the patient sits on each but-tock, thrust abruptly downward on each shoulder. Both sacroiliac and facet pain are usually increased by this maneuver: sacroiliac pain when the maneuver is per-formed with the weight on the affected side; facet pain when the maneuver is per-formed with the weight on either side.

Conclude with the patient lying down.

9. If the distinction between posterior longitudinal ligament, facet, sacroiliac, and muscular low back pain remains uncer-tain, attempt the following manipulations and palpations:

a. Help the patient assume the supine posture illustrated in Figure 9–12. This po-sition is generally as comfortable as any. Encourage the patient to relax and not to stiffen against pain, but merely to report the pain. Assure the patient that you will stop the maneuver at the point of pain.

b. When the patient is quite relaxed and appears to understand, attempt to flex the patient's hips and low back maximally as illustrated in Figure 9–13. This maneuver does not increase posterior longitudinal ligament pain and may decrease it, it may

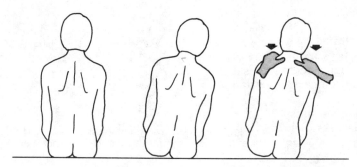

Fig. 9–11. Manipulation of the sacroiliac joints.

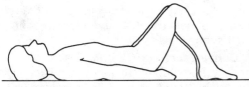

Fig. 9-12. Supine position for low back examination.

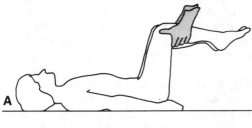

A

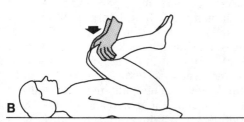

B

Fig. 9-13. *A* and *B*, manipulation in lumbosacral flexion.

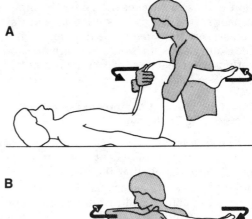

A

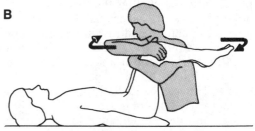

B

Fig. 9-14. *A* and *B*, manipulation of lumbosacral spine in lateral bending.

increase or decrease facet pain, it will have no effect on sacroiliac pain, and may or may not increase muscle pain.

c. Return the patient's hips to 90° flexion and hold this position until the patient can again relax and report the degree of residual pain. Then laterally bend the lumbosacral spine in each direction, as illustrated in Figure 9-14. This maneuver will have no effect on posterior longitudinal ligament pain, will usually increase facet pain in either or both directions, will usually have no effect on sacroiliac pain, and will usually increase muscle pain when bending away from the affected muscles.

d. Help the patient to lie on one side and apply torque to the lumbosacral spine as illustrated in Figure 9-7. Then perform the same manipulation with the patient lying on the opposite side. This maneuver will have no effect on posterior longitudinal ligament pain, it will usually increase facet and sacroiliac pain, and it will have no effect on muscle pain.

e. Help the patient to lie prone and repeat the palpation which was performed

standing. Deep palpation may be more effectively accomplished with the patient relaxed in the prone position.

10. Attempt the classic straight leg raising maneuver. Except in the very limber, the pelvis begins to tilt by 70° straight leg raising. Thus, straight leg raising to 70° bilaterally will often increase the back pain of the facet syndrome and the sacroiliac sprain. This pain will augment again if the leg is quickly lowered. While this pain may radiate into the thighs, it will usually not radiate into the leg and foot, and will not be worsened at 70° by dorsiflexion of the ankle (which places an additional stretch on the sciatic nerve).

The classic straight leg raising maneuver will not affect the posterior longitudinal ligament pain of early disc syndrome, but will, of course, augment the nerve root pain of the late disc syndrome, and the nerve root pain of chronic facet syndrome. Again, dorsiflexion of the ankle with the leg at the point of nerve root pain will worsen that pain.

11. Test cutaneous sensation to pinprick and light touch over the knees, the legs, and the dorsum, and lateral plantar aspects of the feet. L_3 dysfunction will decrease sensation over the knee, L_4 dysfunc-

tion will decrease sensation over the inner aspect of the leg, L_5 dysfunction will decrease sensation over the dorsum of the foot, and S_1 dysfunction will decrease sensation over the lateral plantar aspect of the foot. (See figure 9–6.)

The Treatment of Musculoskeletal Soft Tissue Low Back Pain

Acute Stage.

1. When pain of recent onset is disablingly severe, whether the result of a disordered facet, disc, sacroiliac joint, or myofascial structure, bed rest in a position of comfort is fundamental. Two positions are usually fairly comfortable: supine with hips and knees flexed, or on the side with hips and knees flexed. Bathroom privileges are allowed, but other ambulatory activities are not recommended at this stage.

2. Heat or cold may be applied to the back for analgesia 15 minutes at a time as many times as the patient wishes throughout the day.

3. *Isometric* and *passive* lumbosacral flexion exercises should be done for 1–2 minutes at a time at least once hourly, during waking hours. (See Figure 9–15.) Patients must attempt these exercises from the outset and begin this recommended regimen as soon as the exercises are accompanied by *only a slight* increase in pain.

4. Oral anti-inflammatory medication may be prescribed for any of the condi-

tions. See Chapter 18. They are most likely to seem of benefit when given for the acute facet syndrome.

Convalescent or Chronic Stage.

1. When pain of the acute low back has diminished such that cautious movement is relatively pain-free, or when the patient's complaint is of chronic low back pain, an *active* exercise program becomes fundamental. For all conditions, we encourage cautious walking and the performance of *active* as well as *passive flexion* exercises. For chronic pain syndromes which are not associated with the narrow canal or spondylitic nerve root syndrome, and for the convalescent stage of the myofascial and sacroiliac pain syndrome, we recommend *active* unilateral and bilateral *extension* exercises in addition. (See Figure 9–16.) Chronic back disorders are most likely to remain in remission when extensors as well as flexors are well conditioned. Myofascial pain usually emerges from pain in the extensor muscles and tendons. For whatever reasons, working as well as stretching exercises of musculotendinous pain disorders in chronic or convalescent stages has seemed to us to be of benefit. Particularly unilateral extension exercises create some sacroiliac joint play

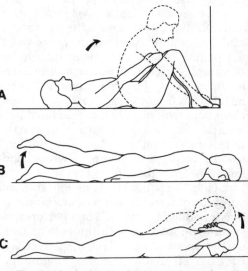

Fig. 9–16. Active low back exercises. *A,* active lumbosacral flexion. Flexion exercise begins by merely touching the knees, and progresses to as full a sit-up as possible. *B,* and *C,* active lumbosacral extension exercise. Extension exercise begins with B and progresses to C as possible.

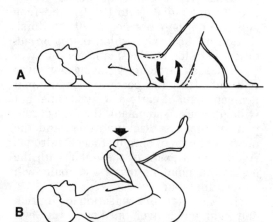

Fig. 9–15. Isometric and passive lumbosacral flexion exercises. *A,* isometric (pelvic tilt). *B,* passive flexion.

which has seemed to us to be of benefit for disorders of the sacroiliac joint.

Active exercise is never recommended for the acute disc syndrome, whether with or without nerve root pain. However, in our view, the chronic disc syndrome—like the chronic facet syndrome—is likely to remain stagnant without exercise. While weight lifting and those sports requiring sudden movements that apply large levering forces on the low back are curtailed, we urge those with chronic disc or facet pain—whether accompanied by nerve root pain or not—to walk or swim daily, and to perform active flexion and extension exercises for maximum trunk muscle conditioning.

All patients with chronic back pain are taught the principles of back care. (See Appendix to this chapter.)

2. Chronic low back pain can often be temporarily relieved by heat or cold application, passive flexion exercises, and aspirin grains 10 every 4 hours.

3. Oral anti-inflammatory medications, as such, are probably not useful at this stage.

4. Occasionally, a chronic focal myofascial pain will yield to a local injection of corticosteroid or lidocaine, or to simple needling.

5. A sacroiliac support may allow reasonably comfortable activity during convalescence or during exacerbations of a chronic pain problem. We prefer the sacroiliac support to the classically recommended lumbosacral corset for L_4-L_5 and L_5-S_1 disorders as, in our opinion, the sacroiliac support gives adequate support to the L_4-L_5 and L_5-S_1 functional units without preventing the slight lumbosacral flexion which is optimal for low back stability or weakening the back and abdominal muscles by too extensive immobilization, which we believe are disadvantageous effects of the classically prescribed lumbosacral corset. (See Figure 9-17.)

When to Refer a Patient with Low Back Pain to an Orthopaedist. Patients should be referred to an orthopaedist in the following circumstances:

1. When the diagnosis of the pain is obscure, the patient should be referred within an interval of time humanely dependent upon the degree of disability.

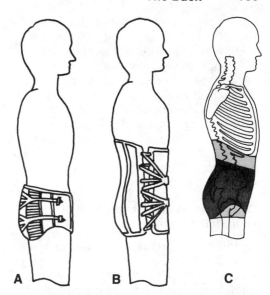

Fig. 9–17. Comparison of the sacroiliac support to the lumbosacral corset. *A*, sacroiliac support. *B*, lumbosacral corset. *C*, levels stabilized by the two devices.

2. When bone pain is suspect, the patient should be referred within the week.

3. When a disc or facet syndrome, with or without nerve root symptoms, but without objective nerve root dysfunction, fails to improve after 8 weeks' compliance with a conservative regimen, the patient should be referred within the next week.

4. When nerve root dysfunction is objectively evident, the patient should be referred within 1–3 weeks.

5. When the narrow canal syndrome is suspect, the patient should be referred within 1–3 weeks.

6. When facet or myofascial pain are associated with spondylolisthesis which increases during any period of observation, the patient should be referred within 1–3 weeks.

Scoliosis — Lateral Curvature of the Spine

Etiology and Prevalence

The etiology of scoliosis is often classified in two groups: *nonstructural* or *reactive scoliosis* includes those caused by a short leg, uneven muscle spasm, poor posture, or hysteria; *structural scoliosis* includes those having congenital bone defects, metabolic or paralytic conditions, and the so-called idiopathic scoliosis.

Idiopathic scoliosis comprises the largest group and occurs in approximately 20–30/1000 adolescent children. It is now recognized as an inherited disorder, characterized by dominant polygenic inheritance with incomplete penetrance, and a 25% kindred incidence. However, the mechanism linking genotype with phenotype is not understood.

Classification and Description of Idiopathic Curves

Idiopathic curves are classified by age: *infantile,* from birth to 3 years of age; *juvenile,* from 3 to 10 years of age; and *adolescent,* from 10 years through the full growth period. In the adolescent group, the incidence of significant curves is much higher in girls (90%), and the right thoracic curve is the most prevalent.

Spinal curves are described by the convexity and level of the arcs at their apices. The most common curve and one which often develops rapid progression is the right thoracic-left lumbar curve. Figure 9–18 illustrates a right thoracic-left lumbar curve as it will appear when looking at the patient's back. The major curve is the thoracic, and the minor curve the lumbar.

Any number of combinations of curves are encountered. (See Figure 9–19.)

Lateral curvature is accompanied by rotation of the vertebrae. The bodies of the vertebrae rotate toward the convexity of the curve. Hence, as seen from the upper surface of the vertebrae, a clockwise rotation will accompany a right thoracic curve, causing a rib hump to protrude on the right side of the thorax, and a counterclockwise rotation will accompany a left lumbar curve causing a rotational prominence of transverse processes to protrude on the left side of the lumbar back. These curves and rotations are most evident when a person bends forward to touch the toes. (See Figure 9–18.)

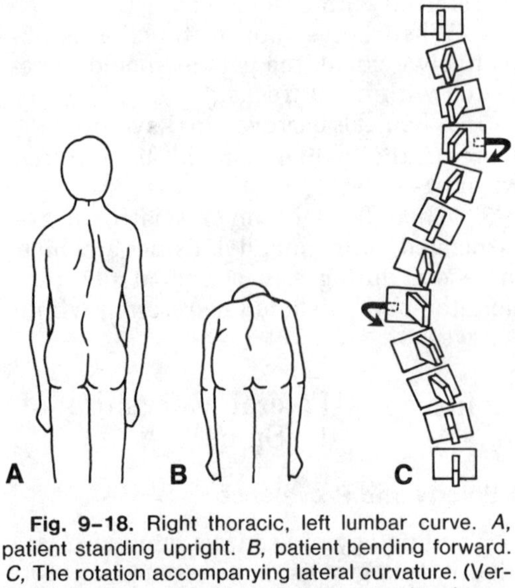

Complications of Scoliosis

The structural thoracic constraints produced by moderate and severe curves constitute a restrictive pulmonary disease. Untreated, people so afflicted will manifest ventilatory insufficiency, suffer repeated episodes of penumonia, and eventually are likely to die in respiratory failure.

Any curve, whether mild or severe, creates abnormally wearing forces on discs and facets, and may lead by early middle age to the pain and peripheral neuropathy of intervertebral disc degeneration and degenerative joint disease.

The Therapeutic Postulates

Concepts of therapy have been in flux for years, dramatically so over the past 2–3 years. In our opinion, all therapeutic regi-

Fig. 9–18. Right thoracic, left lumbar curve. *A,* patient standing upright. *B,* patient bending forward. *C,* The rotation accompanying lateral curvature. (Vertebral bodies rotate toward the convexity, hence clockwise rotation accompanies right thoracic curve, and counterclockwise rotation accompanies left lumbar curve, as viewed from overhead.)

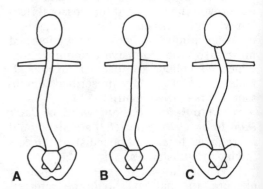

Fig. 9–19. Example of the variety of curves. *A,* left thoracolumbar. *B,* left lumbar. *C,* Right cervicothoracic, left thoracolumbar.

mens derive from one of two general postulates, which we like to call the *pessimistic postulate,* and the *optimistic postulate.* Advocates of both postulates agree that once a curve has progressed to 20–25°, the natural course of the disease is constant progression until adolescent growth ends. They differ, however, over the question of prevention.

Pessimistic Postulate. The pessimists postulate two diseases, a stable mild scoliosis, and an inexorably progressive scoliosis. They judge the progressive disease probably to be uninfluenced by bracing, and certainly to be uninfluenced by exercise. They expect surgical stabilization will be required for most—if not all—persons with a progressive curve shortly before the end of the adolescent growth period. They generally recommend surgery when the curve reaches 30–35°. Though the unique drawbacks of surgery include the constrains on function of a fused spine, incomplete correction inherent in the current procedures, late breakage of the stabilizing rod, and respiratory failure and death during surgery or early in postoperative convalescence, the pessimists weigh these evils against the evil of the disease itself and feel forced to endorse the surgery.

Optimistic Postulate. The optimists postulate a spectrum of diseases, small categories of which either remain stable and mild without treatment, or progress inexorably, and the major categories of which progress, but much less if treated with bracing and/or exercise.

Recognition of Scoliosis

The health evaluation of children should always include an examination of the spine and the general posture. A regular routine inspection from the head down to the feet, or from the feet up to the head is efficient and less likely to miss an early curve. The early detection of scoliosis, as indeed of all posture problems (kyphosis, lordosis), is critical if the optimistic therapeutic postulate is correct.

An effective screening examination will consider the following questions:

1. Are the shoulders level?
2. Are the scapulae evenly spaced from the vertebrae and level?
3. Do arms hang with equal space between the elbows and the sides?
4. Are iliac crests even?
5. Are hips equally prominent?
6. Is the trunk even, when the person bends forward to touch the toes?
7. Are leg lengths equal?
   a. Measure *true leg length* from the anterior-superior iliac spine to the distal medial malleolus.
   b. Measure *apparent leg length* from the umbilicus to the distal medial malleolus.
8. Are any other members of the family scoliotic?

A standing anteroposterior x-ray of the full spine must be made whenever there is suspicion of scoliosis.

Measurement of the Curves

Both optimists and pessimists base their therapeutic decision upon the quantitative severity of the curve. The Cobb technique for quantifying the degree of a curve is a commonly accepted method. (See Figure 9–20.)

The Optimistic Therapeutic Regimen

For nearly 20 years, we have been advocates of the optimistic postulate. In our experience, a home exercise program, taught and monitored in our physical therapy department—if begun when curves are less than 15–20°—has seemed to stop or retard progression of curves, as compared to the natural course of the disease. However, we have made no disciplined study to prove or disprove our clinical impression. Dr. Walter P. Blount, who has designed and studied the influence of the Milwaukee Brace, and members of the scoliosis team from Children's Hospital Medical Center in Boston, who designed and for the past 2–3 years have been working with the Boston Brace, have stated that the effectiveness of wearing braces seems much greater when the children are also participating in an exercise program. See Blount and Moe, 1973, Chapter 5, and Manual for "The Boston Brace System" Workshop, Chapter 7. Some arguments against exercise have stressed the non-compliance of children and parents. In our program, compliance has been the rule when the physician, the therapist, the parent, and the child have agreed about the nature of

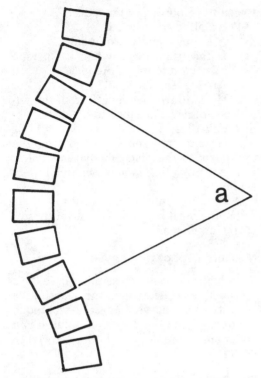

Fig. 9–20. The Cobb technique for quantifying the degree of a curve. Lines are extended from the vertebra at either end of the curve that inclines most toward the concavity. The line from the superior vertebra parallels its upper margin, and the line from the inferior vetebra parallels its lower margin. The angle (*a*) is the measurement of the curve.

the disease and the value of exercise treatment.

Treatment based upon the optimistic postulate is team treatment: the child, the parents, the primary physician, the orthopaedist, the physical therapist, the orthotist, and occasionally a social worker or clinical psychologist conspire together to retard the progression of the curve. The regimen begins with an initial evaluation by a physician and physical therapist. Occasionally, insights bearing on the resilience of the child and the family may cause the primary physician to request an evaluation by a social worker and/or clinical psychologist. These professionals then meet with the child and the parents, and the goals and means to achieve them are detailed and agreed upon.

Each exercise program is individualized according to the child's needs, and include mobilizing and strengthing movements, el-

evation, postural training, and breathing exercises. A physical therapist experienced in working with scoliotic children must be employed.

Mobilizing and Strengthening Movements. The child is encouraged to be physically active, avoiding only contact sports. All else equal, the prognosis for athletic children is far better than for sedentary children.

Intervertebral ligaments, paraspinous muscles, the tensor fasciae latae, the hamstring muscles, the iliopsoas, the gastrocnemius and soleus and pectoral muscles tend to become contracted. The physical therapist looks for these contractures and teaches stretching exercises to combat those that are developing.

Corrected posture can be actively held only when paraspinous, gluteal, and abdominal muscles are strong and the child

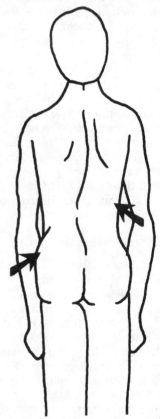

Fig. 9–21. Elevation—the fundamental exercise. Children are taught to pull away from a brace or from the therapist's hands. *Arrows* designate the points against which a Boston brace or therapist's hands will press.

is consciously able to direct their activity. The physical therapist teaches exercises to strengthen and heighten the child's awareness of these muscles.

Elevation. This fundamental exercise is taught by showing the child how to "stand tall"—how to activate muscles that reduce the curves and lengthen the axis of the trunk. This exercise is easiest to learn in a brace, but our physical therapists teach it to children with curves less than 15–20° who do not yet require bracing. (See Figure 9–21.)

Posture Training. Elevation is a specific aspect of posture training which is practiced as such during exercise periods. In addition, children are made aware of their tendencies to lumbar lordosis and dorsal kyphosis and are taught actively to correct these tendencies.

Breathing Exercises. These are essential to maintain adequate thoracic motion and decrease the tendency to develop restrictive pulmonary disease which other wise is the rule for progressive scoliosis.

A detailed description of the Milwaukee exercise regimen may be found in Chapter 5 of Blount and Moe, 1973.

We require 15 minutes daily for concentrated exercise and continuous attention to posture throughout each day. We have found regular follow-up necessary to maintain the child's and parents' interest, to help with the inevitable personal distress that may demoralize the child or the parents, to detect changing needs and to modify the regimen accordingly, and to detect special problems that may require specific technical assistance. After the patient and parents have learned the basic program, we have them follow with a physical therapist every 2–3 months, and with a physician every 6–18 months. An x-ray of the spine must be taken prior to each visit with the physician.

If the primary physician is knowledgeable, and a physical therapist well experienced with scoliosis is available, an orthopaedist need not be involved at the outset. An orthopaedist particularly interested in scoliosis must become involved when a curve exceeds 15°, and when a lesser curve increases (most likely during periods of rapid growth). At these stages, bracing will invariably be necessary.

Primary physicians who wish to guide their patients through the preventive program we have outlined should study the first five chapters of Blount and Moe, 1973, should observe the work of an experienced physical therapist, and should formalize a preventive regimen with the physical therapist. The physician should watch for publications by the Boston group.

Appendix

The following is a modification of the instruction sheet given patients who suffer back pain by the physical therapy department of Group Health Cooperative of Puget Sound:

Back Care

Our experience tells us that back pain is not cured by professional care alone; a painful back usually improves when it is well cared for by its owner 24 hours a day.

The most helpful thing we can do for your back is to show you how to take care of it yourself by learning new ways to stand, to sit, to lift, and even to sleep or rest. Take special note of the sleeping and resting positions below since it is possible to strain your back just by resting it improperly. A well-positioned rest can be a very effective pain reliever.

At your doctor's request, the therapist may give you certain exercises to be done every day. The exercises are specifically designed to stretch and strengthen the muscles that support your back. You can combine daily exercise, good posture and sensible body mechanics in your own effective back care program.

Home Treatments Using Heat and Cold

Hot Moist Towels:	Cover towels with plastic and wrap in a blanket. Apply to painful area for 15–20 minutes.
Commercial Hot Packs:	Cover with several layers of dry towels. Apply for 10–20 minutes.
Tub Bath:	Bath should be as warm as possible, for 10–20 minutes.
Strong Needle Shower:	Warm as possible, for 5 minutes.
Electric Heating Pad:	Set heat on *low* for 10–20 minutes. *Use extreme caution!* Do *not* sleep all night with pad on-pressure on the pad can cause burns.
Moist Ice Towels:	Fold a wet towel in quarters and freeze in your freezer. Place in a pillowcase to prevent ice burn; apply for 10–20 minutes.
Ice Massage:	Make ice in a small paper cup, rub ice direct over painful area for 5–15 minutes or until area becomes numb.
Ice Bag:	Place ice bag on painful area, 10–20 minutes.
Commercial Cold Pack:	Place in warm moist towel before applying to prevent ice burn. Apply 10–15 minutes.

By applying the illustrated suggestions, you can decide what works best for your back problem. Make back care a part of your daily routine to minimize strain and avoid possible injury. Consult with your doctor or your therapist regarding exercise, special activities, an increase in pain, or a change of symptoms.

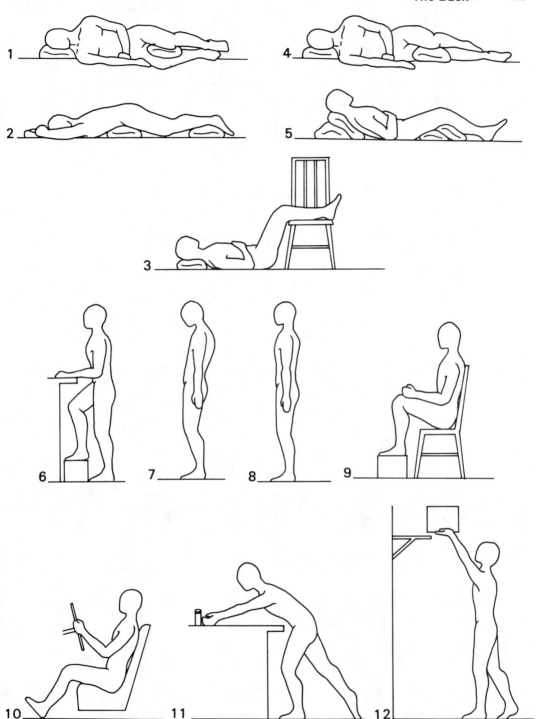

Fig. 9-A. *1–5.* Recommended resting or sleeping positions. *6.* Whenever possible, bend one knee when standing. *7.* Poor posture increases back strain. *8.* Good posture reduces strain. Keep your back straight. *9.* Sit with knees higher than hips. *10.* Try moving the car seat forward so that knees are bent. *11, 12.* When reaching forward or overhead keep your back straight and put one leg out behind you.

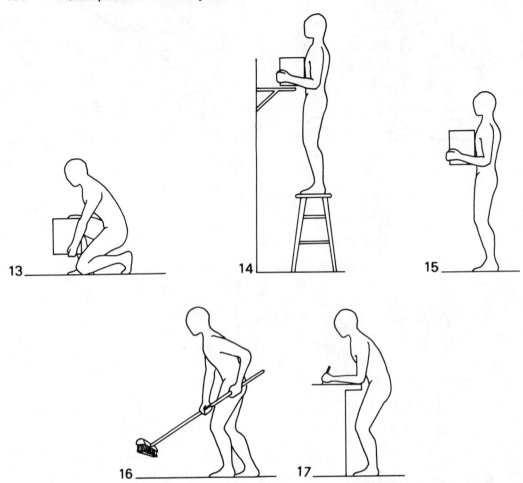

Fig. 9-A *13.* When lifting, bend hips and knees, keeping back straight; keep object close to you and lift with your legs. *14.* Avoid lifting overhead by using a stool or ladder. *15.* When carrying, hold object close to you. *16, 17.* In daily activities involving bending or stooping, bend your knees. Avoid twisting.

CHAPTER 10

Fractures and Dislocations of the Spine

Essential Anatomy

The peculiarities of the various functional units of the spine and a general description of their controlling and supporting soft tissues have been outlined in Chapters 1 and 9. This section summarizes three points important to the basic study of spine fractures and dislocations.

1. From early school age to the end of life, the functional units of the normal spine articulate with one another in ways which create an alternation of two lordotic with two kyphotic curves. The lordotic segments, the neck and lumbar back, are the most mobile: the cervical spine moves quite freely in all three planes of motion (flexion-extension, lateral bending, and rotation), and the lumbar spine moves quite freely in the sagittal and frontal planes of motion (flexion-extension and lateral bending). The kyphotic segments, the dorsal spine and the sacrum, are the least mobile: the dorsal spine moves only in the transverse plane (rotation), and the sacrum, being a solid bone, does not move at all except in very slight play at its articulations with the pelvis.

The junctions between the most mobile and the least mobile segments of the spine are the points at which angulating-twisting forces are greatest. Hence, the most disrupting dorsolumbar injuries tend to involve the functional units D_{12}–L_1 and L_1–L_2. Though, by this rule, the cervical units C_6–C_7 and C_7–T_1 should be the most vulnerable, the great mobility of all the cervical units and the angular forces generated by the mass of the head subject all cervical units to a nearly equal vulnerability: the chances of the moment determine the point at which maximum force will apply.

2. The spinal cord ends variably at the 1st or 2nd lumbar vertebra, and the cauda equina, composed of all lumbar and sacral nerve roots, ends near the end of the spinal canal, in the sacrum. Thus, the fractures and dislocations which can injure the cord itself are all those above the 3rd lumbar vertebra.

3. The two sympathetic chains are closely approximated to the bodies of the vertebrae. Thus, fractures of the bodies of D_{12}, L_1, and L_2, which bleed anteriorly, may irritate the sympathetic chains bearing preganglionic neurons to the intestine and result in very troublesome paralytic ileus.

Presumption of Unstable Injury and Methods of Transportation

Neck and back pain following injury by forces of great or unknown degree should be suspected to represent an unstable fracture or dislocation of danger to the cord. This suspicion should become a presumption when the individual is reluctant to move, complains of dysesthesias, or demonstrates weakness or paralysis of any extremity, or when deep palpation over and on either side of the spine demonstrates distinct tenderness.

Once the presumption is made, the patient should be moved only in ways that prevent further motion of the injured functional units. While the cervical spine can be fairly well stabilized during transport by manual or halter traction, immobilization on a fracture board is probably safer. Any space between the back of the neck and the fracture board should be filled with some folded material (for example, a sweater or towel), and supports to prevent rotation and lateral bending should be placed on both sides of the head and neck (preferably sandbags or some equally stable makeshift equivalent). An adequate fracture board must be wide enough to accommodate the patient's shoulders and long enough to support the length of the spine, including the occiput and pelvis. An ideal fracture board extends the length of the patient. The patient should be firmly strapped onto the board.

Essentials of Assessment and Diagnosis

In nearly all cities and many towns of the United States today, rescue squads are so well trained and equipped that patients are quite safely transported to hospitals. However, paradoxically, not all hospitals are so well prepared to receive them. Many primary clinicians encounter an unstable spine injury once in 5 years at most, in contrast to the stable injuries which they encounter once a week at least. Some clinicians may discount the patient's danger and proceed as with stable injuries; others, though aware of the patient's danger, may not know exactly how to proceed, and in the stress of an emergency, may fabricate a disastrous plan. We urge strict adherence to the following assessment plan:

1. Without moving the patient, assess the vital functions and provide all necessary support. When a patient suspected of an unstable neck injury appears to need ventilatory support, introduce an oropharyngeal airway and try to effect adequate ventilation through a mask. When at all possible, the neck should be stabilized before attempting to introduce any endotracheal airway. When an endotracheal airway must be introduced before the neck can be stabilized, methods must be employed, by those who can, which do not hyperextend the neck.

2. Assess neurologic function without moving the spine: If the patient is conscious and able to communicate, test light touch sensation in all fingers and over both surfaces of the feet, test vibratory sensation in both ankles, and ask the patient to move fingers and toes and test the plantar cutaneous reflex; if the patient is unconscious or unable to communicate, one can only look for involuntary movements and test the plantar cutaneous reflexes. The unconscious patient with evidence of head injury must be presumed to have an unstable neck injury as well, until disproved by complete cervical x-rays. When paralysis is evident, the level of paralysis should be determined as accurately as can be done without moving the spine. Attention to the following neuro-anatomic facts will suggest a safe and useful exam:

a. Control of the diaphragm is mediated through segment C_4.

b. Control of the deltoid and occasionally cutaneous sensation in the thumb are mediated through segment C_5.

c. Control of the thenar eminence and cutaneous sensation in the thumb, index, and middle fingers are largely mediated through segments C_6 and C_7.

d. Control of the intrinsic muscles to the fingers and cutaneous sensation to the fourth and fifth fingers are mediated through segments C_8 and T_1.

e. Intercostal ventilatory movements are mediated through segments T_2 through T_{10}.

f. The quadrantal abdominal cutaneous reflexes are mediated through segments T_7 through L_1.

g. Cutaneous sensation to the chest from the sternal angle to the xiphoid is mediated through segments T_2 through T_6.

h. Cutaneous sensation to the abdomen from the xiphoid to the anterior-superior iliac spines is mediated through segments T_7 through T_{11}.

i. Cutaneous sensation to the inguinal and femoral regions is mediated through segment T_{12} and L_1.

j. Cutaneous sensation to the anterior and lateral thighs is mediated through segment L_2 and L_3.

k. Cutaneous sensation to the medial aspect of the lower leg is mediated through segment L_4.

l. Cutaneous sensation to the lateral aspect of the lower leg is mediated through segment L_5 and S_1.

m. Cutaneous sensation of the dorsum or dorsomedial aspect of the foot is mediated through segment L_5.

n. Cutaneous sensation to the heel and the lateral aspect of the foot is mediated through segment S_1.

o. Cutaneous sensation to the genitals is mediated through segments S_2 through S_4.

p. Ability to stiffen the knee and elevate the patella by contraction of quadriceps muscle is mediated through segments L_3 and L_4.

q. Control of extension and flexion of the great toe is mediated through segments L_5 and S_1 respectively.

Based on those neuro-anatomic facts, we recommend the following exam:

a. Note whether ventilation is active and, if active, whether it employs the intercostals or the diaphragm, or both (C_4 and T_2 through T_{10}).

b. While feeling the deltoid, ask the patient to move the arm 1–2″ away from his side (C_5).

c. Test light touch to the fingers (thumb, C_5–C_6; index and middle fingers, C_6–C_7; ring and fifth fingers, C_7–C_8, and T_1).

d. Ask the patient to oppose the thumb and fifth fingers (thenar eminence, C_6; hypothenar eminence, C_8).

e. Test light touch to the chest (T_2 through T_6).

f. Test light touch to the abdomen and attempt to elicit the quadrantal abdominal cutaneous reflex (upper quadrants, T_7 through T_{11}; lower quadrants, T_{12}–L_1).

g. Test light touch to the anterior lateral thighs (L_2–L_3).

h. While feeling the quadriceps and watching the patella, ask the patient to

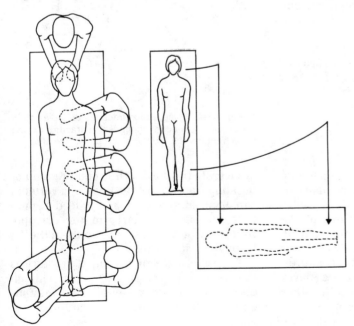

Fig. 10–1. Transferring the patient with a spine injury.

stiffen the knee (L₃–L₄).

   i. Test light touch to the medial aspect of the calf (L₄).

   j. Test light touch to the dorsomedial aspect of the foot (L₅).

   k. Test light touch to the lateral aspect of the foot (S₁).

   l. Ask the patient to extend and flex the great toe (L₅–S₁).

A surgeon's therapeutic choices will be strongly determined by the history of the paralysis: whether since the patient's first examination a paralysis has appeared, progressed, remained stable, or regressed. Thus, a clearly recorded and accurate initial examination is critical.

3. Once vital functions are assessed and neurologic function is assessed, obtain a lateral x-ray of the injured segments while keeping the patient immobile on the fracture board. Complete x-rays should be deferred until stability is assured.

4. Hospital immobilization of the unstable injury must be directed by a well-experienced physician. He will employ some variant of a Stryker frame for all spine injuries and, in addition, some form of head and neck traction for cervical injuries.

5. The patient must not be moved from the fracture board to the Stryker frame until that experienced physician is present, and until adequate personnel are present to lift the patient safely: one person for the head, two or four for the trunk, and one for each leg. The patient's arms are crossed over the chest during the transfer. (See Figure 10–1.)

Compression Fractures of the Bodies of the Vertebrae (See Figure 10–2)

Axial compression forces, depending upon their magnitude and the resilience of the bony architecture, can produce wedge compression or bursting fractures of the vertebral bodies. Unless accompanied by a violent posterior rupture of a disc and/or more extensive associated fractures, wedge compression fractures are never complicated by a cord injury. On the other hand, the posterior fragments of a burst fracture may be so displaced as to contuse

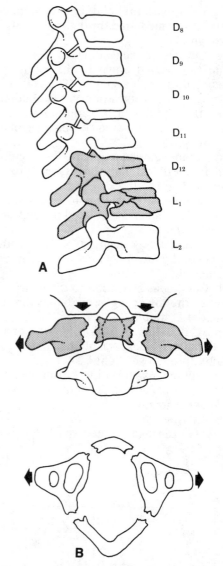

Fig. 10–2. Compression fractures of bodies of the vertebrae. *A*, wedge compression fracture of D₁₂. Burst fracture of L₁. *B*, burst fracture of the atlas.

or lacerate the cord. While compression or bursting fractures of the body of a vertebra can occur at any level, and indeed at multiple levels, particularly in the osteoporotic, they occur most commonly in the T₁₂ through L₂ segments.

A special case of the burst fracture is the fracture of the ring of Atlas. Though disruption of the vertebral ring may be extreme, cord damage is by no means invariable.

Fractures of the Posterior Elements of the Vertebrae, Shearing Fractures of the Bodies of the Vertebrae, and Dislocations of the Vertebral Units (See Figure 10–3)

In the neck, these injuries occur most commonly at the C_5–C_6 segment, though—as pointed out in the anatomic section of this chapter—injuries are almost as common at other levels. In the dorsolumbar spine, these injuries occur most commonly at the T_{12} through L_2 segments. While in the cervical region, the spinal cord segments correspond to the vertebral segments, this correspondence is not maintained in the lower levels: the thoracic segment of the cord extends between C_7 vertebra and D_{10} vertebra, the lumbar segments between D_{10} and D_{12} vertebra, the sacral and coccygeal segments between D_{12} vertebra and L_2 vertebra. (See Figure 10–4.) Thus, unstable spine injuries across T_{12} through L_2 segments will injure the sacrococcygeal segments of the cord.

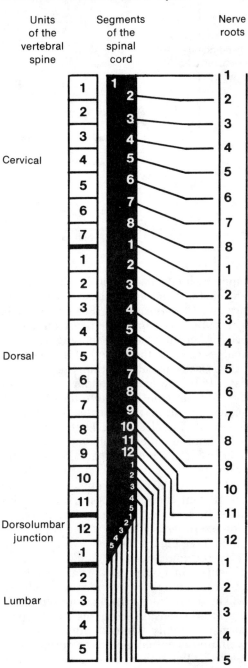

Fig. 10–4. Relationship of cord segments to vertebral segments.

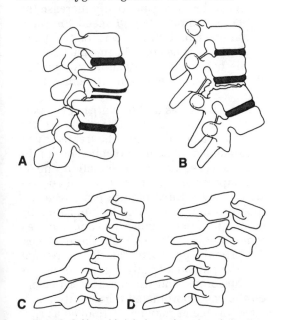

Fig. 10–3. Unstable injuries to the spine. *A,* fracture of the superior facet with disruption of the intervertebral disc and both longitudinal ligaments. Lumbar spine. *B,* fracture of the superior facet, with shearing fracture of the vertebral body. Thoracic spine. *C,* subluxation of the cervical spine. *D,* dislocation of the cervical spine.

Treatment of Spine Fractures

Wedge compression fractures without associated disc rupture require supportive and rehabilitative treatment only. These

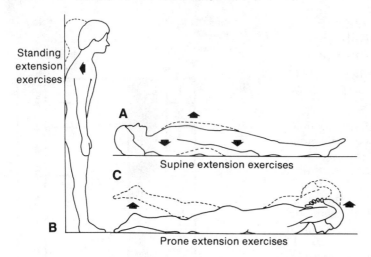

Fig. 10-5. Extension exercises.

injuries should be treated by the primary physician. A pathologic basis for the fracture must be considered. (See Chapter 20). The patient is kept at bed rest on a firm bed and given necessary nursing care and analgesics until the period of severe pain has passed—usually within the first 5–7 days. Paralytic ileus secondary to sympathetic chain irritation and to the effects of analgesics often complicates the first 2 weeks of convalescence. That neurogenic ileus and the patient's reluctance to strain may result in a rectal impaction and eventual intestinal colic. Liberal use of stimulant laxatives from the outset will spare the patient those unnecessary added insults. As soon as pain allows, active extension exercises are begun in the supine position. (See Figure 10-5.)

By the middle of the 2nd week, most patients can resume sitting and cautious walking, though any tendency to slump will augment the pain. Once upright, more vigorous extension exercises can be performed, initially while standing against a wall, and eventually from the prone lying position. Patients with a dorsal kyphosis will be best able to effect the extension exercises from the standing position against a wall, but they can do the exercises from the prone position with enough pillows under the chest and abdomen. Ex-

tension exercises must be continued until normal movement is possible without pain. Exercises should be done to the point of fatigue, but short of a worsening of pain. They should be repeated at least four times a day and preferably more. While the exercise may be easy to describe, instruction and encouragement by an attentive tactful physical therapist can greatly increase the patient's compliance and speed the rehabilitation. Eventual recovery of full painless activity is usual, but can—particularly in the osteoarthritic—take many months. Rarely, a permanent pain problem will result.

Burst fractures and fractures of the posterior elements and dislocations of the facet and disc joints must be treated by an orthopaedist or neurosurgeon. These injuries often require open reduction and/or decompression laminectomy, and/or fusion. They always require prolonged immobilization, and when complicated by cord injury, they require long and complex rehabilitation. Through all these stages, the primary physician can do the patient and the patient's family a great service as an interpreter and troubleshooter (except on the best-coordinated rehabilitation services, problems may be overlooked as specialists deal with their unique responsibilities).

CHAPTER 11

The Hip

Essential Anatomy

Like the upper extremities, the lower extremities make their attachment to the body axis through their articulation with a bony "girdle." However, the hip joints differ from the shoulder joints in three respects:

1. While the shoulder girdles are attached to the body axis by muscles and the rather mobile sternoclavicular joints, and are thus capable of movement independent from the body axis, the hip girdles are attached to the body axis by the abdominal and erector spinae muscles, and by the unyielding ligaments of the essentially immobile sacroiliac joints, and are thus capable of movement only with the body axis. These movements are the movements of the lumbosacral spine: anterior tilting, posterior tilting, lateral tilting, and very slight rotation.

2. While the articular surface of each shoulder girdle is a relatively flat surface, and each shoulder joint is thus entirely dependent upon muscles and ligaments for its stability, the articular surface of each hip girdle is a deep cup, and each hip joint thus is inherently stable during weight-bearing with little help from its ligaments, and with its muscles more responsible for postural than for articular stability.

3. The articular surface of each hip girdle is a weightbearing surface and is thus much more vulnerable to the wearing effects of use than is the articular surface of each shoulder girdle.

Six anatomic details are necessary for an understanding of hip disorders:

1. The general structure of the pelvis.
2. The structure of the hip joint and upper third of the femur.
3. The innervation of the hip joint.
4. The muscles controlling the hip joint.
5. The bursae of the hip joint.
6. The relationship of the hip joint to the major nerves and vessels to the extremity.

The General Structure of the Pelvis

The pelvis is a closed ring formed by the rather rigid articulations of two *coxal bones,* and the *sacrum.* Their three joints are the two *sacroiliac joints* and the *pubic symphysis.* The great stability of the sacroiliac joints derives from the tension of their ligaments and the locking orientation of their facets. Five ligaments bind each sacroiliac joint (see Figure 11–1):

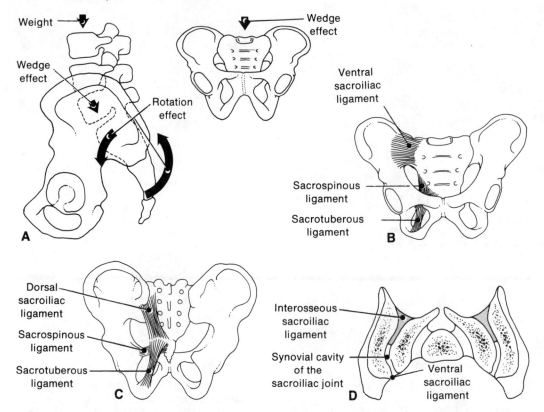

Fig. 11–1. Forces and stabilizing ligaments at the sacroiliac joint. *A*, forces acting at the sacroiliac joint. *B*, anterior view of the stabilizing ligaments. *C*, posterior view of the stabilizing ligaments. *D*, coronal section of the sacroiliac joint.

1. The *interosseous sacroiliac ligament* which forms the fibrous portion of the joint, posterosuperior to the synovial portion of the joint.

2. The *dorsal sacroiliac ligament* which passes from the lower third of the sacrum diagonally upward across the joint to the posterior iliac spine and merges with the interosseous sacroiliac ligament as it crosses the joint.

3. The *ventral sacroiliac ligament* which bridges the margin of the joint anterior to the synovial portion of the joint.

4. The *sacrotuberous ligament* which passes from the lower third of the sacrum diagonally downward to the ischial tuberosity.

5. The *sacrospinous ligament* which passes from the lower third of the sacrum laterally to the *ischial spine.*

Note that the orientation of the sacrotuberous ligaments allows them to oppose the weight of the body on the anterosuperior end of the sacrum, preventing it from rotating the sacrum around the fulcrum of the sacroiliac articulation. Note also the keystone mechanism of the sacroiliac articulation. As the body weight wedges the sacrum more tightly between the coxal bones, the interosseous ligaments pull the coxal bones more tightly against the sacrum. These wedging forces and the levering forces of the sacrotuberous ligaments are chiefly responsible for the great stability of these weightbearing joints.

Pregnancy hormones impart an elasticity to these ligaments which allows for greater play at the sacroiliac joints. This increased elasticity also weakens the ligaments, however, making them more vulnerable to sprain. While sudden axial forces can sprain these ligaments in any individual, some pregnant women are likely to suffer sprains merely from the forces of normal ambulation.

The pubic *symphysis* is stabilized by a

fibrocartilagenous disc, the *interpubic disc,* and by two ligaments which merge into it, the *superior pubic ligament,* and the *arcuate pubic ligament.* While these ligaments and the interpubic disc are strong, the location of the hip joints adds a major contribution to the stability of the pubic symphysis. The weight of the body forces the pelvic ring onto the lower extremities at points on the ring where that force will tend to close the pubic symphysis. (See Figure 11-2.) Hence, the structure of the sacroiliac joints and the orientation of the hip joints cause balanced weightbearing so to strengthen the pelvic ring that it becomes as strong as its bony components.

Each coxal bone is composed of three parts: the pubis, the ischium, and the ilium. Each of these parts emerges from a separate center of ossification and all fuse into a single bone by early adolescence. Each ilium articulates with the sacrum, and each pubis articulates with its opposite pubis at

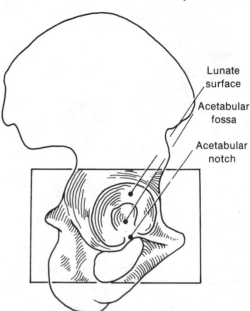

Fig. 11-3. Acetabulum.

the pubic symphysis. Each ischium forms a separate ring with each pubis, called the obturator foramen. Within the architecture of these ischiopubic rings, lies the strength of the anterior half of the pelvic ring. Each part participates in the formation of the acetabulum. The superior ramus of the pubis and the body of the ischium form its anterior and posterior walls, and the body of the ilium forms its superior wall. The posterior and superior walls are particularly prominent and substantial. Inferiorly, the anterior and posterior walls end before they meet, forming between them the *acetabular notch,* which merges with the superolateral border of the obturator foramen. The surface of the acetabulum is composed of two parts, an incomplete marginal ring of hyaline cartilage, the *lunate surface,* surrounding the central rough *acetabular fossa,* which merges with the acetabular notch as it breaks across the lunate surface inferiorly. (See Figure 11-3.)

Three cartilagenous epiphyses are clinically important: the iliac crest, the anteroinferior iliac spine, and the ischial tuberosity. They begin to ossify by midadolescence and do not fuse to the coxal bones until the mid- to late twenties. (See Figure 11-4.)

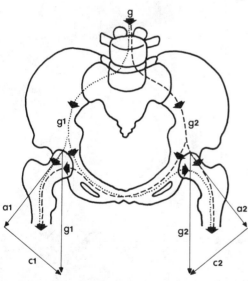

Fig. 11-2. Schematic representation of lines of force across the pubic symphysis as a consequence of the wedge effect created by the orientation of the pelvic-femoral articulations. Vector diagrams resolve the distribution of gravitational force (g) at each articulation ($g_1 = g_2 = \frac{1}{2}$ g) into two components, axial ($a_1 = a_2$) into each extremity, and compressive ($c_1 = c_2$) into the pubic symphysis. Compressive forces neutralize each other and thereby stabilize the pubic symphysis, and augment the axial component ($a_1 = a_2$) such that the total force distributed to each extremity = $g_1 = g_2 = \frac{1}{2}$ g during stable two-extremity stance.

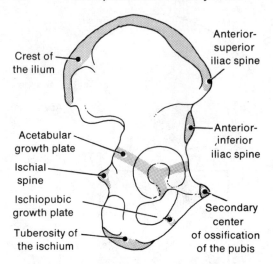

Fig. 11–4. Growth plates and secondary centers of ossification of the coxal bone.

The Walls of the Hip Joint and Upper End of the Femur

The walls of the acetabulum are deepened by a fibrocartilagenous extension called the *acetabular labrum*. The labrum terminates inferiorly with the termination of the anterior and posterior walls at the acetabular notch. The circle of the acetabular cup is completed by the *transverse acetabular ligament* which bridges the acetabular notch and blends with each end of the labrum. (See Figure 11–5.) The labrum and the transverse acetabular ligament extend beyond the hemisphere of the femoral head. Thus, they hold the femoral head in the acetabulum, much as the annular ligament holds the radial head in articulation with the capitulum of the humerus. The labrum must be ruptured before the femoral head can be dislocated out of the acetabulum.

The capsule of the hip joint extends from the margin of the labrum and the transverse acetabular ligament distally to attach to the femur as follows: superiorly—to the medial surface of the greater femoral trochanter; anteriorly—to the intertrochanteric line; inferiorly—to the base of the neck just superior to the lesser trochanter; posteriorly—to the neck of the femur at about the junction of its middle and distal thirds. The fibrous membrane of the capsule blends with the labrum and transverse acetabular ligaments proxi-

mally and with the periosteum of the femur distally. The synovial membrane of the capsule extends from the peripheral borders of the lunate surface and transverse acetabular ligament over the labrum to pass distally with the fibrous membrane to its femoral attachments, at which point it reflects back along the neck of the femur to attach to the peripheral border of the cartilage of the head of the femur. From the central border of the lunate surface and transverse acetabular ligament, it re-

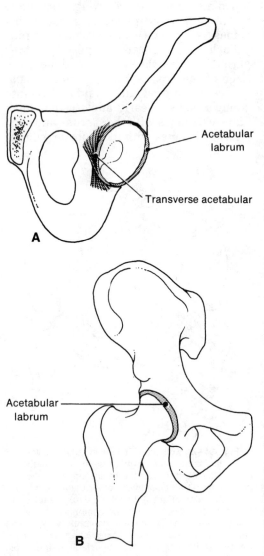

Fig. 11–5. Fibrocartilaginous rim of the acetabulum. *A,* the two structures of the rim. *B,* restraining apposition of the fibrocartilaginous rim to the femoral head.

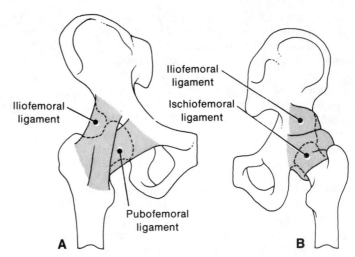

Fig. 11–6. Ligaments of the hip joint. *A,* anterior view. *B,* posterior view.

flects over the fibrovascular tissue of the acetabular fossa and notch along the *ligament of the head of the femur* to attach to the central border of the cartilage of the head of the femur, surrounding the rough *fovea* of the head of the femur. Arthrocentesis takes advantage of the broad extension of the capsule and synovial space along the anterior surface of the femoral neck.

The capsule of the hip joint is stabilized by four ligaments (see Figure 11–6):

1. The *zona orbicularis*—a circumferential ligament which thickens the fibrous membrane of the capsule near the base of the neck of the femur.

2. The *iliofemoral ligament*—a very strong ligament, consisting of two parts, which give it the shape of an inverted Y. It makes its broad proximal attachment to the anterior and posterior surfaces of the body of the ilium. Its posterior portion rotates medially as it reflects anteriorly over the anterior surface of the hip joint to attach to the anterior surface of the greater femoral trochanter, and its anterior portion extends directly distally to the intertrochanteric line. The anterior portion resists extension and the posterior portion resists internal rotation.

3. The *pubofemoral ligament*—a rectangular ligament which passes transversely from a broad proximal attachment to the body of the pubis, posterior to the iliofemoral ligament, to merge some of its fibers with the anterior limb of the iliofe-

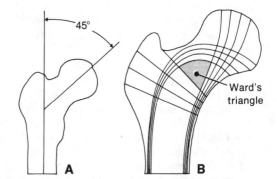

Fig. 11–7. Architecture of the upper end of the femur. *A,* neck of the femur angulates medial to the axis of the femoral shaft. *B,* trabecular architecture parallels the lines of tension and compression.

moral ligament, and to attach the remainder of its fibers to the inferior surface of the femoral neck. It resists abduction.

4. The *ischiofemoral ligament*—a broad ligament extending in three parts from the posterior surface of the body of the ischium across the posterior surface of the hip joint to the posterosuperior portion of the base of the neck, where it merges with the greater trochanter. It is a thin ligament which is ruptured by posterior dislocation of the hip.

The architecture of the femur presents five features which are of particular clinical importance:

1. The neck of the femur angulates about 45° medial to the axis of the shaft of the femur. (See Figure 11–7.) This angulation causes weight to apply shearing forces

to the neck of the femur which resolve into curving lines of tension and compression. The trabecular architecture of the upper end of the femur is correspondingly oriented to bear optimally those forces of tension and compression. This correspondence is a dramatic illustration of a fundamental law of bone architecture: form accommodates to meet force. (See Figure 11–7.) Strong, relatively straight trabeculae extending from the superior surface of the head of the femur to the thick cortical bone of the inferior border of the neck of the femur, and the medial surface of the shaft of the femur resist the forces of compression. Strong arcuate trabeculae extending from the inferior border of the head and neck of the femur to the thick cortical bone at the outer border of the femur resist the forces of tension. Somewhat weaker trabeculae extending from the inferior border of the neck of the femur to the greater trochanter resist weaker forces of compression and tension. Between these three trabecular groups lies a structurally weak cancellous zone called Ward's triangle.

2. *The lateral placement of the hip joints* necessitates that strong abducting forces apply to the upper end of the femur during single extremity weightbearing in order to maintain the erect posture. Thus, the abductors are subject to considerable wear and tear. (See Figure 11–8.)

3. The blood supply to the head of the femur is carried largely by arteries that pierce the capsule and run toward the head between the neck of the femur and the synovial membrane. An inconstant artery accompanies the ligament of the head of the femur into the fovea of the head. Thus, intracapsular fractures of the neck of the femur (the proximal two-thirds is entirely intracapsular) are likely to tear across the major blood supply and result in aseptic necrosis of the head of the femur. The fractures at the base of the neck, being largely extracapsular, are less likely to cause this complication.

4. *Two trochanters and one tuberosity* provide the surfaces for attachment of most of the muscles of the hip. The *greater femoral trochanter* forms the upper pole of the body of the femur and provides

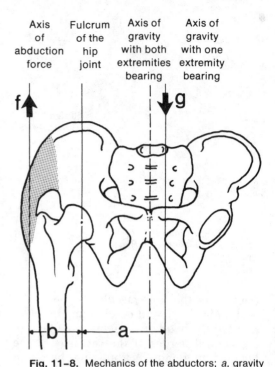

Fig. 11–8. Mechanics of the abductors; *a*, gravity moment arm, one extremity bearing; *b*, abduction moment arm of bearing extremity; *g*, force of gravity (weight); *f*, abduction force. (fb = ga, $f = g\frac{a}{b}$, f = g $\frac{3}{1}$ = 3g; if g = 150 pounds, f = 3 × 150 pounds = 450 pounds.)

attachment for most of the abductors and external rotators (gluteus medius and minimis, piriformis, and obturator internus and externus). The *lesser femoral trochanter* arises at the inferior angle of the body and neck of the femur and provides attachment for the strongest hip flexor, the iliopsoas. The two trochanters merge posteriorly as the *intertrochanteric crest*. On the posterior surface of the body of the femur, just distal from the greater trochanter, arises a low axial ridge called the *gluteal tuberosity,* to which attaches the gluteus maximus, the major extensor of the hip.

5. The head and trochanters of the femur develop as epiphyses which begin to ossify in childhood: the head of the femur (often called the capital femoral epiphysis) begins to ossify during the first year of life, the greater trochanter begins to ossify in preschool years, and the lesser trochanter

in early school years. All fuse with the metaphysis in adolescence, the capital epiphysis fusing last. Like any epiphysis, these are vulnerable to traumatic separation, but the capital femoral epiphysis is also vulnerable to slippage during average play. See later discussions in this chapter.

The Innervation of the Hip Joint

Branches of the lumbar and sacral plexuses innervate the hip joint. These are largely constituted by neurons from the 2nd through the 5th lumbar segments. Several of the branches originate from the obturator nerve. The fact that other branches from the obturator nerve innervate the anterior portion of the knee joint fits with the characteristics of pain referral from the hip: hip pathology often presents as anterior knee pain, and vice versa.

The Muscles Controlling the Hip Joint

Numerous short and long muscles control the hip joint. While many contribute to more than one movement, it is convenient to think of them as abductors, flexors, adductors, extensors, and rotators. For our purposes, a thus simplified summary of the complex material will be adequate.

1. The primary abductors are the *gluteus medius,* and *gluteus minimis.* (See Figure 11-9.) Both take origin from the wing

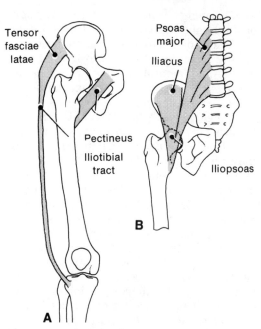

Fig. 11-10. Flexors of the hip. *A,* primary hip flexors during walking. *B,* strongest hip flexors.

of the ilium, and both insert upon the superior surface of the greater femoral trochanter. Both are innervated by the superior gluteal nerve which usually emerges from the sacral plexus proximal to the sciatic nerve. It is predominantly composed of fibers from the 4th to the 5th lumbar nerve roots. Painful foci will develop in these muscles and their attachments to the greater femoral trochanter, and these foci are the commonest cause of the abductor myofascial pain syndrome.

2. Anterior to the primary abductors is the *tensor fasciae latae muscle* which merges its tendinous fibers with the tendinous fibers of the gluteus maximus, to form the iliotibial tract down the lateral aspect of the thigh to its merger with the lateral patellar retinaculum of the knee. (See Figure 11-10 and 11-12.) It acts with the *pectineus* as a primary hip flexor during walking. The *pectineus* originates from the superior ramus of the pubis and inserts on the posterior surface of the back of the femur, just inferior to the base of the lesser trochanter. The tensor fasciae latae is innervated by the superior gluteal nerve. The pectineus is innervated by the femoral nerve and the obturator nerve, both of

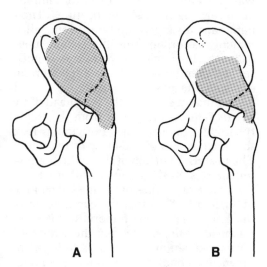

Fig. 11-9. Abductors. *A,* gluteus medius. *B,* gluteus minimus.

which emerge from the anterior division of the lumbar plexus. Those fibers which innervate the pectineus originate predominantly from the 2nd and 3rd lumbar segments. The femoral artery and vein lie on the pectineus muscle in the femoral triangle.

Though a weak hip flexor, the *rectus femoris* may contract strongly when kicking. Of its two ileal origins, its origin from the anteroinferior iliac spine is clinically important, as it may be avulsed by kicking movements during adolescence, when the spine is still an unfused epiphysis. (See Figure 11–26.)

The strongest flexor is the double-bellied muscle, the *iliopsoas,* the psoas portion of which originates from the bodies and transverse processes of the lumbar vertebrae, and the iliacus portion of which originates from the anterior surface of the wing of the ilium. Both portions merge to insert upon the lesser femoral trochanter. (See Figure 11–10.) Both portions are innervated by branches of the femoral nerve which are composed of fibers originating predominantly from the 2nd through the 4th lumbar segments. It is brought into action when flexion must be performed with particular forcefulness, as is necessary for kicking. It crosses the hip joint just lateral to the pectineus muscle. The femoral nerve lies upon it.

3. The primary adductors of the hip are the three adductor muscles, the longus, brevis and magnus, and the gracilis. Though they arise separately, it is enough to remember that the group arises in an arc from the anterior surface of the body of the pubis, through the lateral surface of the inferior ramus of the pubis and the contiguous ischial ramus, to the ischial tuberosity. The three adductors insert upon the linea aspera on the posterior surface of the shaft of the femur, and the gracilis inserts upon the tibia just distal to the medial condyle. The three adductors lie layered upon one another, the longus most anteriorly, the magnus most posteriorly, and the brevis in between. The gracilis lies medial to the three adductors, as the most medial muscle in the thigh. (See Figure 11–11.) They are all innervated by the obturator nerve. The most posterior portion of the adductor magnus is inner-

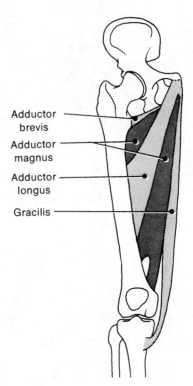

Fig. 11–11. Adductors of the hip (anterior view).

vated by the tibial portion of the sciatic nerve. Like the flexors, they are largely controlled by the 2nd through the 4th lumbar segments.

4. Like the flexors, the extensors of the hip are of two kinds, those employed for walking, and those employed for climbing or for arising from sitting postures. Those dominant during walking are four, all of which take origin from the ischial tuberosity: the long head of the biceps femoris, the semitendinosus, the semimembranosus, and the posterior portion of the adductor magnus. While the long head of the biceps femoris originates from the ischial tuberosity, the short head originates from the linea aspera of the body of the femur. The posterior portion of the adductor magnus inserts on the adductor tuberosity on the posterior surface of the medial condyle of the femur. The other three muscles cross the knee, the biceps femoris to insert on the head of the fibula, and the semitendinosus and semimembranosus to insert on the medial condlye of the tibia. (See Figure 11–12.) All these muscles are innervated by the sciatic nerve which is composed of

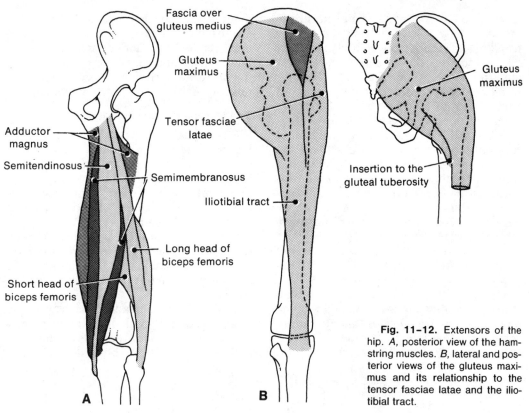

Adductor magnus

Semitendinosus

Fascia over gluteus medius

Gluteus maximus

Tensor fasciae latae

Semimembranosus

Iliotibial tract

Long head of biceps femoris

Short head of biceps femoris

Gluteus maximus

Insertion to the gluteal tuberosity

A

B

Fig. 11–12. Extensors of the hip. *A,* posterior view of the hamstring muscles. *B,* lateral and posterior views of the gluteus maximus and its relationship to the tensor fasciae latae and the iliotibial tract.

fibers originating from the 4th lumbar through the 3rd sacral spinal segments.

Those muscles brought into play for climbing and rising from sitting postures are the *gluteus maximus* and, again, the posterior portion of the *adductor magnus.* Because they also flex the knee, the biceps femoris, semitendinosus, and semimembranosus can hardly dominate such actions. The gluteus maximus arises from the wing of the ilium, the sacroiliac joint, and the sacrum, and inserts largely into the iliotibial tract. A lesser deep portion inserts upon the gluteal tuberosity of the body of the femur. See Figure 11–12. The gluteus maximus is innervated by the inferior gluteal nerve, which emerges from the anterior division of the sacral plexus or from the sciatic nerve itself. It is predominantly composed of fibers from the 5th lumbar and 1st sacral spinal segments.

5. In the depths of the buttocks, extending across the posterior surface of the hip joint are the short or pure external rotators of the hip: *within the pelvis,* the *piriformis*

originates from the anterolateral surface of the sacrum, emerges through the greater sciatic notch, and passes laterally and downward to insert on the medial surface of the greater femoral trochanter; the *obturator internus* originates from the inner surface of the obturator membrane, emerges through the lesser sciatic notch, angulates sharply over that border of the ischium, and passes laterally and upward to insert on the medial aspect of the greater femoral trochanter. *Outside the pelvis,* the *obturator externus* originates from the outer surface of the obturator membrane and passes upward and laterally to insert upon the medial surface of the greater femoral trochanter; the two *gemelli* originate from the ischium to either side of the lesser sciatic notch, the superior from the ischial spine, and the inferior from the ischial tuberosity, to pass laterally with the obturator internus and merge with its tendon; the *quadratus femoris* originates from the ischial tuberosity and passes laterally to insert on the intertrochanteric crest. (See Figure 11-13.) The piriformis is innervated by a branch from the middle trunk of the anterior division of the sacral plexus, composed of fibers from the 1st and 2nd sacral spinal segments. The obturator externus is innervated by branches from the obturator nerve which emerge from the lumbar plexus, composed of fibers from the 3rd and 4th lumbar spinal segments. The remainder of the short external rotators are innervated by branches from the sacral plexus, one of which innervates the obturator internus and superior gemellus, and the other of which innervates the inferior gemellus and quadratus femoris.

The pectineus and iliopsoas muscles externally rotate the hip, while they flex the hip.

There are no pure internal rotators. Among the abductors, flexors, adductors, and extensors are muscles that also apply some force that internally rotates: the gluteus minimus internally rotates while ab-ducting, the tensor fasciae latae internally rotates while flexing, the gracillis internally rotates while adducting, and the semitendinosus and semimembranosus, and the posterior portion of the adductor magnus internally rotate while extending.

The Bursae of the Hip Joint

Five bursae are of clinical interest: (See Figure 11-14.)

1. The psoas or iliopectineal bursa lies between the iliopsoas muscle and the anterior surface of the hip joint. Occasionally, it communicates with the synovial space of the hip joint.

2. The trochanteric bursa lies between the skin and the broad superficial tendon of the gluteus maximus as it merges with the iliotibial tract over the greater femoral trochanter.

3. The gluteal bursa lies posterior to the greater femoral trochanter, between the superficial tendon of the gluteus maximus and the greater femoral trochanter.

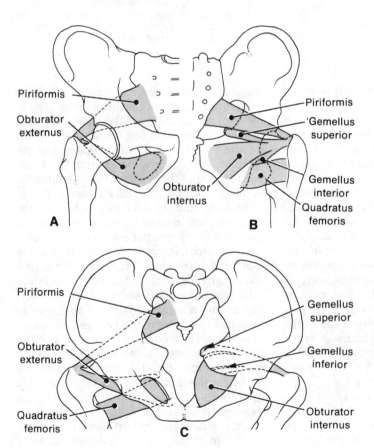

Fig. 11-13. Pure external rotators. *A*, anterior view. *B*, posterior view. *C*, superior view.

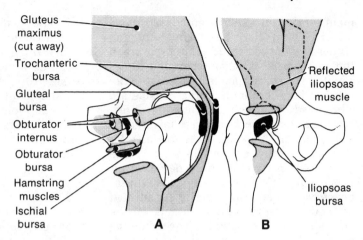

Gluteus maximus (cut away)

Trochanteric bursa

Gluteal bursa

Obturator internus

Obturator bursa

Hamstring muscles

Ischial bursa

Reflected iliopsoas muscle

Iliopsoas bursa

A   **B**

Fig. 11-14. Bursae about the hip joint. *A*, posterior view. *B*, anterior view.

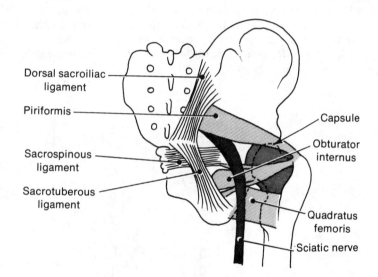

Dorsal sacroiliac ligament

Piriformis

Sacrospinous ligament

Sacrotuberous ligament

Capsule

Obturator internus

Quadratus femoris

Sciatic nerve

Fig. 11-15. Relationship of the sciatic nerve to the posterior aspect of the hip joint and the external rotators.

4. The *ischial bursa* lies over the origin of the hamstring muscles from the ischial tuberosity.

5. The bursa of the *obturator internus* lies between the tendon of that muscle and the margin of the ischium over which it turns as it emerges from the pelvis through the lesser sciatic foramen.

The Relationship of the Hip Joint to the Great Vessels and Nerves of the Lower Extremity

The sciatic nerve emerges from the sacral plexus through the greater sciatic notch, between the piriformis and the obturator internus. In the sciatic notch, it is vulnerable to a crushing injury by a pos-

teriorly dislocated femoral head. (See Figure 11-15.)

The femoral artery, vein, and nerve enter the thigh over the iliopsoas and pectineus muscles. In this free anterior position, cushioned by the iliopsoas and pectineus muscles, they are not likely to be injured by hip displacements.

Non-Traumatic Afflictions of the Hip Joint

General Clinical Characteristics

By definition, *afflictions of the joint* eventually inflame the joint capsule and its synovial lining, and the resultant synovitis produces a joint effusion. The ligaments of the hip are so oriented (see above under "The Walls of the Hip Joint and Upper End of the Femur") that pressure in the joint space is least when the hip is slightly flexed, adducted, and externally rotated. Pain terminals in the capsule are stimulated by stretch and thus joint pressure, and their threshholds are lowered by inflammation. As pointed out above under "The Innervation of the Hip Joint," some of the neurons which these nerve terminals excite constitute a part of the obturator nerve, which also is partly constituted by neurons from pain terminals in the anterior aspect of the knee. The following general clinical characteristics of hip joint afflictions derive from these anatomic and pathologic facts. During the course of a particular affliction, they emerge in the following order (see Figure 11–16):

1. The pain pattern. The pain of hip joint affliction is felt in the groin, anteromedial thigh, and the knee.

2. The effect of movement. Pain is intensified by, and thus eventually restricts abduction, internal rotation, and extension of the hip joint. Slight restriction of internal rotation may be the earliest sign of hip joint pathology. The range of internal rotation is most reliably tested with the patient lying prone and the knee flexed to 90°.

3. The posture of the joint. Flexor spasm is the reflex response to hip joint pain. In time, this reflex posture becomes uncorrectable as muscles and ligaments on the flexor aspect of the joint shorten. The flexion posture may be masked by a compensating lumbosacral lordosis. If this compensating lordosis is ablated by full flexion

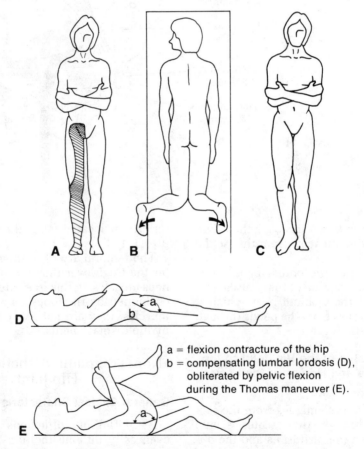

a = flexion contracture of the hip
b = compensating lumbar lordosis (D), obliterated by pelvic flexion during the Thomas maneuver (E).

Fig. 11–16. Characteristics of hip joint pain. *A,* location of the pain: Initial location over the groin and/or anterior aspect of the knee; referral of pain along the anterior aspect of the thigh, and eventually into the leg as well. *B,* painful manipulation. *C,* posture of the joint. *D* and *E,* Thomas maneuver.

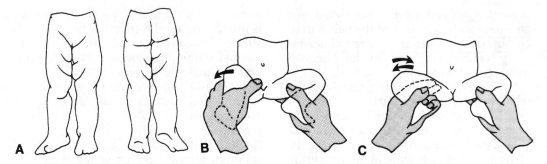

Fig. 11-17. Physical characteristics of congenital hip dislocation (the right hip is dislocated). *A*, asymmetry of skin folds characteristic of congenital hip dislocation: anterior and posterior views. *B* and *C*, manipulation: with the hip flexed to 90°, range of abduction may be restricted (*B*), or recurrent dislocation and relocation may be produced by alternate abduction and adduction (*C*). This movement in and out of the joint will be detected as a click, readily palpable over the outer aspect of the hip.

of the opposite hip across the abdomen (the Thomas maneuver), the flexion contracture of the afflicted hip will be revealed.

While those characteristics emerge universally among adults and children who suffer hip joint afflictions, other unique characteristics herald some of the hip joint afflictions of children. These unique characteristics will be described in context. The particular hip joint afflictions, their diagnosis and treatment are described in order, from birth to old age.

Congenital Dislocation of the Hip

Congenital hip dislocation is the most common affliction of the hip joint to present during the first 3 years of life. Girls are more likely to be afflicted than boys. The development of the acetabulum and the head of the femur appear to be interdependent. Any circumstance that changes their anatomic relationship, subluxates the hip and will change the development of the two structures. How the subluxation occurs in the first place continues to be debated. Two disparate postulates define the debate:

1. The femoral head is subluxated by some force during intrauterine development;

2. The development of the joint is polygenically determined to yield a joint capsule, acetabular labrum, and transverse acetabular ligament that are so lax as to be incapable of retaining the developing head in the acetabulum, while yielding an ilio-

psoas muscle that is so taut as to block the return of the subluxated head to the acetabulum.

However the subluxation occurs, the resultant abnormal ("dysplastic") bony structures and their lax supports fail to form a stable joint. Uncorrected, a permanent dislocation will result. At any point in this abnormal developmental process, the adductors may or may not shorten.

Infants born with the acetabular and capital femoral dysplasias may or may not demonstrate dislocation at birth, but the majority will dislocate by 3 months of age. Whether the predislocation phase can be identified remains debated. Once the dislocation occurs, one or more of the following signs are manifest (see Figure 11-17):

1. The infant may not move the affected extremity as much as the normal extremity.

2. The affected extremity may appear short in comparison to the normal.

3. The affected extremity may be externally rotated as compared to the normal.

4. The gluteal, inguinal, and knee folds may be bilaterally asymmetrical.

5. Since the adductors may or may not shorten, abduction to the frog-leg position may or may not be restricted.

6. During alternate abduction and adduction of both hips with the hips flexed to 90°, the head of the femur of the dysplastic joint may repeatedly slip in and out of the acetabulum. This movement of the abnormal hip may be perceived as a palpable or audible click.

When one or more of these signs are

evident, dysplasia must be suspected, and an anteroposterior x-ray of the pelvis must be obtained. Evidence of three abnormal x-ray features will confirm the diagnosis (see Figure 11–18):

1. The curve of the inner margin of the femoral neck and the curve of the inner margin of the obturator foramen normally lie in the same arc, called Shenton's line. When the femur is displaced out of articulation with the acetabulum, the curves may no longer lie on the same arc.

2. When the femur is laterally luxated, its malposition is obvious when related to a vertical line dropped from the superior lip of the acetabulum perpendicular to a line drawn through the center of both acetabula. This vertical line is called Perkin's line. The beak of the neck of the normally articulating femur lies well medial to this line, while the beak of the neck of the luxated femur lies closer to, or lateral to this line.

3. When an acetabulum is dysplastic, the slope of its superior margin, *the acetabular angle,* will be increased. The normal acetabular angle decreases with age from an upper limit at birth of about 40° to an upper limit at 2 years of age of less than 30°. Radiologists and orthopedists refer to chronologic tables before judging the normality of an acetabular angle.

Treatment. We recommend that the

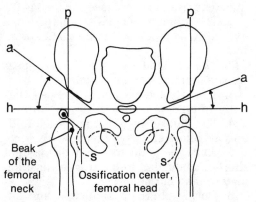

Fig. 11–18. X-ray characteristics of congenital hip dislocation. (1) The arc of Shenton's line (*s*) is discontinuous on the dislocated side. (2) The beak of the femoral neck and the ossification center of the femoral head (if present) are displaced laterally and upward toward or beyond Perkin's line (*p*), and Hilgenreiner's line (*h*). (3) The angle between the acetabular line (*a*) and Hilgenreiner's line (*h*) is increased.

congenital dislocations be treated by an orthopaedist as the therapeutic choice is subtle. Closed reduction is usually accomplished without anesthesia. Occasionally, open reduction is necessary. The reduction is maintained by restraining the hip in a posture that seats the head of the femur well against the acetabulum. Classically, the hip was immobilized in plaster at 90° flexion, full abduction and full external rotation. Of very recent years, it has become increasingly apparent that this position places a stress upon the pericapsular arteries to the hip joint which too often has led to their occlusion and a consequent avascular necrosis of the head of the femur. At present, therapeutic opinion remains in flux and a variety of positions are chosen, all of which avoid strain on the capsule. We currently immobilize the hip at 90° flexion, 20° less than full abduction, and in neutral rotation which places the heel of the foot within or just lateral to a sagittal plane through the hip joint. When the reduction holds throughout a fairly wide range of motion, we immobilize with a soft splint like a bulky diaper. When the reduction is lost within a narrow range of motion, we immobilize in a rigid splint or plaster. The chosen posture is held until the acetabular angle becomes normal and the acetabular lip is forming well.

Pyogenic Arthritis of the Hip

Pyogenic infection is the second most common affliction of the hip joint during the first 3 years of life. The infecting organism is usually one of four: *Staphylococcus, Streptococcus, Pneumococcus,* and *Hemophilus influenzae.* Untreated infections, if they do not lead to a fatal septisemia, will destroy the hip joint.

Characteristic Clinical Features are the Following:

1. The onset is rapid, a full-blown syndrome usually developing over 24 hours.

2. The child is febrile, usually appears acutely ill, even prostrate, or delirious.

3. The erythrocyte sedimentation rate is rapid, and the leukocyte count is elevated.

4. The afflicted hip is flexed to nearly 90°, and the infant resists all efforts to move the hip in any direction away from this position.

5. Early in the course of illness, x-rays show nothing but the soft tissue outline of an externally rotated hip, classically referred to as "soft tissue swelling."

This disease is a justification for a classic principle of pediatric diagnosis: orthopaedic infection must be intentionally considered when seeking the cause of fever of hidden origin. Note the objective subtlety of this disease. The child may present simply as an acutely ill febrile child who resists or cries when moved. The flexor spasm of the hip will be the only clue pointing to this disease, among all the possible causes for fever of hidden origin. When such a clue suggests the disease, the hip must be aspirated. Recovery of pus confirms the diagnosis.

Treatment. The disease is an emergency and must be treated without procrastination.

1. Any material obtained from the joint must be submitted immediately for Gram stain, culture, and determination of sensitivity.

2. As soon as the joint has been aspirated and pus sent for culture, intravenous antibiotics should be started. We recommend ampicillin 200 mg./kg./24 hours, and dicloxacillin 25 mg./kg./24 hours be given in four divided doses 6 hours apart. Each dose should be given over 15 minutes within 1 hour of its reconstitution. These antibiotics should be maintained until the course of illness and the report of sensitivities dictate a change. Appropriate antibiotics should be continued for at least 2 weeks. When remission is brisk, the oral route may be used during the 2nd week.

3. An orthopaedist must be consulted on the day of admission, as surgical drainage is often indicated.

Non-Specific or Transient Synovitis

This self-limited synovitis of non-specific form is most prevalent among children between 3 and 5 years of age. Etiology is unknown, but unrecognized injuries and viral infections have been postulated. It must be differentiated from pyogenic arthritis and Perthes' disease. When suspicion of pyogenic arthritis remains, the joint must be aspirated. The distinction from Perthes' disease is ultimately made by x-ray. The children are followed closely as a normal x-ray at the first visit does not rule out Perthes' disease.

Characteristic Clinical Features are the Following:

1. The onset of the illness is not so dramatic as pyogenic arthritis, but usually not so insidious as Perthes' disease. The child is usually brought to the physician after 1–2 weeks of limping and complaint of pain.

2. An articulate child will complain of pain in the groin, anterior aspect of the thigh, and sometimes the knee.

3. A low-grade fever, a slight leukocytosis, and a moderate increase in erythrocyte sedimentation rate may be evident.

4. The affected hip is usually flexed, and the child will resist efforts to move the hip rapidly or to move it to extremes of internal rotation, abduction, and extension.

5. X-rays show nothing but the soft tissue outline of an externally rotated hip.

Treatment.

1. Anteroposterior x-rays of the pelvis and lateral x-rays of both hips must be obtained. If the characteristics of Perthes' disease are not evident, rest is advised, and any necessary ambulation should be non-weightbearing, with crutches.

2. Aspirin is given by mouth 65 mg./kg./24 hours in four divided doses.

3. Full weightbearing ambulation is tried when full range of motion is painless. If ambulation is painless, the child is allowed to resume normal activity.

4. Parents are instructed to bring the child back to clinic in 2 months, or sooner should pain return.

5. X-rays of the hip are repeated when the child returns after the 2-month interval. If x-rays are normal at this time, range of motion full and painless, and weightbearing painless, the diagnosis of non-specific synovitis is confirmed, and the child is discharged.

Perthes' Disease

Children between 3 and 10 years of age may suffer an obliteration of the blood supply to the head of one femur. Consequently, the head of the femur undergoes an avascular necrosis. What leads to the obliteration of the blood supply is not known, though recent evidence suggests that increased intracapsular pressure of the effusion of a traumatic or non-specific synovitis may be the initiating process. Eventually, granulation tissue grows into the necrosed head, absorbs the dead bone, and replaces it with new viable bone. The entire process of necrosis and reconstruction takes 2 to 2 ½ years. The ultimate shape of the new femoral head will reflect the extent of disease, the remodeling capacity of the hip, and the treatment during the *reconstructive phase.*

Characteristic Clinical Features are the Following:

1. The disease may afflict children between 3 and 10 years of age, but greatest incidence occurs in children between 5 and 10 years of age.

2. The onset is insidious. Medical advice may not be sought until 6–8 months beyond the first emergence of symptoms.

3. The afflicted child will be noted to limp intermittently. Limping will be most evident after exertion and least evident after rest.

4. The articulate child will complain of pain in the groin, the anterior aspect of the thigh, and sometimes the knee.

5. Some degree of flexor spasm or even contracture will be evident, and the child will resist all efforts to move the hip to full abduction, internal rotation, and extension.

6. Two or more months after onset of symptoms, anteroposterior x-rays of the pelvis and lateral x-rays of both hips will show increased density of the affected head, and eventually a mottled distortion of the head.

Treatment. Current treatment is based upon a fairly recent clarification of the factors that play a part in the molding of the head of the femur. It appears that the contour of the reconstructed femoral head will most closely approach the normal if the head has been kept well centered in the acetabulum throughout the reconstructive process. The femoral head is best centered when the hip is abducted and internally rotated. A number of braces have been designed to accomplish this end. Occasionally, complete coverage of the femoral head cannot be obtained by position alone. Surgical procedures to improve coverage have recently been proposed: Various osteotomies of the femur and the Salter osteotomy of the acetabulum.

The primary practitioner must make the diagnosis and, as soon as the diagnosis is made, must refer the patient to an orthopaedist. Non-specific synovitis and early Perthes' can be indistinguishable. When the distinction is obscure, the primary practitioner must treat for non-specific synovitis and follow the child until the course of the illness and the appearance of repeated x-rays confirm one or the other. Since the outcome of Perthes' disease seems to depend predominantly upon events in the reconstructive phase, absolute non-weightbearing in the early necrotic phase is probably not so essential as has been classically presumed. Hence, the fairly liberal treatment protocol outlined for non-specific synovitis is acceptable until the diagnosis becomes clear.

Slipped Femoral Epiphysis

Perhaps as the consequence of an unknown disorder of the epiphyseal plate, some children between 10 and 14 years of age may sustain a slippage of the capital femoral epiphysis posteriorly and inferiorly. While the disease has seemed to be most prevalent among extremely obese children, or unusually tall, lean children who have experienced a rapid acceleration of growth, these correlations are not absolute. The etiology remains unknown, but some observers continue to suspect an unproved pituitary dysfunction. The condition usually becomes abruptly symptomatic during violent exertion, but it may emerge insidiously.

Characteristic Clinical Features are the Following:

1. A child is brought to clinic after suffering the abrupt onset of pain during violent exertion, or after several days of limping.

2. Pain is classically felt in the knee and the thigh, and not in the hip. Indeed, in a busy practice, the knee may be examined, the hip ignored, and the diagnosis missed.

3. Flexor spasm may or may not be evident.

4. Internal rotation is nearly impossible.

The extremity tends to lie in external rotation, and the child often walks with the foot turned outward.

5. With the child supine, as the hip is flexed, it will tend to rotate externally, until the knee points outside the line of the body. In the normal person, as the hip is flexed, it will remain in neutral rotation, and the knee will point toward the chest.

6. Anteroposterior x-rays of the pelvis, and frog-leg lateral x-rays of each hip will by comparison usually demonstrate the slippage. When these views do not demonstrate a suspected slippage, the technically more difficult true lateral view must be taken. If a line is drawn on either lateral projection along the superior margin of the neck, through the head of the femur, about one-third of the sphere of the femoral head will usually lie above the line. When less of the sphere of the suspected hip than of the normal hip lies above the line, early slippage can be presumed. (See Figure 11-19.)

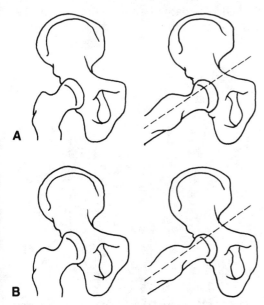

Fig. 11-19. X-ray evidence of slipped femoral epiphysis. *A*, anteroposterior and frog-leg lateral views of normal hip. (The frog-leg lateral view shows one-third or more of the sphere of the epiphysis to lie above a line tangent to the superior margin of the femoral neck.) B, anteroposterior and frog-leg lateral views of the hip showing early epiphyseal slippage. (Anteroposterior view may show little change from normal. Frog-leg lateral view may show less than one-third of the sphere of the epiphysis to lie above a line tangent to the superior margin of the femoral neck.)

Treatment. Treatment is surgical. A slipped epiphysis is fixed with pins. To achieve a satisfactory outcome, it is critical that the diagnosis be made before the epiphysis has slipped too far. A primary practitioner must make the diagnosis. Once the diagnosis is made, the child must be put to bed, instructed to ambulate only when necessary for self-care, and then non-weightbearing with crutches, and must be referred promptly to an orthopaedist.

Degenerative Arthritis

A general review of degenerative arthritis will be found in Chapter 18. As outlined in that chapter, degenerative arthritis emerges when a joint is subject to sufficient wear. Sufficient wear for one individual is different from that for another, and similar intensity of usage can lead to one degree of wear in one joint, and to another degree in another. The hip joint is one of the joints most likely to wear from usage. This vulnerability derives from its anatomy. The lateral placement of the hip relative to the central axis of the body causes the hip to act as a fulcrum between the weight of the body and the force of the abductor muscles. As that fulcrum, it bears a force four times the weight of the body. (See Figure 11-20.) Pain terminals in worn cartilage and reactive bone cause pain on weightbearing, and pain terminals in the fibrous and synovial membranes of the joint capsule cause pain with motion and pain at rest. The variation in degree of pain at rest and the degree of limitation of range of motion probably reflect varying degrees of synovitis. Synovitis flares in response to increased cartilage wear or capsular strain. Increased pain at rest may reflect the increased congestion of motionless inflamed fibrous and synovial membranes.

Characteristic Clinical Features are the Following:

1. An older adult complains of pain in the groin, anterior thigh, and sometimes the knee, which becomes more severe during and after prolonged weightbearing and during prolonged rest. These patients are often kept awake by the pain and become fatigued and irritable.

2. These patients may limp in a characteristic fashion which leans the body out

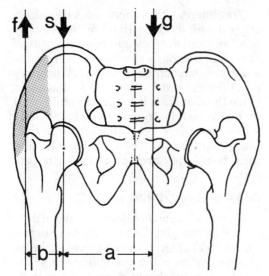

Fig. 11–20. Calculation of force (s) acting on the hip joint during normal gait; a, gravity moment arm, one extremity bearing; b, abduction moment arm of bearing extremity; g, force of gravity (weight); f, abduction force. (fb = ga, $f = g\dfrac{a}{b}$, $f = g\dfrac{3}{1}$ = 3g; if g = 150 pounds, f = 3 × 150 pounds, f = 450 pounds; s = g + f = g + 3 g = 4g, s = 600 pounds.)

over the side of the affected hip. This gait shortens the central moment arm, thereby decreasing the total force on the hip joint. (See Figure 11–21.)

3. Flexor spasm becomes evident within the 1st year of symptoms and increases in degree and becomes frank contracture as the condition persists. Flexor spasm will be manifest by the Thomas maneuver described earlier in this chapter.

4. Efforts to abduct, extend, or internally rotate the hip provoke pain.

5. An anteroposterior x-ray of the pelvis will demonstrate varying degrees of the following destructive changes: narrowing of the joint space—indicative of thinning of the cartilage; irregularity of and cystic and sclerotic changes in the head of the femur and/or acetabulum, and osteophytes at the cartilage margins—all indicative of the reaction of bone to cartilage loss.

Treatment. Physical Therapy. The actively adaptive individual can earn comfort and a delay in the degenerative process by careful compliance with the following physical therapy protocol:

Rest. Progressive wear can be slowed,

and episodes of reactive synovitis can be avoided by decreasing the forces on the hip. The patient must walk less and must use a cane when walking, and heavy patients must lose weight. A cane is used on the side opposite to the affected hip. The proper length of the cane is about 1″ longer than would reach the ground if held in weightbearing grip with the elbow fully extended. Use of the cane on the side opposite to the affected hip decreases the weight which acts on the central moment arm, thus decreasing the total force on the hip, while at the same time allowing an upright gait. Use of the cane on the affected side would decrease the forces on the hip only if the patient leaned out laterally beyond the hip at the same time—a clumsy gait, excessively wearing to the low back as well.

Exercise.

1. Any protective gait, whether with a cane or by leaning out over the hip, will spare the abductor muscles and thus weaken them. Weak abductors will strain and add the pain of abduction strain to the pain of the joint degeneration. To avoid

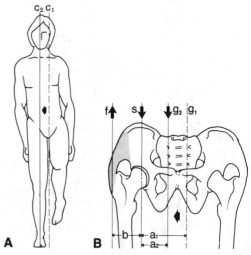

Fig. 11–21. Force (s) acting on a hip joint during leaning gait. *A*, illustrates shift in center of gravity during single extremity weightbearing when the individual leans toward the bearing side. c_1, axis of gravity during erect single extremity stance; c_2, axis of gravity during leaning single extremity stance. *B*, calculation of the force (s); a_1, gravity moment arm, one extremity bearing, erect posture; a_2, gravity moment arm, one extremity bearing, trunk leaning to the bearing side. (fb = g_2 a_2, b = a_2, f = g_2; if g_2 = 150 pounds, f = 150 pounds; s = f + g_2, s = 300 pounds.)

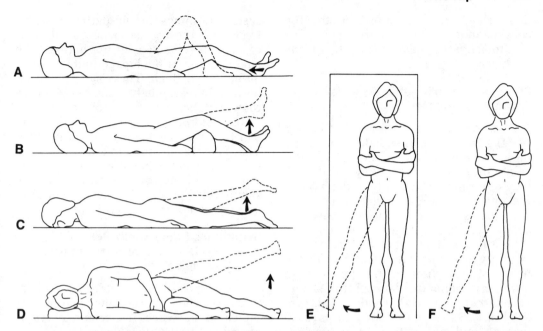

Fig. 11-22. Range of motion and strengthening exercises for the hip. *A,* sliding flexion while supine. (Important during convalescence from hip fractures or surgery.) *B,* quadriceps strengthening. (Important following any period of decreased weightbearing.) *C,* extension against gravity. *D,* abduction against gravity while lying. (Most advanced abduction exercise as it opposes greatest resistance.) *E,* abduction while supine. (Most elementary abduction exercises as it opposes least resistance.) *F,* abduction against gravity while standing. (Intermediate abduction exercise.) (*C–F* are all important during convalescence from all hip disorders.)

this added distress, abduction-strengthening exercises are performed daily. (See Figure 11-22.)

2. Reactive inflammation of the fibrous and synovial membranes of the capsule cause the patient to seek those positions which minimize all stretch upon the hip capsule. Unless this tendency is combatted, the capsule and its ligamentous thickening will shorten, and the range of painless motion will decrease even further. Thus, reversible spasm, and perhaps capsule congestion will become joint contracture. To avoid this further painful restriction, range of motion exercise in abduction and extension is performed daily. (See Figure 11-22.) We advise patients to be instructed in these exercises by a physical therapist.

3. Swimming and bicycling are excellent general conditioning activities which do not add to the wear on the hip joint. Heavy patients in particular should engage in one of those activities, as well as change their diet.

Heat. The analgesic effect of heat de-

creases reactive muscle spasm and thus increases range of motion, which decreases the patient's pain. Moist heat or dry heat over a counterirritant, like methyl salicylate, is most effective. We advise that heat be used prior to each exercise period, and whenever else the patient desires.

Anti-inflammatory Medication. Intra-articular corticosteroids can afford dramatic relief from the pain of a reactive synovitis. However, it must not be used more than three times per year.

Oral medications (aspirin, phenylbutazone, indomethacin, Motrin, and corticosteroids) may also afford relief from exacerbating synovitis. Chapter 18 reviews the use of these medications. Strict compliance with the physical therapy protocol will somewhat protect the patient from reactive synovitis and thus decrease the need for anti-inflammatory drugs.

Surgical Treatment. Inevitably, degeneration will continue, and eventually some patients will not benefit sufficiently from physical therapy and anti-inflammatory medication. These, the primary practitioner should refer to an orthopaedist for consideration of surgical treatment. Today, total hip replacement is the treatment of choice.

Cryptogenic Proliferative Synovial Disorders of the Hip

These diseases are reviewed in Chapter 18. Distinct from rheumatoid arthritis, these all tend to be monoarticular diseases. While they can affect any synovial joint, they occur most commonly in the hip and the knee. Any refractory hip joint pain may represent one of those diseases. A young person presenting with monoarticular arthritis of a joint and no memory of an injury to that joint may well be afflicted by one of these diseases. Any patient with refractory monoarticular arthritis should be referred to an orthopaedist. The synovial diseases respond poorly to physical therapy and anti-inflammatory medication, and a surgical synovectomy is often required.

Infections of the Hip

Adults rarely contract pyogenic arthritis of the hip. Infants are fairly likely to do so. Their affliction is discussed above under "Pyogenic Arthritis of the Hip."

Chronic infection, such as tuberculosis, can occur in the hip joint, even in highly urbanized countries. It presents with all the systemic symptoms of tuberculosis, with the typical hip joint pain syndrome, and sometimes with surrounding subcutaneous abscesses and draining sinuses. X-rays show destructive changes in the head of the femur and/or the acetabulum.

Patients afflicted by infections of the hip must be referred to an orthopaedist promptly.

Periarticular Myofascial Pain Syndromes

All of these syndromes are most prevalent among those of middle age and older. They all may appear abruptly or insidiously, may be immobilizing, or only disturbing, and will refer into the thigh. The most severe and persistent pains will refer into the leg as well. The pain of all these syndromes tends to be a steady ache, most disquieting during sleeping hours, and oc-

casionally intensified by particular activity. Four of the myofascial pain syndromes of the hip refer pain to the buttock, the lateral aspect of the hip, and into the posterior lateral thigh. These syndromes superficially resemble L_4–L_5 and L_5–S_1 nerve root irritations and sacroiliac sprains. Three syndromes refer pain into the groin and the anteromedial aspect of the thigh. They superficially resemble arthritis of the hip joint. The treatment is essentially the same for all the syndromes, and will be summarized in a unified subsection after a discussion of the various syndromes.

Syndromes Superficially Resembling L_4–L_5 and L_5–S_1 Nerve Root Irritation and Sacroiliac Sprain

The pain of all these syndromes will *not* intensify when the sacroiliac joint is manipulated or when the sciatic nerve is placed on stretch. (See Figure 11–23.)

Trochanteric Bursitis. This disorder may be the most common of the pain syndromes of the hip. Pain is felt over the lateral aspect of the hip and thigh. Tenderness is usually well localized over the lateral aspect of the greater femoral trochanter. Visible evidence of inflammation appears very rarely. Occasionally, the pain can inhibit walking; more often, it will inhibit abduction against resistance. Extreme passive flexion and adduction can intensify the pain.

Myotendinous Pain Syndrome of the Buttock and Lateral Thigh. Though this

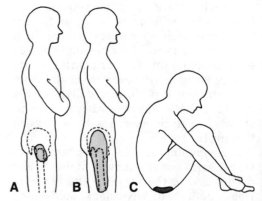

Fig. 11–23. Myofascial pain syndrome superficially resembling S_5 and S_1 nerve root irritation or sacroiliac sprain—zones of tenderness. *A,* trochanteric and gluteal bursitis. *B,* myotendinous pain syndrome of buttock and lateral thigh. *C,* ischial bursitis.

disorder is about as common in our experience as trochanteric bursitis, it is not designated in the standard nomenclature. It represents the cryptogenic myofascial pain process within the tensor fasciae latae, the gluteus medius and minimus, or the iliotibial tract. The distribution and persistence of pain and the response of pain to certain activities are identical to those characteristic of trochanteric bursitis. The distinction from trochanteric bursitis is made only by palpation. Unless the bursa is also involved, tenderness is not evident over the lateral aspect of the greater femoral trochanter. The point of tenderness will be found over any of the three muscles, over the superior pole of the greater trochanter where the gluteus medius and minimus insert, over the tendons of the tensor fasciae latae or gluteus maximus near their merger in the iliotibial tract, or more distally in the upper or middle third of the iliotibial tract itself. The distinction from trochanteric bursitis is important when a local injection of corticosteroid is intended. If such an injection is to be of any benefit, it, of course, must be made precisely into the site of tenderness.

Gluteal Bursitis. This disorder is encountered less often than is trochanteric bursitis. Pain is felt in the buttock and down the posterior aspect of the thigh. Tenderness is evident deeply along the posterior border of the greater femoral trochanter. Full passive flexion and adduction may intensify the pain. Walking, particularly climbing and rising from the sitting position, may intensify the pain.

Ischial Bursitis. This disorder is encountered less often than is trochanteric bursitis. Pain is felt in the buttock and down the posterior aspect of the thigh. Tenderness is usually well localized over the ischial tuberosity. The patient will usually complain that it hurts to sit on the affected side. Rarely, a cystic swelling will be palpable, and rarely inflammation will be visibly evident.

Syndromes Superficially Resembling Arthritis of the Hip Joint

These syndromes can be distinguished from arthritis of the hip only by careful physical examination of hip range of motion, and of the myofascial structures that

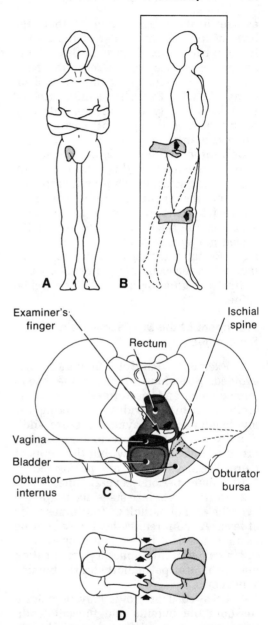

Fig. 11-24. Myofascial pain syndromes superficially resembling arthritis of the hip joint—zones of tenderness and painful manipulations. *A* and *B*, psoas bursitis. *A*, zone of tenderness; *B*, manipulation. *C* and *D*, obturator bursitis. *C*, zone of tenderness by rectal exam (superior view of the pelvis); *D*, manipulation.

can mimic hip pain. (See Figure 11-24.)

Psoas Bursitis. This disorder presents less often than trochanteric bursitis, but more often than gluteal and ischial bursitis. The pain is felt in the groin and down the anterior aspect of the thigh. Walking is invariably inhibited. Tenderness will be evident in the anterior thigh at about the level of the inferior border of the greater femoral trochanter. Efforts to flex the hip against resistance will increase the pain, and passive extension of the hip will increase the pain. Extension can be affected with the patient lying on the opposite side, or by having the patient perform the Thomas maneuver.

Obturator Bursitis. Some physicians deny the existence of this syndrome. Others strongly affirm it. Those who affirm it describe the syndrome quite precisely. Pain is felt in the groin and down the inner aspect of the thigh. Efforts to abduct the flexed hip against resistance increase the pain. Rectal examination reproduces the pain when the examining finger is pressed against the anterior border of the ischial spine.

Treatment of the Myofascial Pain Syndromes

1. Exercise. Painful activities are avoided. Stretching exercises are begun immediately and performed within the limits of pain. Individuals suffering the myotendinous pain syndromes are additionally advised actively to exercise the involved muscles also within the limits of pain. These exercises are performed in 5–10 minute periods several times daily.

2. During the severe stage, ice is applied over the area of pathology four times daily at least. As pain remits, heat may be used as an analgesic if the patient desires.

3. Oral anti-inflammatory medication may be helpful, particularly for the bursitis syndromes.

4. Local corticosteroids may be helpful for both the bursitis and musculotendinous syndromes, if injected precisely into the area of pathology.

5. Should the syndrome persist after 6–8 weeks of compliance with therapy, the patient may be referred to an orthopaedist for confirmation of the diagnosis. However, orthopaedists have no other treatment to offer.

Pelvic Sprains

Sacroiliac Sprains

These sprains have been discussed in Chapter 9.

Sprains of the Pubic Symphysis

These sprains are quite prevalent in pregnant women in their third trimester. Occasionally we have encountered persons who are suffering the syndrome following surgery in the lithotomy position, or who have fallen directly onto the pubis, as does a child when slipping off the pedals of a bicycle which is too large, and landing astraddle the frame. We rarely encounter other individuals so afflicted, and then nearly always after they have sustained injuring forces to the pelvis great enough to sprain one of the sacroiliac joints as well. Characteristic clinical features are the following:

1. Aching pain is usually felt in the perineum and may refer into one or both groins and down the inner aspects of one or both thighs.

2. Weightbearing, particularly the transfer of weight from one extremity to the other, active or passive movement of either or both extremities while sitting or lying, and shifting weight from one buttock to the other will usually abruptly increase the pain.

3. Pressure over the pubic arch with the heel of the hand will always increase the pain, and digital palpation will always find the symphysis itself tender.

4. Unfortunately, sprains sustained in pregnancy usually persist until delivery. Often remission is noted during the first few days after delivery. Occasionally remission does not occur for several weeks after delivery.

Treatment.

1. Activity is kept within the limits of common pain tolerance. Individuals suffering pelvic sprains can resume essential activities sooner if the pelvis is bound by a trochanter belt or sacroiliac support. While these appliances are available in many surgical supply houses, any broad canvas or leather belt that can be drawn tightly about the hips between the iliac crests and the greater femoral trochanters will do. (See Figure 11–25.) These supports decrease the severity of the abrupt pains which are provoked by movement.

2. Ice or heat, and minor analgesics are usually able to ease the persisting aching pain.

3. Healing will occur as fast as it can if

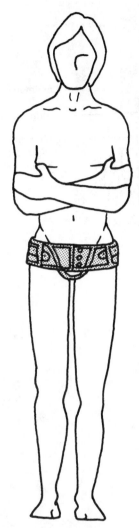

Fig. 11–25. Trochanter belt.

activity is kept within the limits of common tolerance, though anti-inflammatory agents, including local corticosteroid injections, may speed the recovery for some. The oral anti-inflammatory agents should not be used during pregnancy, but may be used when remission is delayed beyond the first postpartum week and the parturiant is not nursing.

Periarticular Myofascial Injuries

These disorders are primarily distinguished from the "pain syndromes" by their immediate relationship to a recognized abrupt injuring force. These forces apply either as blunt or penetrating impact, or as violent stretch. The usual inju-

ries involve one or more of the following muscle groups, and their binding fascial layers:

1. The abductors—gluteus medius and minimis, iliotibial tract.
2. The flexors—sartorius, tensor fasciae latae, rectus femoris, and iliopsoas.
3. The adductors—adductor longus, brevis, and magnus.
4. The extensors—gluteus maximus, adductor magnus, semimembranosus, semitendinosus, long head of the biceps femoris.

Intramuscular Injuries

Contusing and stretching injuries will disrupt collagenous fibers, myofibrils, and blood vessels. Arterial bleeding will produce intramuscular or perimuscular hematomata, usually evident as well-localized swellings. Eventual inflammation will produce generalized swelling of the injured tissues. The hematoma that continues to bleed episodically, usually due to repeated injury, during convalescence, may become a site of new bone formation and result in a variably disabling complication known as myositis ossificans. Inflammation and intramuscular hematoma formation may so increase the tissue pressure in an injured muscle as to cause an ischemic necrosis of that muscle.

Avulsion Injuries

Abrupt contraction of a muscle against strong resistance may cause an avulsion fracture of one of its attachments. These avulsions are by far most likely to occur during adolescence, when the attachments are still ununited epiphyses. (See Figure 11–26.)

Abrupt resisted hip flexion, as may occur when a kick is blocked, may cause one of the following avulsions:

Rectus femoris may avulse its origin from the anteroinferior iliac spine. *Sartorious* may avulse its origin from the anterosuperior iliac spine. *Iliopsoas* may avulse its insertion from the lesser femoral trochanter.

Abrupt opposed hip extension, as may occur during an effort to rise with a weight, or during the splits, may avulse the origin of the *semimembranosus, semiten-*

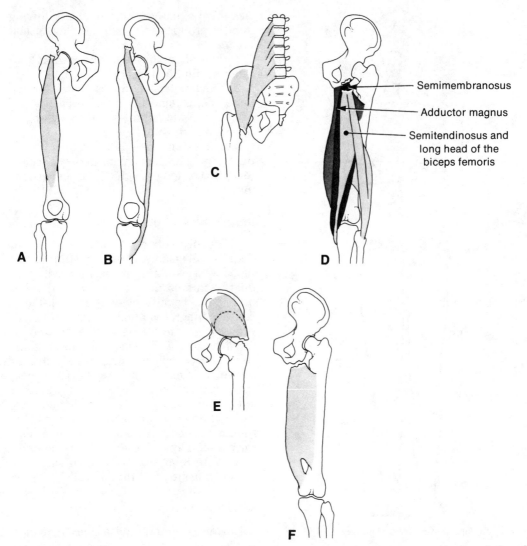

Semimembranosus

Adductor magnus

Semitendinosus and long head of the biceps femoris

Fig. 11–26. Avulsion injuries to the muscles of the hip. *A,* straight tendon of rectus femoris. *B,* sartorius. *C,* iliopsoas. *D,* hamstrings. *E,* gluteus medius and minimus. *F,* adductors.

dinosus, and/or *long head of the biceps femoris* from the ischial tuberosity.

Abrupt opposed hip abduction, as may accompany a fall, can avulse the insertion of the *gluteus medius and minimis* from the greater femoral trochanter.

Abrupt opposed hip adduction or hip extension, as may occur during a fall or the splits, can avulse the origins of the *adductor group* from the inferior ischiopubic ramus and ischial tuberosity.

Characteristic Clinical Features of Myofascial Injuries Are the Following:

1. Pain is localized to the injured muscle and fascia at the outset, but may spread variably with persistence.

2. The injured muscle is uniquely tender. If, following stretch injuries, the attachment points are uniquely tender, avulsion fracture should be suspect.

3. Swelling may be evident over the zone of the muscle, and ecchymoses will appear after 1 or more days, usually in a position gravity dependent to the injured muscle.

4. Voluntary contraction of the muscle is painful and may be inhibited. Indeed, some patients are incapable of contracting an injured muscle, in spite of urgent instruction to do so.

5. Any maneuver that stretches the in-

jured muscle or fascia produces pain.

6. X-rays may show an avulsion fracture of the attachments of a muscle injured by violent stretch.

Treatment

The goals of treatment are reconstruction of the disrupted anatomy, the prevention of myositis ossificans and ischemic necrosis, the earliest possible resolution of inflammation, the prevention of stiffness, and the restoration of strength. The realization of these goals is facilitated by the following therapeutic principles:

1. If within 6 hours of an injury, swelling and tenderness and pain on weightbearing are slight, minimal disruption of muscle tissue and minimal intramuscular bleeding can be presumed. Such injuries require little treatment. Active stretching and working exercises may speed the resolution, and icing or, after the first 48 hours, heat application may decrease any pain at rest.

2. If within 6 hours of an injury, swelling, tenderness, and pain on weightbearing are marked, a major disruption of muscle tissue must be presumed, and the patient must be considered at risk for complications. These patients must be treated as follows:

a. When it is known or suspected that the injuring force was a stretching force, examine for tenderness at the attachment points, and obtain x-rays whenever tenderness is elicited. When x-rays demonstrate avulsion fractures with little separation, the patient may be instructed to avoid weightbearing and intentional contraction of the muscle for 6 weeks. If at that time callus formation is adequate by x-ray, active range of motion and muscle-strengthening exercise and progressive weightbearing may be started. On the other hand, when x-ray demonstrates avulsion fractures with wide separation, the patient must be referred to an orthopaedist who may immobilize the patient in a spica cast, or repair the avulsion by open reduction and internal fixation.

b. When muscle bellies have been injured by whatever mechanism, means must be applied to minimize further intramuscular bleeding or inflammatory swelling: immobilization, elevation when pos-sible, icing, and tight binders. These means should be applied throughout the first 48 hours. The binders must not exceed venous pressure. (Distal to the binder, congestion must not be evident, and capillary return must be normal or at least as brisk as in the twin extremity.)

c. If at any point during convalescence, usually within the first 48 hours, any injured muscle becomes very painful and tense at rest, ischemia must be suspect, and the patient must be referred to an orthopaedist immediately.

d. After 48 hours, gentle active stretching and contracting exercises may begin. These movements should not pass through the point of pain.

e. As pain recedes, the vigor of the stretching and contracting exercises may increase and weightbearing may begin. During the 1st week of convalescence, exercise and weightbearing should be limited to avoid increased muscle pain. After the 1st week, exercises should proceed to the point of fatigue, unless pain becomes unbearable.

f. Athletes must not resume contact sports or sprinting until swelling and tenderness are gone. The bleeding attendant on repeated injuries is most likely to lead to myositis ossificans. Other activity may be resumed as soon as it can be practiced with little increase in pain. The healing period for muscle sprains may be surprisingly prolonged. Restriction of activity for a period of 2 months or more is often necessary following the more severe injuries.

Sprains of the Hip Joint

The forces that sprain the hip joint are the same kind as those that dislocate the joint, but are of lesser magnitude. The injury is presumed to be a stretch or a partial tear of the joint capsule and its reinforcing ligaments. The synovium becomes acutely inflamed, and the injured capsule may bleed into the joint. Patients present with a history of abrupt injury, and clinical findings are identical to those of acute arthritis of the hip.

Treatment

Patients whose range of motion is only slightly restricted may be presumed to have suffered a minor sprain, and after 24–48 hours' rest, may resume weightbearing and begin active range of motion exercises. Patients whose range of motion is severely restricted are presumed to have suffered a major sprain and are taught the restorative regimen employed following the period of immobilization for dislocations.

Dislocations of the Hip Joint

Hip dislocations are most prevalent among the young whose bones are strong and whose activities carry the risk of violent injury. On the other hand, the elderly, whose bones are fragile, are more likely to suffer hip fracture before the injuring force can lever the head of the femur out of the acetabulum.

The hip can dislocate in three directions: posterior, anterior, and central. In our experience, the posterior dislocation is by far the most common, and the anterior and central dislocations about equally rare. (See Figures 11–27 and 11–28.)

Posterior Dislocation

Posterior dislocations are produced by forces which act axially along the femur, while the hip is flexed and adducted, or flexed and in neutral deviation. In today's world, these forces are most commonly encountered in auto accidents when the knees of front-seat riders are driven against the dashboard. When adducted,

the head of the femur is likely to ride over the posterior rim of the acetabulum, as it bursts through the posterior capsule and ischiofemoral ligament. When in neutral deviation, the head of the femur is likely to fracture through the posterior rim of the acetabulum as it bursts through the posterior capsule and ischiofemoral ligament. The less the flexion at the moment of injury, the more likely is the head of the femur to come to rest over the wing of the ilium. The greater the flexion at the mo-

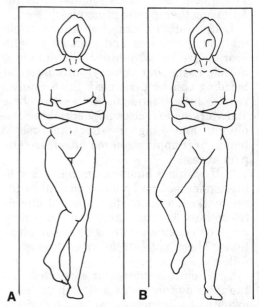

Fig. 11–28. Postures of hip dislocation. *A*, posterior dislocation. *B*, anterior dislocation.

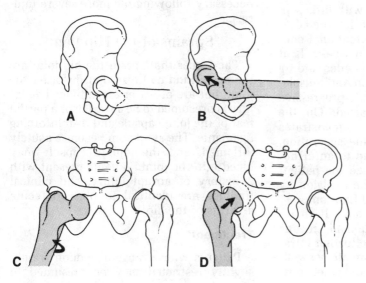

Fig. 11–27. Dislocation of the hip. *A*, normal articulation. *B*, posterior dislocation. *C*, anterior dislocation. *D*, central dislocation.

ment of injury, the more likely is the head of the femur to come to rest in the greater sciatic notch. Displacement into the greater sciatic notch is very likely to contuse or lacerate the sciatic nerve. However the dislocation occurs, the acetabular labrum is invariably torn or avulsed with a portion of the acetabular rim.

Individuals who have suffered a posterior dislocation usually present with considerable pain in the buttock and posterior thigh, and with the injured extremity shortened, and the hip flexed, adducted, and internally rotated. An anteroposterior x-ray of the pelvis and a true lateral of the hip will confirm the dislocation, and will show any accompanying fracture of the acetabulum. However, acetabular fractures are not usually obvious; some will be identified only by the most meticulous examination of the x-rays. As soon as a posterior dislocation is suspected, sciatic nerve function must be tested. Dorsiflexion of the ankle is impossible if the sciatic nerve has been injured. Examination for active dorsiflexion is a harmless test with which most conscious patients will be quite willing to cooperate.

Anterior Dislocation

Anterior dislocations are produced by violent forces which abduct, externally rotate, and extend the hip. Such forces cause the head of the femur to ride over or through the transverse acetabular ligament and/or burst through the inferior wall of the joint capsule. The head of the femur may come to rest over the pubis, or may lodge in the obturator foramen. Individuals who fall from a height or who fall when skiing out of control are the most likely to suffer these dislocations.

Individuals who have suffered an anterior dislocation usually present with considerable pain in the groin and anterior and medial thigh, and with the injured hip abducted, externally rotated, and often slightly extended. The extremity is typically not shortened.

Central Dislocation

Central dislocations are produced by violent forces that drive the head of the femur through the acetabulum into the pelvis. Such forces may be delivered directly against the greater trochanter while the hip is adducted, or along the axis of the femur while the hip is abducted. These dislocations are usually suffered by those injured in car accidents or in falls from a height.

Individuals who have suffered central dislocations usually present with considerable pain in the groin and anterior and medial thigh, and with the hip slightly adducted and externally rotated. The extremity is typically not shortened.

Complications of Dislocation

1. As indicated, posterior dislocations may be complicated by sciatic nerve injury.

2. Any dislocation may so damage the blood supply to the femoral head as to result in aseptic necrosis of the head.

3. Any dislocation, particularly those that have produced a fracture of the acetabulum, is likely to roughen the weight-bearing cartilage surface and predispose to a premature degenerative arthritis.

Reduction of the Dislocation

With adequate muscle relaxation, posterior and anterior dislocations are usually not difficult to reduce. Indeed, as has occasionally occurred on ski slopes, immediately after an injury, before muscle spasm has developed, a reduction may be accomplished without anesthesia. We employ the following maneuvers for reduction of these dislocations (see Figure 11–29):

Posterior Dislocations:

1. With the patient supine, the hip is flexed to 90°.

2. While an assistant or the kneeling operator's foot stabilizes the pelvis, the operator applies traction from behind the flexed knee in the axis of the thigh.

3. With full traction applied, the operator gently externally rotates the hip, using the lower leg as a lever. This maneuver may immediately effect the reduction. When it does not, gentle alternating external and internal rotation often will.

4. When these maneuvers have not succeeded, reduction may be achieved by gently extending and abducting the hip

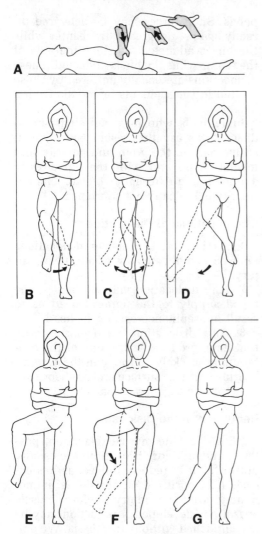

Fig. 11–29. Reduction of dislocations: *A* through *D*, posterior dislocation; *A*, upward traction with hip flexed 90°; *B*, external rotation while continuing traction; *C*, alternate external and internal rotation while continuing traction; *D*, extension and abduction while maintaining traction and external rotation. *E* through *G*, anterior dislocation. (Note the position of the patient at the edge of the examining table.) Maneuver begins with hip and knee flexed to 90°, as in *A*. *E*, hip abducted to nearly 90° while maintaining flexion. *F* and *G*, hip slowly continuously extended, adducted, and internally rotated (performed as one maneuver).

while maintaining traction and external rotation.

5. Reduction is usually rewarded with a heavy click. However, if the posterior rim of the acetabulum has been fractured, this click may not be appreciated. Under these conditions, reduction may be very difficult to perceive.

6. Once reduction is presumed, the hip is extended to the long axis of the body and abducted and externally rotated about 30°.

7. An x-ray is made.

8. If the reduction is confirmed and the fragment of any attendant fracture of the acetabulum is replaced, a hip spica may be applied to hold the hip in straight extension and 30° abduction and external rotation. If a dislocation alone has occurred, immobilization is maintained for 3 weeks. If the acetabulum has been fractured as well, immobilization is maintained for 6 weeks.

9. If closed maneuvers have failed to reduce either the dislocation or an attendant acetabular fracture, open reduction will be required. An attendant acetabular fracture will usually be stabilized by internal methods of fixation.

Anterior Dislocation

1. With the patient supine, the hip and knee are flexed to 90°.

2. The hip is then abducted to nearly 90°, bringing the head of the femur near the inferior acetabular notch and its bridging transverse acetabular ligament.

3. From this position, slow extension, adduction, and internal rotation, effected as a continuous movement, will usually lever the head of the femur through the rent in the inferior wall of the capsule, over the transverse acetabular ligament, back into the acetabulum. Reduction is accompanied by a heavy click.

4. X-rays must be obtained to confirm reduction.

5. Once reduction is confirmed, the hip immediately is adducted, and neutrally or slightly internally rotated for 3 weeks. While this position can be maintained by binding the legs together, we consider this method to be dangerously immobilizing and unnecessarily uncomfortable. A proper hip spica or traction apparatus can accomplish the same end and give the patient more freedom of movement.

Central Dislocation. This dislocation cannot be reduced by simple manipulation. A combination of longitudinal and lateral traction over several days is usually required. Occasionally, open reduction is necessary. The goals are to place the head of the femur back into articulation with the weightbearing superior surface of the acetabulum, and to maintain the position until the acetabular fracture heals. Healing of the acetabulum usually requires at least 6 weeks.

Rehabilitation

1. During the period of immobilization, active range of motion of the knee and ankle and exercises to maintain strength of the other extremities must be practiced many times daily.

2. When immobilization can be discontinued, active range of motion of the hip must be practiced many times daily. (See Figure 11-22.)

3. Graduated weightbearing should not be started until range of motion is near-normal. X-rays must be obtained prior to starting weightbearing to rule out aseptic necrosis of the head of the femur. Full weightbearing is usually re-established about 2 months after immobilization has been discontinued.

The Role of the Primary Practitioner

1. The primary practitioner must complete the emergency resuscitation and initial evaluation: (a) Support vital function; (b) search for attendant injuries; (c) obtain proper x-rays; (d) test for sciatic nerve function in cases of posterior dislocation; (e) obtain intravenous pyelogram and urethrogram if attended by open pelvic fractures. (See below under "Treatment" for "Fractures of the Pelvis.")

2. If safe anesthesia can be effected and an orthopaedist is some time distant, a manually tactful primary practitioner should attempt the reduction of posterior and anterior dislocations, without waiting for the orthopaedist.

3. An orthopaedist must become initially involved (a) if reduction of posterior or anterior dislocations cannot be accomplished, or (b) if acetabular fragments remain displaced following reduction of a posterior dislocation, and (c) in all cases of central dislocation.

4. Since aseptic necrosis and degenerative arthritis can complicate any hip dislocation, an orthopaedist must eventually become involved some time during the 1st week, if only by telephone.

5. Follow the patient's convalescence with the orthopaedist, assuming responsibility for chronic and intercurrent medical problems and advising adaptations in the rehabilitative process better to fit with the patient's idiosyncrasies.

6. In many cases which have required the services of an orthopaedist, particularly in rural areas, final rehabilitation may be most economically managed by the primary practitioner.

Fractures of the Hip

Fractures of the hip are most prevalent among the osteoporotic. Hence, elderly women, who as a group are more predisposed to osteoporosis than young women or men of any age, are by far the most likely to suffer hip fractures. Correlatively, the forces that produce these fractures are often slight—a fall like that from which a youth would promptly arise to continue violent play, or merely a sudden twist as may apply to a weightbearing extremity when trying to avert a fall, or as may apply to a non-weightbearing extremity when working at cross purposes with a health worker who is trying to roll the individual over in bed, or to get the individual into or out of bed or a chair.

As discussed above (pages 177–178), the architecture of the upper end of the femur is superbly suited to resist the forces of weightbearing. However, it is not so suited to resist twisting and shearing forces from other directions. The zone of Ward's triangle, which is crossed by the weakest and fewest of the trabeculae, is the least capable of resisting such forces, and is thus the most vulnerable to fracture. Hip fractures are classified into two large groups: intracapsular and extracapsular. (See Figure 11-30.) The importance of this distinction derives from the vascular anatomy of the head and neck of the femur, summarized above on page 178. Intracapsular fractures, the subcapital and transcervical fractures, are likely to disrupt the blood supply to the head of the femur, resulting in avascular necrosis of the head of the femur. Extracapsular fractures, the trochanteric fractures, will not do this.

Most fractures, whether intra- or extracapsular, are unstable and variably dis-

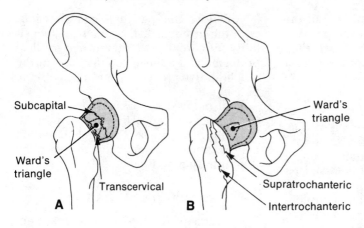

Fig. 11-30. Fractures of the hip. *A*, intracapsular. *B*, extracapsular.

placed. Rarely, a fracture will be firmly impacted so firmly as to withstand weight-bearing. Most of the impacted fractures are intracapsular fractures.

Characteristic Clinical Features Are the Following:

1. An elderly person has fallen or twisted a hip.

2. Usually such a person will not bear weight, and is carried to the clinic. Rarely, a person with an impacted fracture may have walked about in pain for several days before consulting.

3. Pain is referred to the groin and front of the thigh.

4. If the patient tries to move the extremity, the effort will usually be promptly stopped by severe pain. However, those with impacted fractures may move fairly well, though with pain.

5. The injured extremity is usually shortened and externally rotated, although impacted fractures may not be. (See Figure 11-31.)

6. Anteroposterior pelvis and true lateral hip x-rays will demonstrate the fracture. Impacted fractures may be rather obscure, and will be missed unless x-rays are carefully inspected. The only clue to an impacted intracapsular fracture may be an abrupt change in the arc of curvature of one of the borders of the neck. (See Figure 11-32.)

Treatment

Rarely a young person with an extracapsular fracture may be treated by 2-3

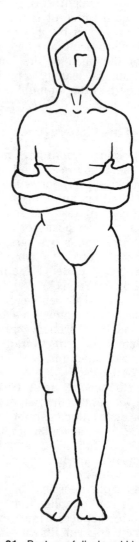

Fig. 11-31. Posture of displaced hip fracture.

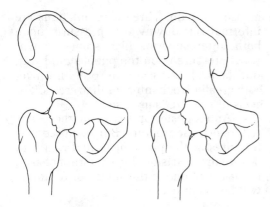

Fig. 11–32. X-ray evidence of the impacted fracture. The curve of the superior and/or inferior borders of the neck of the femur may be discontinuous. (Note the normal curves are represented by dotted lines.)

months traction in bed, or a fairly agile person with an impacted fracture may be treated with non-weightbearing activities for 2–3 months. The vast majority of these fractures are treated surgically. Surgical alternatives include nailing, with or without a plate, or replacement of the head of the femur with a prosthesis, either of the old Moore variety, or the more recent total hip replacement.

The Role of the Primary Practitioner

1. The primary practitioner must complete the initial evaluation. (a) Suspect the diagnosis and obtain proper x-rays. (b) Identify the fracture, whether intra- or extracapsular, and whether displaced or impacted. (c) Identify the patient's other health problems and assess the anesthetic and surgical risks. (d) Transmit this information to an orthopaedist.

2. Admit the patient to bed and immobilize the extremity for comfort, either in Buck's traction or a Thomas' splint. (See Figure 11–33.)

3. Follow the patient's convalescence with the orthopaedist, assuming responsibility for chronic and intercurrent medical problems, and advising adaptations in the rehabilitative process better to fit with the patient's idiosyncrasies.

4. Assume full responsibility for the patient's final rehabilitation when, as is most likely in rural areas, it is economically best for the patient.

Fractures of the Pelvis

Fractures of the pelvis, unless pathologic, are invariably caused by violent forces like those generated by a motor vehicle accident or a fall from a height. These fractures are of two varieties, *closed ring fractures* and *open ring fractures*. (See Figure 11–34.) For the shape of a rigid ring to be distorted, it must be disrupted at two points. Hence, all uncomplicated single fractures are closed ring fractures, and all open ring fractures are either double or multiple fractures, or single fractures complicated by an associated disruption of one

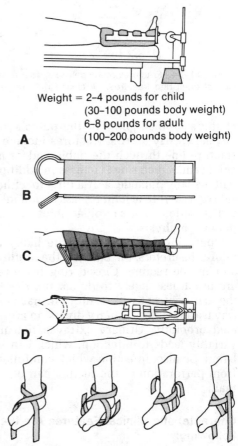

Weight = 2–4 pounds for child
  (30–100 pounds body weight)
  6–8 pounds for adult
  (100–200 pounds body weight)

Fig. 11–33. Traction methods for emergency immobilization of hip and thigh injuries. *A*, Buck's traction using "Buck's boot." *B*, Thomas' splint. *C* and *D*, Thomas' splint applied using "Buck's boot." (While tape can be used to apply traction to the leg, a non-adhesive high-friction appliance is more comfortable and less likely to injure the skin. The "Buck's boot" illustrated in *A* and *D* is made in four sizes and can be procured from a surgical supply house.) *E*, application of cravat for traction in the field. When applied, circulation in the foot must be closely monitored.

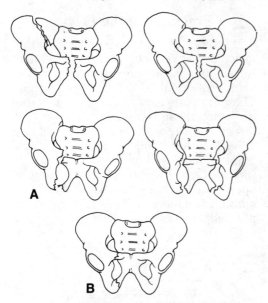

Fig. 11–34. Fractures of the pelvis. *A,* four examples of open ring fractures. *B,* closed ring fracture.

of the sacroiliac joints or the pubic symphysis. Nearly all ring fractures include a fracture line through the pubic and/or ischial rami. Open ring fractures in addition will usually include a fracture to either side of a sacroiliac joint or, less commonly, a dislocation of a sacroiliac joint, or the pubic symphysis.

Open ring fractures are quite likely to injure the ureters, the bladder, the urethra, and/or the rectum. Closed ring fractures are much less likely to do so. Injuries to the urinary tract will result in urinary extravasation unless urinary diversion is created promptly. Urinary extravasation invariably leads to infection, which can be lethal. So also, infection which can follow from perforation of the rectum can be lethal.

Characteristic Clinical Features Are the Following:

1. An individual who has been involved in a violent accident, if conscious, will complain of pain which often girdles the hips or localizes unilaterally in a buttock or groin.

2. Any effort, active or passive, to move the lower extremities will increase the pain.

3. Manipulations of the pelvis will in-crease the pain. Three manipulations are informative: downward pressure upon both anterosuperior iliac spines, downward pressure upon the pubic symphysis, and central compressive pressure over both greater trochanters or iliac crests. The heels of the hands are used.

4. Anteroposterior x-rays of the pelvis will reveal the fracture. Single closed ring fractures of the pubic or ischial rami can be obscure; occasionally, an abrupt change in the arc of one of the obturator foramina will be the only clue.

Treatment

1. Closed ring fractures may be treated simply with bed rest and gentle active range of motion exercises until pain has diminished sufficiently to allow partial weightbearing. Usually, partial weight-bearing is possible within 1 week. Weight-bearing will then continue progressively until it is painless, and the patient can then be discharged. Rehabilitation of patients with closed ring fractures is often facili-tated by a trochanter belt or a sacroiliac support as the patient so supported can often proceed with ambulation sooner.

2. Evaluation of any pelvic fracture will require an investigation of the bladder and urethra and the rectum. The vesicourethral evaluation may be simply accomplished by urinalysis unless suspicion of vesico-urethral disruption is strong as should be the case in the face of any open ring frac-ture, the patient's complaint of painful ur-gency, or blood in the urethral meatus. Such circumstances contraindicate void-ing and necessitate direct investigation by intravenous pyelogram and urethrogram. Evaluation of the rectum may be simply accomplished by digital rectal examina-tion. Unusual rectal tenderness or a pal-pable rent or weakness imply a rectal per-foration. When findings seem equivocal, a proctoscopic examination is necessary. When these investigations give evidence of vesicourethral or rectal disruption, a urologic or general surgeon must be con-sulted immediately.

3. Reduction and immobilization of open ring fractures of the pelvis is usually deferred to an orthopaedist. The principles are the following:

a. Straight traction on an extremity on

the fractured side, using heavy weights, sometimes up to 50 pounds, is usually necessary to draw the fractured side—which is invariably displaced proximally—downward into apposition with the normal side of the pelvis.

b. A pelvis that has been levered open by the forces of the injury can be closed by a pelvic sling, which suspends the pelvis from an overhead bar. The degree of compression upon the pelvis which such a sling can apply can be varied by varying the distance between the two sides of the sling.

c. The pelvis which has been compressed into overlapping alignment may be opened outward into normal alignment by lateral traction. Lateral traction can be accomplished in one of two ways: (1) A traction pin can be placed through both greater trochanters and weights applied on each side of the patient to apply laterally directed forces to the pelvic ring; or (2) a simpler and perhaps less traumatic method for the patient may be to immobilize both lower extremities in full-length casts, and to attach them to a bar which extends from knee to knee. Once the plaster has hardened fully, forces may then be applied at the ankles to adduct them toward one another. Such forces will then lever over the fulcrum of the bar to create abductive forces at the hips, thus tending to open the pelvis back into reduced alignment.

4. Rehabilitation of open ring fractures should begin immediately with active range of motion of the ankles and strengthening exercises of the upper extremities. The immobilization of the pelvis must usually continue for 6 weeks before it would be sufficiently stable to allow discontinuation of the immobilization and the beginning of the next phase of rehabilitation. The next phase of rehabilitation will include active assisted range of motion exercises in bed, graduating eventually to partial weightbearing as range of motion and strength return, and gradually to full weightbearing as pain and strength allow.

The Role of the Primary Practitioner

1. The primary practitioner must complete the emergency resuscitation and initial evaluation. (a) Support vital functions. (b) Search for attendant injuries. (c) Obtain proper x-rays. (d) Obtain urinalysis and/or intravenous pyelogram and urethrogram, and perform rectal and any indicated proctoscopic examination. (e) Transmit this information to an orthopaedist and, if necessary, to a urologist or general surgeon.

2. Admit the patient to bed and immobilize both extremities in Buck's traction to increase the patient's comfort.

3. Follow the patient's convalescence with the orthopaedist and any other surgeons as may be involved, assuming responsibility for chronic and intercurrent medical problems, and advising adaptations in the rehabilitative process better to fit with the patient's idiosyncrasies.

4. Assume full responsibility for the patient's final rehabilitation when—as is most likely in rural areas—it is economically best for the patient.

CHAPTER 12
The Thigh and Knee

Because the knee is a weightbearing hinge joint, the strength and coordination of its controlling muscles are major determinants of the stability of the knee, and thus of its usefulness and vulnerability to wear. Hence, rehabilitation from any knee disorder places the major emphasis upon the restoration of strength to these muscles. Correlatively, injuries to these muscles or to the shaft of the femur, from which several of these muscles originate, and along which all bridge their forces, will immediately disable the knee and can, with poor management or bad luck, permanently do so. Therefore, it has seemed to us properly emphatic and most efficient to include these two regions, the thigh and the knee, in the same chapter.

Essential Anatomy

The Thigh

The Shaft and Condyles of the Femur.
The *shaft* of the femur extends from the trochanters to the condyles. It is triangular in cross section, with the apex, the *linea aspera*, directed posteriorly. It is slightly bowed with an anterior convexity. It inclines from the trochanters to the condyles

in slight adduction, causing the normal stance to be slightly "knock kneed." The linea aspera provides insertion for the adductors and extensors of the hip, and with the anterior surface of the midshaft and trochanteric region, provides origin for the extensors of the knee. As the shaft approaches the condyles, it broadens laterally and medially, and the ridges of the linea aspera diverge to merge with the supracondylar ridges. These ridges outline a triangle to which no muscles attach, called the *popliteal surface*. (See Figure 12-1.)

The *condyles* of the femur present semilunar cartilagenous articular surfaces inferiorly and roughened epicondylar surfaces medially and laterally. Anteriorly, these condyles merge to form the *patellar articular surface,* and posteriorly they are separated by the *deep intercondylar fossa.* The condylar end of the femur angulates with the shaft of the femur such that the plane of the condylar articular surfaces is horizontal when the shaft is inclined in adduction. (See Figure 12-1.)

The Controlling Muscles of the Knee.
Extensors. The major extensor of the knee is the quadriceps muscle which forms the

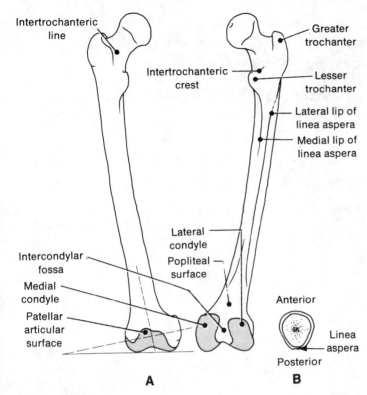

Intertrochanteric line

Intertrochanteric crest

Greater trochanter

Lesser trochanter

Lateral lip of linea aspera

Medial lip of linea aspera

Lateral condyle

Popliteal surface

Intercondylar fossa

Medial condyle

Patellar articular surface

Anterior

Posterior

Linea aspera

A

B

Fig. 12–1. The femur. A, anterior and posterior views. B, cross section, midfemur.

anterior bulk of the thigh. Its four parts and their origins are the following (see Figures 12–2 through 12–4): The *rectus femoris*, the most anterior of the four, originates by two tendons from the ilium, a straight tendon anteriorly from the anterior inferior iliac spine, and a reflected tendon posteriorly from the posterior ridge of the acetabulum. That the straight tendon and anterior inferior iliac spine are vulnerable to injury when kicking from a position of hip extension has been pointed out in Chapter 11.

The *vastus medialis* lies deep to the rectus femoris proximally and emerges distally to create the medial curve of the distal thigh. It takes a long curving origin which extends from the intertrochanteric line anteriorly along the length of the inner lip of the linea aspera posteriorly. Its medial location and the direction of its fibers cause it to apply medially- as well as proximally-directed forces to the patella during the last 15° of extension. The importance of this action will become apparent in the discussion of chondromalacia patellae and recurrent patellar dislocation.

The *vastus lateralis* creates the lateral bulk of the thigh. It takes a long curving origin which extends from the inferior aspect of the greater trochanter anteriorly along the length of the outer lip of the linea aspera posteriorly.

The *vastus intermedius* lies deep to the other three portions of the quadriceps, and merges distally with the vastus medialis and lateralis. It takes a long broad origin from the anterior surface of the femur.

All four parts of the quadriceps muscle *insert* upon a common tendon called the *quadriceps tendon*, which attaches to the upper border of the patella and merges to either side with the patellar retinacula (see below). While this tendon is the only attachment for the rectus femoris to the patella, the three vasti make direct attachment to the patella as well: the medialis to the medial border, the lateralis to the lateral pole, and the intermedius to the upper border, deep to the quadriceps tendon.

All the extensors are *innervated* by branches of the femoral nerve, composed of neurons from the 2nd through the 4th lumbar segments.

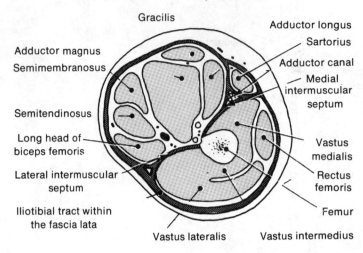

Gracilis

Adductor longus

Sartorius

Adductor canal

Medial intermuscular septum

Adductor magnus

Semimembranosus

Semitendinosus

Long head of biceps femoris

Lateral intermuscular septum

Iliotibial tract within the fascia lata

Vastus medialis

Rectus femoris

Femur

Vastus lateralis

Vastus intermedius

Fig. 12–2. Cross section of the midthigh.

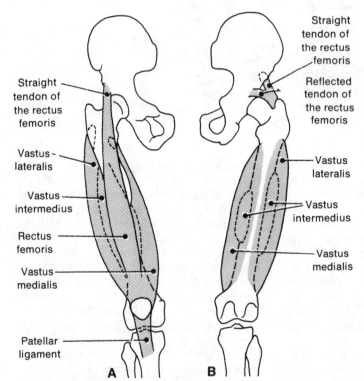

Straight tendon of the rectus femoris

Straight tendon of the rectus femoris

Reflected tendon of the rectus femoris

Vastus lateralis

Vastus intermedius

Rectus femoris

Vastus medialis

Vastus lateralis

Vastus intermedius

Vastus medialis

Patellar ligament

A   B

Fig. 12–3. The quadriceps muscle. *A*, anterior view. *B*, posterior view.

Flexors. The chief flexors of the knee, except the weak sartorius, were described in Chapter 9 as they also, except for the sartorius, are extensors of the hip. These strong chief flexors are the *gracilis,* the *semitendinosus,* the *semimembranosus,* and the *biceps femoris* muscles. (See Figures 11–11, 11–12, and 12–4.) The long head of the biceps femoris, and the other three muscles take origin from the ischial tub-erosity. The short head of the biceps femoris takes origin from the distal third of the lateral lip of the linea aspera. At about the upper border of the popliteal surface of the femur, these muscles diverge, the biceps femoris and its tendon proceeding laterally to insert into the head of the fibula and lateral tibial condyle, the gracilis, semitendinosus and semimembranosus, and their tendons proceeding medially, the

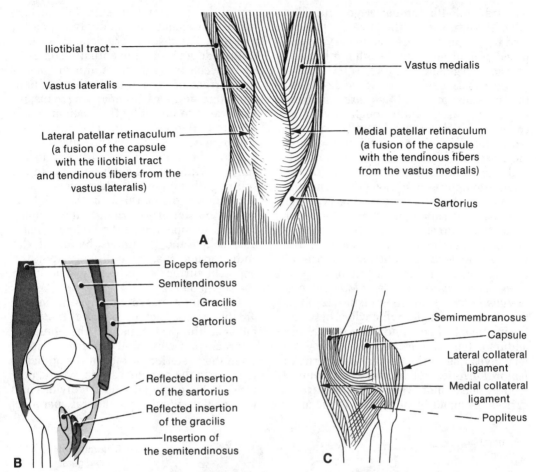

Iliotibial tract

Vastus lateralis

Lateral patellar retinaculum
(a fusion of the capsule
with the iliotibial tract
and tendinous fibers from the
vastus lateralis)

Vastus medialis

Medial patellar retinaculum
(a fusion of the capsule
with the tendinous fibers
from the vastus medialis)

Sartorius

A

Biceps femoris
Semitendinosus
Gracilis
Sartorius

Reflected insertion
of the sartorius

Reflected insertion
of the gracilis

Insertion of
the semitendinosus

B

Semimembranosus
Capsule
Lateral collateral
ligament
Medial collateral
ligament
Popliteus

C

Fig. 12-4.   Tendinous expansions merging with capsule of the knee joint. *A*, anterior view showing the patellar retinacula. *B*, anterior view showing the tibial insertion of the sartorius, semitendinosus, and gracilis medially, and the fibular insertion of the biceps femoris laterally. *C*, posterior view showing the relationship of the semimembranosus to the capsule medially and posteriorly. The medial head of the gastrocnemius overlies posterior to the semimembranosus tendon—not illustrated.

gracilis and semitendinosus to insert into the medial aspect of the shaft of the tibia just inferior to the attachment of the patellar ligament to the tibial tubercle, and the semimembranosus to insert upon the posterior aspect of the medial tibial condyle and to merge some of its fibers with the joint capsule medially and posteriorly. The *sartorius* originates upon the antero-superior iliac spine, and spirals superficially across the anterior thigh to insert with the gracilis and semitendinosus upon the medial aspect of the shaft of the tibia.

The knee flexors have other actions as well. The gracilis is an adductor and internal rotator of the hip, as well as a flexor of the knee. The semitendinosus and semi-

membranosus are extensors and internal rotators of the hip, as well as flexors of the knee. The biceps femoris is an extensor of the hip, as well as a flexor of the knee. With the knee flexed, the knee flexors can serve as rotators of the leg: the gracilis, semitendinosus and semimembranosus internally rotate the leg; the biceps femoris externally rotates the leg.

The *sartorius*, along with all the anterior muscles of the thigh, is innervated by branches of the femoral nerve containing neurons from the 2nd-4th lumbar segments.

The *gracilis*, with all the adductors of the hip, is innervated by branches of the obturator nerve, containing neurons from the 3rd and 4th lumbar segments. The other three flexors of the knee are innervated by branches of the sciatic nerve, composed of neurons from the 5th lumbar and 1st sacral segments.

The Fascia Lata. (See Figure 12-2.) All the muscles of the thigh are enclosed within the fascia lata, a tough unyielding covering which merges laterally with the tendinous fibers of the iliotibial tract, and merges internally with the medial and lateral intermuscular septa, which divide the thigh into anterior and posterior compartments. As this fascial covering will not yield, extravasation of enough blood or tissue fluid into either of the two compartments of the thigh will tamponade the vessels and lead to ischemic necrosis of the muscles in that compartment.

Relationships of the Major Muscles and Nerves in the Thigh. (See Figure 12-5.) In the *femoral triangle,* which lies between the inguinal ligament and the sartorius and adductor longus muscles, the femoral artery gives rise to the *deep and superficial femoral arteries.* Each artery is accompanied by one or more veins. The deep artery carries the major blood supply to the mus-

cles of the thigh, and the superficial artery carries the major blood supply to the leg and foot. The *deep artery* penetrates deep to the adductors and eventually comes to lie between these muscles and the posterior surface of the femur. In this location, the artery and its accompanying veins are vulnerable to injury by the fragments of a fractured femoral shaft. The superficial artery passes deep to the sartorius muscle, within a fascial canal called the adductor canal, formed by the fascia lata and a splitting of the medial intermuscular septum. In the distal third of the thigh, it passes posteriorly around the femur, through an opening in the adductor magnus, called the tendinous hiatus of the adductor magnus, to lie directly upon the popliteal surface of the femur, anterior to the sciatic nerve.

The *sciatic nerve* emerges from the greater sciatic notch to enter the thigh between the piriformis and the obturator internus muscles, and courses distally upon the posterior surface of the adductor magnus to the popliteal space, where, posterior to the popliteal artery, it divides into its medial *tibial* and lateral *peroneal*

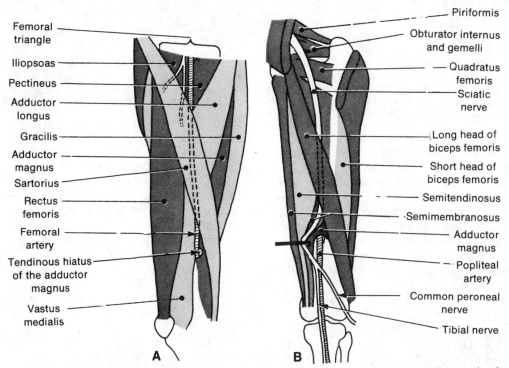

Fig. 12-5. Relationships of the major vessels and nerves in the thigh. *A,* anteromedial view. *B,* posterior view.

branches. As it passes through the thigh, its branches innervate the biceps femoris, the semitendinosus, the semimembranosus, and the posterior portion of the adductor magnus.

As the *femoral nerve* enters the thigh deep to the inguinal ligament, it lies just lateral to the *femoral artery* with which it extends into the *femoral triangle*. While still in the femoral triangle, it divides into numerous muscular branches, which innervate the anterior muscles of the thigh.

The Knee

The Tibiofemoral and Patellofemoral Articular Surfaces and Their Relative Motions. The general structure of the condyles of the femur was described above. The condyles of the tibia are platforms widened out from the tibial shaft. (See Figure 12–6.) Their superior surfaces present two slightly concave cartilagenous articular plates, separated by depressions anteriorly and posteriorly, called *intercondylar areas*, and by a central *intercondylar eminence* which bears the medial and lateral *intercondylar tubercles*.

Four anatomic and dynamic facts determine the relative motions of the articular surfaces of the tibiofemoral joint (see Figure 12–7):

1. The semilunar cartilagenous articular surfaces of the femoral condyles are rounded half-discs of continuously varying arcs.

2. The circumference and radius of the lateral femoral condyle are shorter than those of the medial femoral condyle.

3. The articular surface of the tibial condyles is relatively flat.

4. The center of flexion and extension forces acting upon the tibia is eccentric to the centers of the varying arcs of the condyles.

As determined by these facts, the tibial and femoral articular surfaces move upon one another both by rolling and by gliding motions, and the medial condyle rolls fewer degrees than the lateral condyle, and glides farther than the lateral condyle. Since the friction of gliding is more wearing than the friction of rolling, barring an injury to the lateral articular surfaces, the

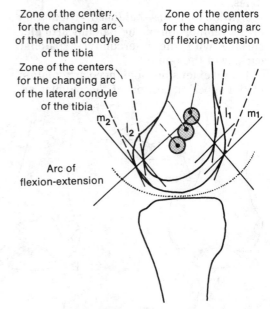

Zone of the centers for the changing arc of the medial condyle of the tibia

Zone of the centers for the changing arc of flexion-extension

Zone of the centers for the changing arc of the lateral condyle of the tibia

Arc of flexion-extension

Fig. 12–7. Schematic illustration demonstrating the angular relationships that necessitate a greater degree of gliding motion by the medial condyle and a greater degree of rolling motion by the lateral condyle. The center of the arcs of flexion-extension is nearer to the center of the arcs of the medial femoral condyle than to the center of the arcs of the lateral femoral condyle. Thus, more rolling motion is necessary to keep the lateral condyles in alignment than to keep the medial condyles in alignment. The more rolling motion is necessary, the less gliding motion is necessary. ($l_1 > m_1$; $l_2 > m_2$.)

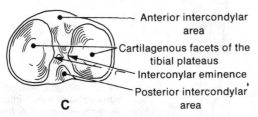

Intercondylar eminence

Medial plateau of the tibial condyles

Lateral plateau of the tibial condyles

A **B**

Anterior intercondylar area

Cartilagenous facets of the tibial plateaus

Interconylar eminence

Posterior intercondylar area

C

Fig. 12–6. The proximal condyles of the tibia. *A,* anterior view. *B,* posterior view. *C,* superior view.

medial articular surfaces should wear faster than the lateral. The truth of that logical probability is manifest on x-rays of the knees of the elderly, which usually show the medial articular interval to be narrower than the lateral.

The *patella* is a triangular sesamoid bone. Its apex inferiorly attaches to the patellar ligament, and its base superiorly attaches to the quadriceps tendon and muscle. Its inner cartilagenous surface is wedge-shaped and accommodates to the intercondylar patellar articular surface of the femur. From full flexion to full active extension, the contact surfaces of the patellofemoral articulation of the ideal knee shift as follows (see Figure 12–8):

1. Full flexion—the medial portion of the patellar surface articulates with the lateral aspect of the medial condyle.

2. Early extension—balanced articulation of the inferior portion of the patellar articular surface with both femoral condyles.

3. Midextension—balanced articulation of the midportion of the patellar articular surface with the intercondylar patellar surface of the femur.

4. Full extension—balanced articulation of the superior portion of the patellar ar-

ticulation with the intercondylar patellar surface of the femur.

When the orientation of the quadriceps muscle and the patellar ligament are set at an angle with one another, the summation vector of the quadriceps muscle and the patellar ligament causes a lateral shift of the patella during extension. (See Figure 12–9.) With this shift, the lateral portion of the patellar articular surface and the medial aspect of the lateral condyle become the contact surface between mid- and full extension. Since the same forces are applying to a smaller contact surface, the pressure on that surface is greater and the wear should be greater. Thus, this shift is thought to contribute to the development of chondromalacia patellae. (See section with this title, below.)

The Menisci. The two menisci are fibro-cartilagenous wedges that rim and cushion each tibiofemoral articulation. (See Figure 12–10.) The circumference and radius of the medial meniscus are greater than those of the lateral meniscus. The ends of the lateral meniscus attach to the intercondylar eminence, and the ends of the medial meniscus attach to the intercondylar areas. Their outer rims attach to the synovial membrane of the articular capsule.

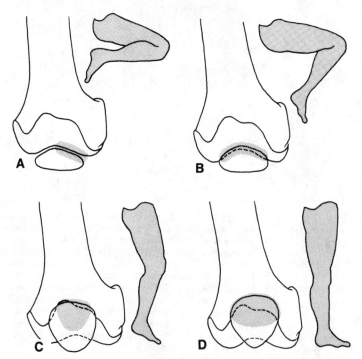

Fig. 12–8. Changing relationships of the patellofemoral articulation during knee motion. *A,* full flexion. *B,* early extension. *C,* midextension. *D,* full extension.

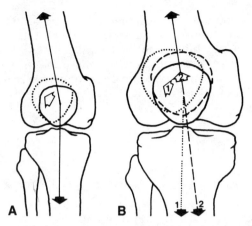

Fig. 12–9. Effect upon patellar motion during extension, of an angular orientation between the axis of the quadriceps action vector and the axis of the patellar ligament resistance. *A,* the resultant change in patellofemoral articulation between mid- (*solid line patella*) and full (*dotted line patella*) extension. *Solid arrows* indicate the two vectors. The *open arrow* indicates the resultant vector. *B,* vectors illustrated for two hypothetical patellar ligament insertions. *Solid line* indicates the quadriceps action vector, and the patellar position in midextension. *Dotted* and *dashed lines* indicate the two patellar ligament orientations (*1* and *2*) and corresponding patellar positions at full extension. *Solid arrows* indicate the several vectors. *Open arrows* indicate the resultant vectors for insertions 1 and 2.

During all motions of the tibiofemoral articulations upon one another, the tibial weightbearing points shift slightly: during flexion and extension, because those motions are accomplished by rolling as well as gliding; and during rotation. (See Figure 12–11.) These motions create wedging forces between the tibial and femoral condyles which tend to move the wedge-shaped menisci in directions which partially accommodate to the shifts in the weightbearing points. In addition to these passive accommodations, certain attachments of the menisci to other knee structures allow for active accommodation as well (see Figure 12–12):

1. The medial collateral ligament pulls the medial meniscus posteriorly during flexion and internal rotation of the femur, and anteriorly during extension and external rotation of the femur.

2. The meniscofemoral ligament pulls the posterior segment of the lateral meniscus medially during external rotation of the femur.

3. The popliteus muscle pulls the lateral meniscus posteriorly during flexion or during external rotation of the femur.

The lateral meniscus is least firmly attached to the joint capsule, thus is more free to pivot around the central attachments of its ends than is the medial meniscus which is bound not only to the synovial capsule but also to the fibrous capsule as well, and the ends of which are attached anteriorly and posteriorly in the intercondylar areas, rather than centrally about the intercondylar eminence. The great mobility of the lateral meniscus and its active accommodation to flexion and external rotation may account for the fact that it is injured much less often than is the medial meniscus.

The Fibrous Capsule and the Ligaments of the Tibiofemoral and Patellofe-

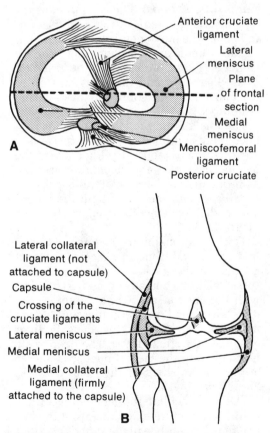

Fig. 12–10. Relationship between the menisci, the capsule, and the ligaments of the knee. *A,* superior view of the menisci and cruciate ligaments. *B,* posterior view of a frontal section of the knee through the middle third.

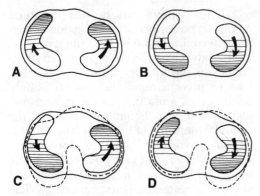

Fig. 12–11. Shifts in tibial weightbearing points and passive accommodations of the menisci during flexion-extension and rotation. *Shading* indicates weight distribution. *Arrows* indicate accommodative passive movements of the menisci. *Longer arrows* over the lateral meniscus symbolize its greater mobility. *A*, full extension. *B*, near full flexion. *C*, Medial rotation of the femur. *D*, lateral rotation of the femur.

moral Articulations. The restraints of the capsule and ligaments of these joints guide and check the movements of their articular surfaces upon one another. The primary clinician should understand the function of six ligaments and their relationship to the capsule of the joint and neighboring structures.

The *medial and the lateral patellar retinacula* are continuations of the fascia lata and quadriceps tendon to either side of the patella. They merge with and reinforce the anteromedial and anterolateral aspects of the fibrous capsule. They limit the lateral and medial movements of the patella. (See Figure 12–4.)

The *medial collateral ligament* extends in two layers from the medial femoral condyle to the medial tibial condyle. The superficial layer is strong and triangular, with the apex at the medial femoral condyle. The deep layer is thinner and blends more intimately with the capsule than does the superficial layer. The deep layer is attached to the medial meniscus nearer to the femoral than to the tibial condyle. (See Figure 12–10.)

The *lateral collateral ligament* is a thick cord-like structure extending from the lateral femoral condyle to the superior styloid of the fibula. It does not blend with the capsule of the tibiofemoral articulation. The biceps femoris attaches with the ligament to the head of the fibula, and the common peroneal nerve courses around the fibula just inferior to these attachments. Injuries to the lateral collateral ligament are thus likely to injure the biceps tendon and the common peroneal nerve as well. (See Figure 12–13.)

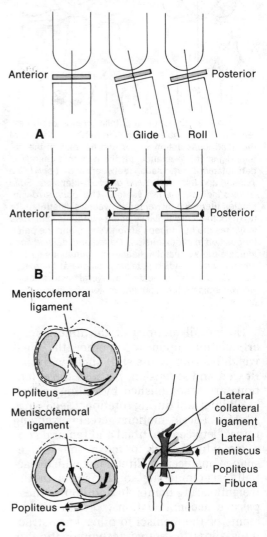

Fig. 12–12. Active accommodations of the menisci during knee movement. *A*, during flexion, the medial meniscus is pulled posteriorly over the medial condyle of the tibia by the medial collateral ligament. During extension, it is pulled anteriorly. The rolling motion of the tibia, rather than the gliding motion, creates these forces on the meniscus. *B*, during rotation, the medial meniscus is pulled posteriorly by internal rotation of the femur, and anteriorly by external rotation of the femur. *C* and *D*, during external rotation of the femur, the movement of the meniscofemoral ligament and the contraction of the popliteus muscle pull the lateral meniscus posteriorly and medially.

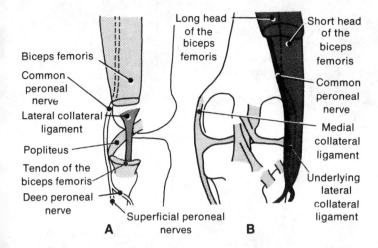

Fig. 12-13. Relationship of the common peroneal nerve to the lateral collateral ligament, the tendon of the biceps femoris, and the proximal end of the fibula. *A*, lateral view. *B*, posterior view.

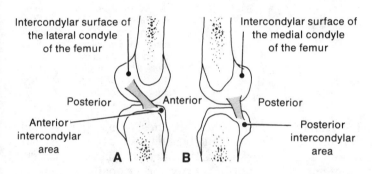

Fig. 12-14. Cruciate ligaments. *A*, medial view of the anterior cruciate ligament. *B*, lateral view of the posterior cruciate ligament.

The *anterior cruciate ligament* extends from the anterior intercondylar area of the tibia posterolaterally to the intercondylar surface of the lateral femoral condyle. The *posterior cruciate ligament* extends from the posterior intercondylar area of the tibia anteromedially to the intercondylar surface of the medial femoral condyle. (See Figures 12–10 and 12–14.)

The collateral and cruciate ligaments are most taut when the knee is in full extension. During flexion, while some of the fibers of every ligament relax, because of their orientation and because of the rolling action between the articular surfaces, some of the fibers of every ligament remain taut. These four ligaments limit joint play as follows:

Lateral angulation—medial collateral ligament followed by the anterior cruciate, followed by the posterior cruciate.

Medial angulation—lateral collateral ligament, followed by the posterior cruciate, followed by the anterior cruciate.

External rotation of the femur—medial collateral ligament and both cruciates together.

Internal rotation of the femur—medial collateral ligament, followed by the anterior cruciate, followed by the posterior cruciate.

The Synovium of the Tibiofemoral Articulation. The continuity of the synovial membrane is difficult to visualize from verbal description. Figure 12–15 illustrates the three-dimensional form of the synovial space and the lines of attachment of the synovium to the articular borders of the femur and tibia. Note that the patellar surface of the synovial capsule is sketched in dotted line. We suggest that the continuity first be studied without trying to imagine the reflections of the membrane off the patella. When the continuity can be visualized without the patella, simply imagine a hole in the anterior membrane wall, with the patella stuck into it.

Three relationships are clinically significant:

1. The synovial space extends as a sin-

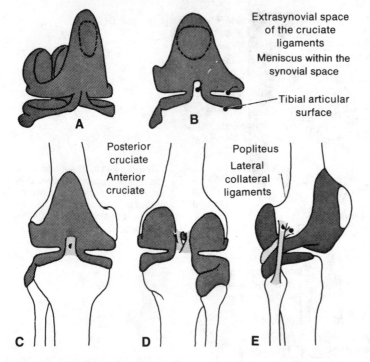

Extrasynovial space
of the cruciate
ligaments

Meniscus within the
synovial space

Tibial articular
surface

Posterior
cruciate

Anterior
cruciate

Popliteus

Lateral
collateral
ligaments

A B C D E

Fig. 12–15. Synovial space of the knee. Diagrammatic cast of the synovial space. *A*, three-quarter anterior view. *B*, full-face anterior view. *C* through *E*, the cast of the synovial space applied to the femur, patella, tibia, and fibula to indicate the margins of attachment of the synovial membrane to those bones.

gle sac superior to the patella, between the femur and the quadriceps tendon, and that single sac divides inferiorly into two sacs, each of which surround one tibiofemoral articulation. Thus, the patellar, the femoral condylar, the intercondylar femoral patellar, and the tibial condylar surfaces form the cartilagenous walls of the synovial space.

2. The menisci are included within the synovial space.

3. The cruciate ligaments are excluded from the synovial space.

The Tibiofibular Articular Surfaces and Their Relative Motions. (See Figure 12–16.) The head of the fibula includes an oval cartilagenous surface, 1–2 cm. in diameter, that faces anteriorly, medially, and upward. It articulates with a complementary cartilagenous surface on the posteroinferior aspect of the lateral tibial condyle. These surfaces glide slightly in all directions within the plane of the articulation.

The Capsule and Ligaments of the Tibiofibular Joint. The joint is surrounded by a synovial-lined fibrous capsule of modest strength. Its restraining influence is augmented by two tough ligaments: the anterior ligament which blends with the articular capsule, and the posterior liga-

ment which extends as a separate thick band medially and upward to the posterior surface of the lateral tibial condyle. The synovial cavity occasionally communicates with the synovial cavity of the tibiofemoral articulation.

Bursae of the Knee. Thirteen bursae have been described about the knee. Of these, five are of particular importance to the primary clinician (see Figure 12–17):

1. The *prepatellar bursa* lies between the patella and the skin.

2. The *superficial infrapatellar bursa* lies between the lower end of the patellar ligament and the skin.

3. The *deep infrapatellar bursa* lies between the lower end of the patellar ligament and the tibia.

4. The *anserine bursa* lies between the common tendon of the gracilis, sartorius, and semitendinosus (the pes anserinus tendon), and the underlying medial collateral ligament.

5. The *bursa of the semimembranosus* lies between the semimembranosus tendon and the medial head of the gastrocnemius. (Compare figure 12–17B with figure 12–4C.) This bursa may communicate with the synovial cavity of the knee joint.

Ossification Centers about the Knee.

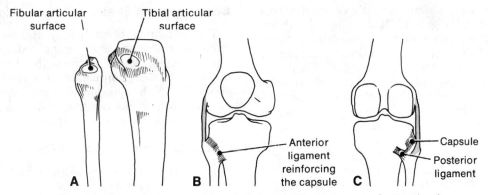

Fibular articular surface   Tibial articular surface

Anterior ligament reinforcing the capsule

Capsule
Posterior ligament

A   **B**   **C**

Fig. 12–16. Tibiofibular joint. *A*, views of the facets. *B*, anterior view. *C*, posterior view.

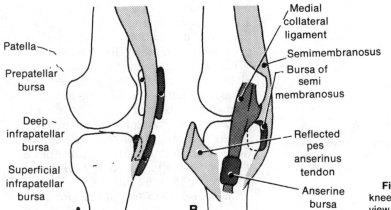

Patella

Prepatellar bursa

Deep infrapatellar bursa

Superficial infrapatellar bursa

Medial collateral ligament

Semimembranosus

Bursa of semi membranosus

Reflected pes anserinus tendon

Anserine bursa

A   **B**

Fig. 12–17. Bursae about the knee. *A*, lateral view. *B*, medial view.

Three ossification centers are of particular clinical importance to the primary clinician (see Figure 12–18.):

1. The *femoral condylar epiphysis* is evident at birth and completes ossification by the 20th year of age.

2. The *tibial condylar epiphysis* is usually evident at birth and completes ossification by the 20th year of age. This epiphysis includes the tibial tubercle as well as the tibial condyles.

3. The *patella* ossifies from a single center which becomes radiologically evident by the 6th year of age. Ossification is completed during puberty.

Disorders of the Thigh

Anteversion of the Femur

This fairly common developmental abnormality usually is noted by a child's parents during preschool years, when it becomes apparent to them that their child

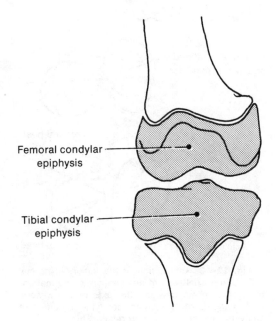

Femoral condylar epiphysis

Tibial condylar epiphysis

Fig. 12–18. Ossification centers of the condyles of the femur and tibia.

has an uncommonly pigeon-toed stance and gait. Figure 12–19 diagrams the abnormality. The earlier the problem is identified, the more likely is non-surgical correction possible. Non-surgical treatment makes use of night external rotation splints, like the Denis Browne splint. Failure to correct results not only in a cosmetic problem, but in increased wear on the weightbearing surfaces of the knees and ankles. The novice should follow the conservative regimen with an orthopaedist. The differential diagnosis of the pigeon-toed stance and gait is reviewed in Chapter 15.

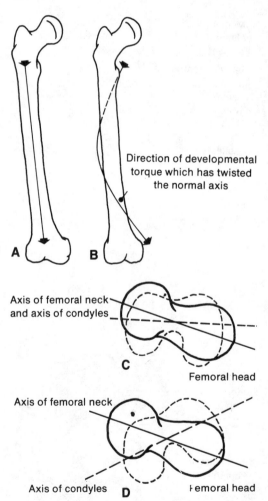

Direction of developmental torque which has twisted the normal axis

Axis of femoral neck and axis of condyles

C

Femoral head

Axis of femoral neck

Axis of condyles D Femoral head

Fig. 12–19. Anteversion of the femur. *A*, normal axis. *B*, the axial twist of anteversion. *C*, normal angular relationship between the axis of the femoral neck and axis of the femoral condyles. *D*, effect of anteversion upon that angular relationship.

Contusions and Strains about the Thigh

The principles of pathology and treatment of contusions and strains about the hip, see pages 195–197, apply without modification to the contusions and strains about the thigh. The muscles most likely to develop myositis ossificans are the adductor muscles and quadriceps.

Fractures of the Shaft of the Femur

These fractures are life-threatening injuries, typically accompanied by considerable bleeding into the thigh, and hypovolemic shock. Forces requisite to produce them are most violent and may impact directly on the surface of the thigh, or may apply torque or angulation to the thigh. Like hip dislocations, they occur most commonly in motor vehicle accidents.

These fractures are nearly always complete and markedly displaced, with overriding angulation and rotation of the distal segment on the proximal. Fractures may be transverse, oblique, spiral, or comminuted, and may be simple or compound. Deep femoral and perforator arteries and veins are usually torn and have bled voluminously into the thigh.

Characteristic Clinical Features.

1. The patient is often injured elsewhere as well.

2. The patient usually develops evidence of circulatory insufficiency within the 1st hour or 2 after injury.

3. Conscious patients will complain of intense thigh pain, which usually refers throughout the extremity.

4. Patients will not move the extremity.

5. The thigh is swollen, and that portion of the extremity below the fracture site is often rotated and angulated.

6. Tenderness, false motion, and crepitation are evident at the fracture site.

7. Anteroposterior and lateral x-rays of the thigh identify the fracture.

Treatment.

1. The patient must be quickly assessed for other injuries.

2. Hypovolemic circulatory failure must be aggressively treated with rapid intravenous infusion of saline and eventually of whole blood.

3. The fracture must be splinted, pref-

erably with a Thomas splint. (See Figure 11–33.)

4. An orthopaedist should be responsible for definitive treatment of the fracture. Straight traction will effect the reduction. Immobilization may be effected externally by supine traction (see Figure 12–20), or internally by an intramedullary rod. The rod cannot be used for comminuted long spiral or compound fractures. Immobilization must continue until the fracture is clinically stable, occasionally as long as 6 months.

5. Rehabilitation begins immediately with ankle exercise and active resisted exercise of the other extremities. Within the 1st month, quadriceps-setting exercises may begin. When the fracture is clinically stable, range of motion exercises and extension and flexion strengthening exercises must begin. Partial weightbearing begins as soon as strength and range of motion allow. Rehabilitation is lengthy and can be discouraging. The services of a physical therapist are usually necessary.

Role of the Primary Practitioner. Primary practitioners must serve their patients in seven ways:

1. Assess for attendant injuries and circulatory failure.

2. Administer intravenous fluids as necessary to restore circulatory competence.

3. Apply a traction splint as noted above.

4. Assess the patient's preinjury health status, discover current medications, and determine the time of the patient's last meal.

5. Admit the patient and notify an orthopaedist.

6. Follow the patient's convalescence, and manage all chronic and intercurrent illnesses.

7. When economically advantageous for the patient, assume responsibility for final rehabilitation after the fracture is clinically stable.

Non-Traumatic Pain Syndromes of the Knee

The Osteochondroses

Like the capital femoral epiphysis, portions of three ossification centers about the knee can undergo an aseptic necrosis of unknown cause. These processes usually begin at some time between the 10th year of age and the completion of growth.

Necrosis within the Tibial Tubercle (Osgood-Schlatter's Disease). The most credible current viewpoint postulates a stress fracture through the growth plate to be the initiating event. The characteristic clinical features are the following:

1. Pain during resisted extension of the knee and pain on kneeling. The onset is usually insidious.

2. Firm swelling and tenderness over the tibial tubercle.

3. A lateral x-ray may or may not show fragmentation of the tibial tubercle. The fragmentation is not evident early in the disease and may persist long after the disease has become asymptomatic. Therefore, the timely diagnosis is not a radiologic diagnosis.

Treatment.

1. The child must be instructed to avoid all activity requiring resisted knee extension—for example, climbing, running, kicking—until pain and tenderness have

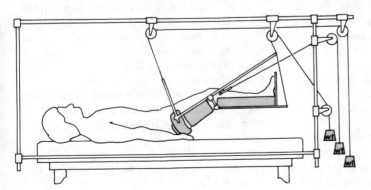

Fig. 12–20. Immobilization of shaft fracture of femur by supine balanced traction (Thomas splint with Pearson attachment).

fully remitted. This restriction usually must apply for 6–8 weeks.

2. When pain is severe, an injection of corticosteroid at the tibial attachment of the patellar ligament can produce a dramatic though incomplete remission of pain.

3. When pain persists after ossification is complete, surgical excision of the tubercle and reattachment of the patellar ligament may be necessary.

Necrosis within the Poles of the Patella (Larsen-Johansson's Disease). The initiating event is unknown. The characteristic clinical features are the following:

1. Pain during resisted extension of the knee and during kneeling. The onset is insidious.

2. Swelling and tenderness over one of the poles of the patella, usually the inferior pole.

3. X-rays may or may not show fragmentation of bone near the affected pole.

Treatment and prognosis are the same as those presented for Osgood-Schlatter's disease.

Necrosis within the Condylar Epiphyses of the Femur (Osteochondritis Dissecans). The initiating event is unknown. The characteristic clinical features are the following:

1. Aching pain in the knee at rest, worsened by weightbearing and causing a limp. The onset is insidious.

2. Physical examination may demonstrate a restriction in range of motion, but usually is otherwise normal. Rarely, an effusion will be evident.

3. Eventual extrusion of a fragment of the affected epiphysis will cause periodic locking.

4. Healing rarely restores a normal x-ray, and if the disease has affected a weightbearing arc, the patient may develop degenerative changes in that knee sooner than otherwise.

5. Anteroposterior, lateral, and "skyline" x-rays of the knee will usually demonstrate the characteristic radiopaque lesion.

Treatment. As the prognosis is unpredictable, the patient should be referred at the outset to an orthopaedist. A decrease or elimination of weightbearing may be prescribed, and the knee may be immobilized in plaster. Any loose body will be removed. Nothing can be done to insure restoration of a normal articular surface across the necrotic area.

Bursitis and Other Myofascial Pains

Prepatellar and Superficial Infrapatellar Bursitis. The prepatellar and superficial infrapatellar bursae are, to the knee, what the olecranon bursa is to the elbow. As such, they are vulnerable to the same forms of bursitis as is the olecranon bursa. The chronic form was classically called "housemaid's knee." The clinical characteristics, treatment, and prognosis of the various forms of prepatellar and superficial infrapatellar bursitis are identical to those of olecranon bursitis. The reader is referred to the discussion of olecranon bursitis in Chapter 5.

Deep Infrapatellar Bursitis and Anserine Bursitis. Weightbearing exercise of a duration and vigor to which an individual may be unaccustomed is occasionally followed by an acute inflammation of the deep infrapatellar bursa or anserine bursa, or both. Thus, the antecedent circumstances and the courses of these diseases are identical to those of subacromial bursitis (see Chapter 3).

Characteristic clinical features are the following:

1. Usually an adult complains of knee pain which began within 1 day of uncustomary weightbearing exercise.

2. An intense aching pain is present at rest and is worsened by resisted extension or flexion.

3. The pain is felt in the knee and may refer into the hip, thigh, and/or lower leg.

4. Swelling may be evident, and tenderness will be elicited deep to the patellar ligament, just superficial to its tibial attachment, or over the pes anserinus tendon. (See Figure 12–17.)

Treatment.

1. The patient is instructed to minimize weightbearing and to avoid resisted extension (no climbing, jumping, running, squatting).

2. The patient is encouraged to apply ice packs over the inflamed bursa four times daily.

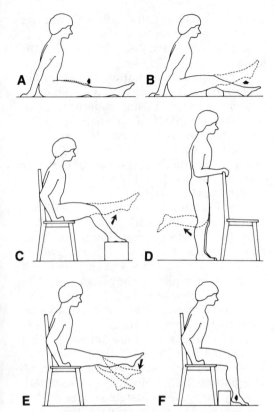

Fig. 12-21. Restorative knee exercises. *A*, isometric quadriceps exercise. *B* and *C*, isotonic quadriceps exercises. *D*, gravity-resisted isotonic flexion exercise. *E*, gravity-assisted isotonic flexion exercise. *F*, isometric flexion exercise.

3. Quadriceps-setting exercise is begun as soon as pain allows. (See Figure 12-21.)

4. Range of motion and full quadriceps drill are begun, as soon as pain and tenderness are fully remitted. (See Figure 12-21.)

5. A corticosteroid injection into the inflamed bursa can yield a dramatic remission. Oral anti-inflammatory agents may be prescribed, but these are less constantly and dramatically effective than is the local corticosteroid injection. (See Chapters 17 and 18.)

Baker's Cyst. An effusion into the semimembranous bursa results in a mass behind the knee which is called Baker's cyst. Because this cyst is rarely more than slightly tender, and often is accompanied by pathology that predisposes to a chronic effusion into the knee joint, and because the semimembranous bursa often communicates with the synovial cavity of the knee joint, it has been concluded that a common cause of Baker's cyst, rather than a primary inflammation of the bursa itself, is a passive collection in a communicating semimembranous bursa of a chronic joint effusion, caused by some pathology of the knee joint: arthritis, chondromalacia patellae, chronic meniscus tear, persistent capsulitis associated with instability secondary to a ligament tear.

A syndrome suggestive of primary acute semimembranous bursitis has been rarely encountered in our practice.

Characteristic clinical features are the following:

1. Patients complain of a mass behind the knee which may or may not be slightly tender, and of variable knee pain and dysfunction, which may suggest some other knee disorder.

2. A fluctuant mass, often 5 × 5 cm. in dimensions, is palpable on the medial side of the popliteal fossa, when the patient lies prone with the knee extended.

3. Clear serous fluid is readily aspirated from the cyst, causing it to collapse.

4. X-rays may or may not show evidence of degenerative arthritis.

Treatment.

1. The diagnosis is confirmed by aspiration, which removes the mass and usually relieves the patient greatly. Patients often fear that these masses may be malignant tumors.

2. The search for the cause of a chronic knee joint effusion: Inquire for more detail about knee symptoms, note range of motion, test patellar and tibiofemoral stability, examine for chondromalacia patellae and for meniscus tear, and x-ray for evidence of degenerative arthritis. Perform an orthopaedic review of systems, a general orthopaedic examination, and a sedimentation rate, should any points of history suggest a generalized arthritic disorder. (See below, "Protocols for the Evaluation of the Symptomatic Knee," and "Evaluation of the Non-Traumatic Painful Knee.")

3. When the underlying disorder is obvious, and its treatment is within the limits of primary practice, proceed appropriately. (See relevant sections in this text.) When no underlying disorder can be found, or when, if found, its treatment

requires specialty expertise, refer the patient to an orthopedist or rheumatologist, as appropriate.

Other Myofascial Pains. Non-traumatic knee pain may be associated only with tenderness of a collateral ligament, a flexor tendon, the quadriceps tendon, or the patellar ligament. In such cases, swelling is rarely evident, and tenderness is not confined to the area over a bursa, and the pain is usually not as immobilizing as is acute bursitis. When a careful examination demonstrates characteristics that fit that clinical picture, we diagnose a myofascial pain syndrome. Treatment is identical to the treatment of bursitis, except that any local injection of a corticosteroid is infused around the affected ligament or tendon. *Caution:* This wastebasket diagnosis, though very useful in primary practice, must be made with caution. An x-ray must have been made to exclude osteochondritis and neoplasia and an examination of the back and hip must have been made before this diagnosis can be entertained, and persistent knee pain in the absence of any diagnostic findings must be referred to an orthopaedist for evaluation.

Chondromalacia Patellae

Degeneration of patellar cartilage and occasionally of the articulating femoral cartilage as well is a common cause of knee pain in vigorous persons of any age. Individuals who have suffered direct impact injury to the patella or repeated lateral patellar dislocations may develop the disorder as a result of direct injury to the cartilage. However, the majority of persons who develop chondromalacia patellae have not experienced any recognized injury to the patella, and while wear appears to worsen the disorder, what starts it for the majority is not known. The lateral motion postulate was summarized above under "The Tibiofemoral and Patellofemoral Articular Surfaces and Their Relative Motions."

Characteristic Clinical Features.
1. A vigorous person complains of pain typically in the anteromedial aspect of the knee, abruptly worsened by efforts to climb, and particularly to descend, and gradually worsened by prolonged sitting

with the knees constrained in flexion, as occurs in most theater seats.

2. The patient may also complain of the knee suddenly giving way.

3. The knee examination is usually entirely normal, except for an occasional effusion, a pathognomonic tenderness under the lateral borders of the patella, and a pathognomonic pain when the patella is pressed upward along the patellar articular surface of the femur, while the extensor apparatus is lax. (See Figure 12–22.)

Treatment.
1. Many young adults maintain a flirting relationship with the disorder. They interrupt their most vigorous climbing or running activities with relatively inactive periods. While they never develop their full potential as athletes, they also keep the disorder somewhat at bay.

2. Other young adults are dissatisfied with such a compromise. They pose the greatest challenge to the clinician. When the patient first presents, the primary clinician should advise no climbing, running, or squatting, until pain has fully remitted. Usually such a remission occurs within 4–6 weeks. Hopefully, during that time, cartilage healing will have proceeded to a

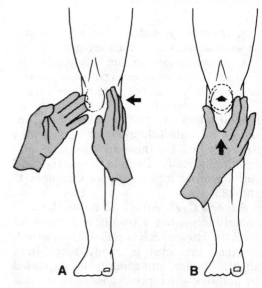

Fig. 12–22. Chondromalacia patellae. Examination for characteristic tenderness. *A,* palpation of the lateral margin of the patella. *B,* compression and elevation of the patella.

point that will allow pain-free resumption of the sport.

3. If young adults' sports are seasonal, they may manage to participate through the season without great handicap, provided they minimize patellar wear out of season. These adults should be advised to maintain condition out of season by swimming or bicycle riding, as these excellent conditioning activities are least wearing to the patellofemoral joint.

4. When such measures prove inadequate, the patient should be referred to an orthopaedist. Various surgical procedures have been designed to decrease the wear on the patellofemoral joint.

Degenerative Arthritis

The generalizations presented in Chapters 11 and 18 concerning degenerative arthritis apply as well to degenerative arthritis of the knees. Degenerative arthritis is most likely to develop in those who are genetically predisposed, or those whose articular surfaces have been disrupted—as may follow osteochondritis or a fracture of the tibial plateau, or misaligned—as may follow a malunion of a supracondylar or shaft fracture of the femur, or exposed to uncushioned weightbearing after removal of a torn meniscus.

Characteristic Clinical Features.

1. An older person or a young person who has suffered knee injury in earlier years complains of knee pain which is abruptly worsened by weightbearing, and may be gradually worsened by prolonged quiescence. If the degeneration has become complicated by loose bodies, the patient may complain of locking. Nearly all complain of moments when the knee gives way.

2. The knee may be distorted by bony spurs, or angulated due to an unequal wearing of the plateaus.

3. An effusion is nearly always evident. (See below, "Examining for Effusion," for a summary of the signs of knee joint effusion.)

4. Range of motion is often limited to an arc somewhat short of full extension and full flexion.

5. If the degeneration has followed from a ligament injury, the knee may be unstable in one or more directions of play. (See below under "Examination of the Collateral and Cruciate Ligaments" for a summary of the tests for instability.)

Treatment.

1. Patients must be taught how to minimize further wear.

a. Weightbearing should be minimized by decreasing the time on one's feet, and by using a cane in the opposite hand, as advised for arthritis of the hip.

b. A strong quadriceps muscle, through its control of the anterior capsule of the joint can greatly increase the stability of the knee, and thus protect it from the added wear of excessive joint play. The patient must be taught the proper execution of quadriceps exercises and must be instructed to perform these exercises to the point of fatigue, at least twice daily for life. (See Figure 12–21.)

c. Bracing with a knee cage may allow some individuals to engage in more weightbearing activity with less discomfort. A surgical supply house will provide a patient with a properly fitted knee cage.

2. Remissions from acute exacerbations may be accelerated by use of corticosteroid injections or oral anti-inflammatory drugs. (See Chapter 18 for review of the use and limitations of these agents.)

3. Ice or heat may be used for their analgesic effect during painful periods. Ice is usually more helpful during acute inflammatory relapses. Otherwise, heat is usually more helpful.

4. Patients should be referred to an orthopaedist when one's best efforts to implement a conservative regimen have failed to yield satisfactory results, when loose bodies are evident, or when a knee is unstable. Orthopaedists are gaining more experience with total knee replacements. Results may eventually prove as satisfactory as are the current results with total hip replacement.

Other Forms of Arthritis

Whenever a patient presents with an acute monoarticular arthritis, *pyogenic arthritis* must be excluded before any other consideration. (See below, "Protocols For

Evaluation of the Symptomatic Knee" and see Chapters 18 and 19.) Infection is excluded by arthrocentesis and Gram stain and culture of the aspirated fluid. Treatment is as advised in Chapter 19.

Rheumatoid arthritis, gout, pseudogout, gonococcal arthritis, and the less common forms of synovial disease are the other causes of monoarthritic arthritis of the knee. These disorders and their differentiation are reviewed in Chapter 18.

Knee Injuries

Injuries to the Extensor Apparatus

The quadriceps muscle and tendon, the patella, the patellar ligament, the patellar retinacula, and their associated bursae constitute the extensor apparatus. The contusions and strains of the quadriceps muscle were discussed earlier in this chapter. The following forces disrupt the extensor apparatus at the knee:

Direct Impact Forces. These forces are typically generated when an individual falls onto the knee or is hurled into a dashboard.

1. Contusions of the quadriceps tendon at its insertion on the patella and/or its merger with the patellar retinacula are fairly uncommon, as the area is not as exposed to impact as are the more distal structures of the knee. The injury presents as an indistinctly circumscribed swelling above the patella, which may be associated with fluctuance if bleeding has occurred into the suprapatellar bursa. Pain inhibits active extension.

2. Injuries to the patella and prepatellar bursa. Direct blows to the patella may contuse the patellar cartilage or fracture the patella. Such fractures are usually comminuted and may or may not be displaced. (See Figure 12–23.) The prepatellar bursa is always contused when these injuries occur. The bursal contusion presents as a hemorrhage into the bursa. These impact injuries to the patella thus present with circumscribed swelling over the patella and variable pain on lateral compression and manipulation of the patella. Pain may or may not inhibit active extension.

3. Injuries to the insertion of the patellar ligament. Direct blows to the insertion of the patellar ligament will contuse the superficial infrapatellar bursa and the patellar ligament at its attachment to the tibial tubercle, and may produce a comminuted fracture of the tibial tubercle. These injuries present with an indistinctly circumscribed swelling and tenderness over and just above the tibial tubercle. Pain may or may not inhibit active extension.

Indirect Distracting Forces. When extension is applied with abrupt violence, as can occur when kicking, leaping, or landing from a height, the resultant force may strain or rupture the extensor apparatus at some point. Strain is suggested by tenderness over the quadriceps tendon or patellar ligament when the anatomy is palpably intact. Rupture is suggested by one of the following clinical pictures:

1. The quadriceps tendon may be avulsed from its patellar insertion and from its merger with the patellar retinacula. (See Figure 12–23.) Such an injury is rare and presents as a depression just above the patella, a fluctuant mass about the depression reflecting hemorrhage into the suprapatellar bursa, and an inability actively to extend the knee.

2. More commonly, the patella may be fractured. The inferior pole may be avulsed with the patellar ligament, or the patella may fracture into two fairly equal pieces. (See Figure 12–23.) The injury presents with a fluctuant swelling, a palpable

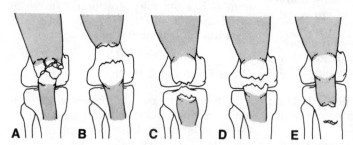

Fig. 12–23. Injuries of the extensor apparatus. *A,* comminuted fracture of the patella. *B,* avulsion of the quadriceps tendon. *C,* avulsion of the patellar attachment of the patellar ligament. *D,* transverse fracture of the patella. *E,* avulsion of the tibial attachment of the patellar ligament.

disruption of the patella, and an inability actively to extend the knee.

3. The patellar ligament may be avulsed from the tibial tubercle. (See Figure 12–23.) This injury prevails with a frequency midway between quadriceps tendon avulsions and distraction fractures of the patella. The injury presents as a distinctly circumscribed swelling about the tibial tubercle, an elevated patella, a palpable tendon defect when the knee is flexed to 90°, fluctuance above the tibial tubercle when hemorrhage has occurred into the deep infrapatellar bursa, and an inability actively to extend the knee.

Evaluation of Injuries to the Extensor Apparatus. When injury to the extensor apparatus is suspected, initial physical examination must be limited to inspection and palpation. Efforts to stress extension or to evaluate range of motion are capable of completing an incomplete rupture of the extensor apparatus and thus convert an injury treatable by closed reduction to an injury requiring open reduction. We induce those patients suspected of an injury to the extensor apparatus to attempt active extension of the knee only when the initial examination and x-ray fail to confirm or exclude a rupture of the extensor apparatus.

When injuries to the extensor apparatus are associated with bursal or knee joint effusion, anteroposterior and lateral x-rays of the knee must be obtained. A tangential view of the patella may show a vertical fracture line, missed by standard anteroposterior and lateral views. However, a tangential view requires that the knee be markedly flexed. Marked flexion may complete the rupture partially produced by distraction force. Hence, tangential views should not be obtained when an injury is suspected to have resulted from distraction forces.

Treatment.

1. When an injured extensor apparatus is intact, and any associated patellar fracture is undisplaced, closed methods of treatment are appropriate and should be applied by the primary practitioner.

a. A simple contusion or strain may be treated by rest and ice packs until active extension is nearly painless. Then quadriceps exercises (see Figure 12–21) and weightbearing to the point of tolerable pain can begin and progress as pain recedes.

b. When the prepatellar bursa is swollen and fluctuant, the bursa should be aspirated.

c. When manipulation of the patella from the sides increases any pain, or an undisplaced fracture of the patella is evident by x-ray, an injury to the patellar cartilage must be presumed, and the knee must be immobilized in full extension in cylinder plaster for 6 weeks. Isometric quadriceps exercise (see Figure 12–21) must be practiced several times daily while the extremity is casted. When the cast is removed, full quadriceps drill and active flexion exercises are begun (see Figure 12–21). Full weightbearing is allowed while the knee is immobilized. When the cast is removed, only partial weightbearing is allowed until at least 30° flexion is free and painless and quadriceps strength approaches that of the normal leg. Only walking is allowed until range of motion and quadriceps strength are fully restored.

2. When the extensor apparatus has been ruptured, either through the quadriceps tendon, through the patella, or by an avulsion of a patellar ligament from the inferior pole of the patella, or from the tibial tuberosity, the knee should be splinted in extension, and the patient referred to an orthopaedist for definitive treatment. Open reduction and internal fixation are usually required.

Recurrent Patellar Dislocation.

Certain anatomic peculiarities of the patellofemoral joint and the extensor apparatus predispose to lateral patellar dislocation when strong isometric extensor forces are applied to a slightly flexed knee (see Figure 12–24).

1. When the anterior eminence of the lateral condyle is relatively flat, it can no longer act as a constraining lateral guide to patellar motion over the patellar articular surface of the femur.

2. When the axis of the patellar ligament angulates laterally from the axis of the quadriceps muscle, a resultant lateral

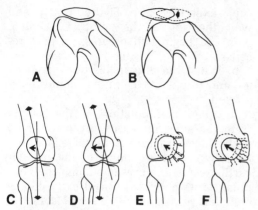

Fig. 12–24. Anatomic peculiarities predisposing to recurrent patellar dislocation. *A*, normal, distal end of femur. *B*, flat anterior eminence of the lateral condyle. *C*, normal lateral vector during active extension. *D*, excessive lateral vector. *E*, normal medial retinaculum. *F*, lax medial retinaculum.

vector tends to move the patella laterally during the last 30° of active extension.

3. When the patellar retinacula are relatively lax during active extension, they present little opposition to forces that tend to displace the patella laterally. When dislocation first occurs, the medial retinaculum is usually torn, eliminating any ability it had to oppose lateral displacement.

When all three peculiarities prevail, recurrent lateral dislocation is very likely.

Characteristic Clinical Features.
Acute Phase.

1. Patients commonly complain that their knee "gave way," "popped out," "dislocated."

2. The patella may still be laterally dislocated when the patient is first seen, but usually it has spontaneously reduced with the patient's first movement after the event. (See Figure 12–25.)

3. Whether the patella is still dislocated or not, the knee joint will almost invariably maifest an effusion of blood.

4. The medial retinaculum will be tender.

Between Recurrences.

1. Manipulation of the patella will show an unusually marked lateral mobility.

2. The patellar ligament may be noted to angulate laterally from the axis of the quadriceps muscle.

3. The patella often moves laterally more than the average during active extension.

Treatment.

The goals of treatment are two: to allow the medial retinaculum to heal strongly without any increase, and ideally, with a decrease in laxity; and to decrease the lateral vector of quadriceps contraction.

The first two or three dislocations can be treated by non-surgical methods, and the primary practitioner should apply them.

1. A persistent lateral dislocation is easily reduced if the patient can be encouraged to inhibit the quadriceps muscle. Once the quadriceps is inhibited, the patella can usually be moved back to normal articulation between the examiner's fingers. Occasionally, the patella will not pass over the lateral condyle in the position of extension. Under those circumstances, the examiner holds the patella as far anteriorly as it will go, while passively flexing the knee. Reduction usually occurs as the knee approaches 30° flexion.

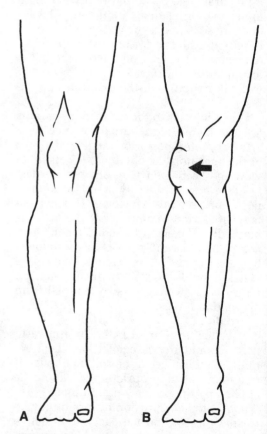

Fig. 12–25. Lateral dislocation of the patella. *A*, normal. *B*, dislocated.

2. A tense hemarthrosis should be decompressed by aspiration. A flaccid hemarthrosis need not be.

3. The extremity is immobilized in full extension in a full-length cylinder cast. As the plaster sets, the examiner displaces the patella slightly in the medial direction and holds it there until the plaster is firmly molded around the displaced patella. This position of immobilization should accomplish two things: give any injured cartilage its best chance to heal, and give the medial patellar retinaculum its best chance to heal strongly and tightly. Immobilization should be maintained for 6–8 weeks.

4. Full weightbearing is allowed in the cast, and isometric quadriceps exercises (see Figure 12–21) are practiced to fatigue several times daily. Once the cast is removed, only partial weightbearing is allowed until flexion is free and painless to 30°, and the quadriceps muscle nearly as strong as that of the normal extremity. Full quadriceps drill and active flexion exercises (see Figure 12–21) must begin as soon as the cast is removed. Quadriceps exercise must be done through the last 15° of extension as only in that arc is the vastus medialis maximally exercised. The stronger the vastus medialis, the greater its resistance to any lateral vectors.

5. An elastic knee support during strenuous activity may add further stability to the patellofemoral joint.

When a patella has dislocated more than three times, in spite of the above regimen, the patient should be referred to an orthopaedist. The orthopaedist will consider some combination of three surgical procedures: releasing some of the inserting fibers of the vastus lateralis, shortening the medial patellar retinaculum, moving the patellar ligament medially.

Sprains and Tears of the Collateral and Cruciate Ligaments.

The direct injuring forces to which the knee is most exposed are a combination of angulating forces which result in an abduction of the leg at the knee, with rotation forces that result in an external rotation of the leg at the knee. (See Figure 12–26.) These forces meet the resistance of the

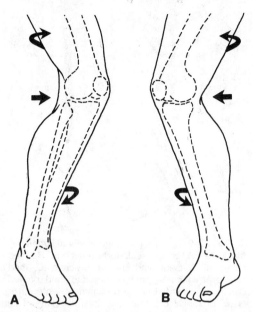

Fig. 12–26. The damaging torces acting on the ligaments of the knee. *A,* forces producing lateral angulation and external rotation of the leg (internal rotation of the thigh). *B,* forces producing medial angulation and internal rotation of the leg (external rotation of the thigh).

collateral and cruciate ligaments in a fixed order. Those structures which first receive the forces are those which are most frequently injured and those which are injured by the least force. Their order of vulnerability is as follows: the medial collateral ligament, the anterior cruciate ligament, the posterior cruciate ligament, and the lateral collateral ligament. (See Figure 12–27.) The knee is rarely injured by the opposite forces, perhaps because these are precisely the forces to which the ankle is most vulnerable.

The sciatic nerve and popliteal artery are at risk whenever a knee has been injured, particularly when it has been grossly angulated.

The knee injuries are discussed below in the order of decreasing frequency and increasing severity. All the injuries are typically athletic injuries. Skiers and all those who compete in team running sports are most vulnerable. However, nonathletes occasionally suffer these injuries when they step unwittingly into depressions, or when their downhill leg slips away from the axis of the body on ice or damp ground.

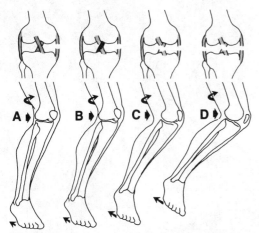

Fig. 12–27. Order of vulnerability of ligaments of the knee. *A,* medial collateral ligament. *B,* medial collateral ligament, and anterior cruciate. *C,* medial collateral ligament, anterior cruciate, and posterior cruciate. *D,* medial collateral ligament, anterior cruciate, posterior cruciate, and lateral collateral ligament.

Sprains of the Medial Collateral Ligament. Characteristic clinical features are the following (see Figure 12–28):

1. All patients will complain of immediate pain at the time of injury. The stoical may add that the pain eased somewhat as they walked about, and that they even resumed their sport for a time.

2. The morning after injury, all patients complain of a painfully stiff knee. Again, the stoics may add that walking about and exercising restored a useful range of motion, decreased the pain, and allowed them to resume their sport.

3. Occasionally, within a few hours after injury, and certainly by next day, a slight fullness will be evident over the medial collateral ligament.

4. The entire ligament will be tender, and often the femoral attachment will be the most tender.

5. Rarely, a serous effusion may appear in the joint between 12 and 48 hours after injury.

6. Stress to the medial collateral ligament will produce pain, but not excessive play. (See "Examination of the Collateral and Cruciate Ligaments.")

7. The remainder of the knee examination will usually be normal, though occasionally an associated meniscus tear will manifest itself by meniscus tenderness and

locking, and rarely sciatic nerve and popliteal artery injury will be suggested.

8. When an adult presents with this clinical picture, an x-ray need not be made. However, undisplaced epiphyseal fractures can present as collateral ligament sprains, thus an x-ray must be made when a child or adolescent presents with such a picture. See Chapter 15 for a fairly detailed discussion of epiphyseal fractures.

Treatment.

1. The stoics may be allowed to continue normal walking and to resume their sport when they are certain pain will not inhibit them and thus expose them to other injuries. Those who are immobilized by pain and stiffness should be supported in a posterior splint for 5–7 days and given

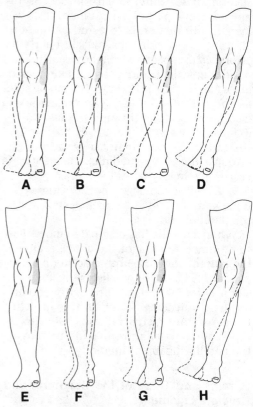

Fig. 12–28. Physical findings characteristic of ligament injuries. *Shaded areas* indicate areas of tenderness. *A* through *D,* knee in 15° flexion. *E* through *H,* knee in full extension. *A* and *E,* medial collateral ligament sprain. *B* and *F,* medial collateral ligament tear. *C* and *G,* medial collateral ligament and anterior cruciate ligament tear. *D* and *H,* lateral collateral ligament, anterior cruciate, and posterior cruciate ligament tear.

crutches for ambulation. (See Figure 12–29.)

2. The stoics may begin active range of motion and resisted quadriceps exercises at once. (See Figure 12–21.) The immobilized should begin isometric quadriceps exercises at once. (See Figure 12–21.)

3. The immobilized are required to remove the splint for active range of motion and resisted quadriceps exercise by the 7th day after injury. Weightbearing may then progress as tolerated.

4. Ice may be applied for comfort during the first 48 hours after injury. Thereafter heat will be safe and may be more comforting. Those modalities are particularly useful prior to exercise.

5. Evidence of locking which cannot be released or of sciatic nerve or popliteal artery malfunction requires a referral to an orthopaedist.

Isolated Tears of the Medial Collateral Ligament. Characteristic clinical features are the following (see Figure 12–28):

1. All patients will complain of immediate pain at the moment of injury, which persists and prevents weightbearing, or causes it to be disablingly awkward.

2. Within a few hours after injury, a joint effusion will usually be evident, and a separate fullness may be visible over the medial collateral ligament. Occasionally, the tear will extend through the capsule. This tear will permit egress of any fluid from the joint, thus preventing the accumulation of an effusion.

3. The entire medial collateral ligament will be tender.

4. Stress to the medial collateral ligament will produce pain and excessive play in abduction. (See "Examination of the Collateral and Cruciate Ligaments.")

5. The remainder of the knee examination will usually be normal. Occasionally an associated meniscus tear will reveal itself by meniscus tenderness and locking, and rarely sciatic nerve and popliteal artery injury will be suggested.

6. In the face of this clinical picture, an x-ray must be made. It may show an avulsion fracture from the medial femoral or tibial condyles, an associated compression fracture of the lateral tibial plateau, a fracture of the femoral condyle, or, in children and adolescents, an epiphyseal fracture.

Treatment. Increasing numbers of orthopaedists are convinced that all unstable knees should be explored, and torn ligaments surgically repaired. In our opinion, such a global view subjects too many people to a needless surgical risk and cost. In our opinion, when instability is barely evident, the knee not tenaciously locked, and sciatic nerve and popliteal artery function are normal, non-surgical treatment leads to optimal results. The primary practitioner should carry out the following regimen:

1. The joint effusion represents a hemarthrosis. When the capsule is tensely distended, the joint should be aspirated, as that decompression will relieve the worst pain. When the capsule remains flaccid, the joint should not be aspirated, as it will offer no further pain relief and carries some risk of infection. As joint bleeding usually continues for a day or two, the knee should be splinted in a posterior splint and examined daily. Recurrence of tense effusion requires repeated aspiration. Such treatment should continue until the effusion is stable and the capsule painlessly lax.

2. Once the effusion is table, and the capsule painlessly lax, the extremity should be x-rayed and immobilized in cylinder plaster in near full extension. (See Figure 12–29.)

3. Full weightbearing is allowed and quadriceps-setting exercises should be performed many times daily throughout the period of immobilization.

4. After 6 weeks, the cast should be removed, and the ligament tested for com-

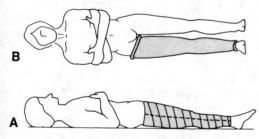

Fig. 12–29. Immobilization of ligament injuries. *A,* posterior splint immobilization of medial collateral ligament sprain. *B,* cylinder cast immobilization of medial collateral ligament tear.

petence. If competent, the patient must begin active range of motion exercises and full quadriceps drill to the point of fatigue, 2–4 times per day. (See Figure 12–21.) On first removing the cast, the patient must limit ambulation to partial weightbearing with crutches. As range of motion and quadriceps strength return, weightbearing may be increased.

When instability is quite obvious, or the knee is locked and cannot be released, or sciatic nerve or popliteal artery malfunction is evident, surgical treatment may well be indicated. The primary practitioner should aspirate a tense hemarthrosis once, apply a posterior splint, and admit the patient to an orthopaedist's care. The usual anesthesia and surgical clearance should be completed and documented.

Tear of the Medial Collateral and Anterior Cruciate Ligaments. Characteristic clinical features are the following (see Figure 12–28):

1. Stress to the medial collateral and anterior cruciate ligaments will reveal a gross instability. (See "Examination of the Collateral and Cruciate Ligaments.")

2. Other characteristics are those of the isolated medial collateral ligament tear with or without associated meniscus and condylar injuries.

Treatment. The ligaments must be surgically repaired. The primary clinician should aspirate a tense hemarthrosis once, x-ray and immobilize the extremity in a posterior splint, and admit the patient to an orthopaedist. The usual anesthesia and surgical clearance should be completed and documented.

Following surgery, the extremity is immobilized in a plaster cylinder for 6–8 weeks. Rehabilitation begins at once and is as outlined for tears of the medial collateral ligament. It may be advantageous to the patient for the primary practitioner to assume responsibility for final rehabilitation.

Tear of the Medial Collateral, Anterior Cruciate, Posterior Cruciate Ligaments (and, Very Rarely, the Lateral Collateral Ligament As Well). Characteristic clinical features are the following (see Figure 12–28):

1. The extremity often lies with the knee obviously abducted, and gross instability can be demonstrated with the least force.

2. The sciatic nerve and popliteal artery are particularly at risk when the extremity is grossly angulated.

3. Other characteristics are those of the medial collateral ligament tear with or without associated meniscus or condylar injuries.

Treatment.

1. Any evidence of sciatic nerve or popliteal artery dysfunction requires immediate referral to an orthopaedist.

2. When the sciatic nerve and popliteal artery function is intact, the primary practitioner may proceed as outlined for the tear of the medial collateral and anterior cruciate ligaments.

Postoperative immobilization and rehabilitation are as outlined for the tear of the medial collateral and anterior cruciate ligaments.

Meniscus Injuries.

Meniscus injuries are generally considered to be caused by rotation of the femur on a fixed tibia while weightbearing. Medial meniscus injuries occur during forceful extension from a position of flexion while the femur internally rotates on the fixed tibia. Lateral meniscus injuries occur during forceful extension from a position of flexion, while the femur externally rotates on the fixed tibia. (See Figure 12–30.) Lateral meniscus injuries occur much less commonly than do medial meniscus injuries. An anatomic basis for this lesser vulnerability of the lateral meniscus is discussed in the anatomic section of this chapter. Sprinting turns during evasive or pursuit running, or a quick turn in heavy snow when skiing, are liable to produce meniscus injuries. Note that in both activities the tibia is fixed while the femur rotates and the joint extends. When angulating forces are added to rotation forces during forceful extension, an ipsilateral collateral ligament and an associated cruciate ligament tear, or a contralateral plateau fracture, may combine with a meniscus tear. The medial meniscus generally tears longitudinally, and the lateral meniscus transversely. (See Figure 12–31.) Locking occurs if, once torn, a fragment of the

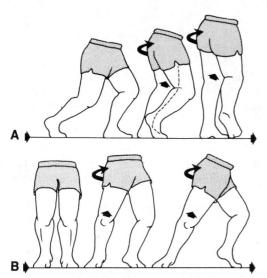

Fig. 12–30. The damaging forces acting on the menisci of the knee. *A,* forces which damage the lateral meniscus. *B,* forces which damage the medial meniscus.

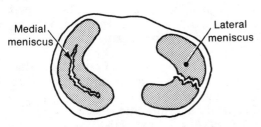

Fig. 12–31. Characteristic orientation of meniscus tears.

meniscus shifts centrally. At some point in the last 20° of extension, the space between the articular surfaces becomes too shallow to accommodate the meniscus fragment. Extension cannot proceed beyond that point.

Characteristic Clinical Features Are the Following:

A meniscus tear may be missed in the acute phase, particularly when associated with other injuries. Those who favor surgery for all unstable knees, base their opinion, in part, upon the fact of the hidden meniscus injury. We rebut this justification with the fact that some meniscus tears heal spontaneously and others rarely displace even though they do not heal, and that removal of the meniscus is inevitably followed, often within 10–15 years, by symptomatic degenerative arthritis in that knee, and therefore that early surgery, ex-

cept for the locked knee which closed manipulations have failed to release, is inappropriate.

The Acute Tear.

1. All patients will complain of immediate pain at the time of injury, which usually persists and prevents weightbearing or causes it to be disablingly awkward.

2. Within a few hours after injury, a joint effusion, representing a hemarthrosis, will usually be evident.

3. Tenderness is confined to the affected joint line, especially in its posterior arc.

4. The knee may be locked or lack full extension.

The Chronic Tear.

1. Most patients give a history of a previous knee injury, followed by repeated moments of giving way or locking. Occasionally, the patient will present when the knee is locked.

2. Occasionally, patients will add that with certain movements they will feel a clicking inside the joint.

3. Often, the affected joint line is tender.

4. A serous effusion may slightly distend the joint.

5. Rotary movements of the knee with the knee flexed may produce an audible or palpable click over the affected joint line.

6. A variety of provocative tests may reveal the tear. We recommend the Mc Murray test and the Apley test. (See below under "Examination for Meniscus Injury.")

Treatment. When suspecting a meniscus tear, the primary practitioner should proceed as follows:

1. Aspirate a tense hemarthrosis.

2. Manipulate to release a locked knee if necessary.

Occasionally, straight traction for several minutes with the knee as near full extension as is painless, will be rewarded by a reduction of a displaced meniscus fragment and return of painless full extension. When this maneuver fails, a less benign maneuver can be tried: Fully flex the knee and rotate the leg internally when dealing with a medial meniscus tear, and externally when dealing with a lateral meniscus tear. While maintaining the rotation, extend the knee with a firm controlled motion, not with a jerk. Release the rotation at the moment resistance is encountered. Reduction may be accompanied by a click and will be followed by a return of painless full extension. This maneuver may release the knee at the first attempt. If it does not, it may be repeated once or twice, but not more, as the maneuver itself can extend the meniscus tear.

3. If released, the knee may be immobilized in a posterior splint until the pain and effusion of any synovial reaction has subsided.

4. Rehabilitation should begin immediately as advised for rehabilitation of splinted collateral ligament sprains.

5. The patient must be instructed to report episodes of locking. Should such episodes prove numerous or at any point intolerable to the patient, the patient should be referred to an orthopaedist for consideration of surgical removal of the torn meniscus.

Fractures of the Tibial Condyles.

The same forces that can tear the collateral and cruciate ligaments can fracture the contralateral tibial plateau as well as tear the ipsilateral meniscus. (See Figure 12–26.) The lateral tibial plateau is fractured far more commonly than the medial. Until they tear, the stressed ligaments act as a fulcrum directing compressive forces onto the opposite tibial plateau. If the bone is less resilient than the ligaments, it will fracture before the ligaments tear. Osteoporotic individuals are more likely to suffer plateau fractures than torn ligaments.

Characteristic Clinical Features.

1. All patients will complain of pain immediately at the moment of injury, which persists and prevents weightbearing.

2. Within the first few hours after injury, the joint capsule will become tense with a hemarthrosis.

3. The fractured condyle will be tender and any manipulation which compresses that side of the joint will increase the pain.

4. Ligaments on the opposite side of the joint may or may not be tender.

5. X-ray will reveal the plateau fracture.

Treatment. The joint line must be restored as accurately as possible and, if the knee is locked, it must be unlocked. The primary practitioner should proceed as follows:

1. A tense hemarthrosis must be decompressed by arthrocentesis.

2. If the meniscus has been torn, the knee may be locked. Traction as described above should be employed in an effort to release the knee. If traction fails, no further effort should be made to release the knee.

3. If a fracture is minimally displaced (less than 3 mm.), the extremity should be immobilized in full extension in a plaster cylinder.

a. Immobilization should continue for 3–4 weeks during which isometric quadriceps exercises and active range of motion ankle and foot exercises should be performed several times daily. Thereafter, the cast should be removed, and gravity-assisted range of motion exercises should begin. (See Figure 12–21.)

b. Resisted quadriceps exercises and weight bearing greater than leg weight alone, should be deferred until bony healing is evident by x-ray—usually by 8 weeks.

c. Initial weightbearing must be partial and may graduate as quadriceps strength and range of motion return.

4. If the fracture line is excessively displaced (more than 3 mm.), the extremity should be immobilized in a posterior plaster splint and the patient admitted to an orthopaedist. Closed reduction may succeed for fractures of the entire condyle, but these fracture often, and central compression fractures always, will require open reduction.

5. In either case, the risk of degenerative arthritis is generally increased, and the patient must be warned of this new risk and the chance of mitigating the risk by decreasing weightbearing activity.

Fractures of the Condylar End of the Femur

The anatomic discussion under "Relationships of the Major Muscles and Nerves in the Thigh" (see above) pointed out the intimate relationship between the condylar end of the femur and the sciatic nerve and popliteal artery and veins. This relationship exposes those neurovascular structures to injury when the condylar end of the femur fractures. That fact, the relative rarity of these fractures, and the superficial resemblance of these fractures to any of the other causes of a hemarthrosis oblige the general practitioner actively to consider this injury whenever evaluating a traumatic hemarthrosis, lest an unwary manipulation result in a crippling neurovascular injury. Note how the protocol for the evaluation of the injured knee takes this necessary caution into account (See below under "Evaluation of the Injured Knee.")

Fractures of the condylar end of the femur usually result from axial compression forces, with or without angulation forces. Particularly in battle zones, direct impact of blunt or penetrating missiles is another cause of these fractures. The fractures in adults are of four kinds (see Figure 12–32):

1. and 2. Fractures of the medial or lateral femoral condyle. The axial compression forces, when accompanied by angulating forces, will usually fracture the condyle on the side of the angulation.

3. T- or Y-shaped intracondylar fractures of the femur. Straight axial compression forces may fracture both condyles at once, driving them proximally to each side of the femur.

4. Comminuted fractures. Straight axial compression forces may, and impact forces will almost invariably shatter the distal end of the femur.

Characteristic Clinical Features.

1. Except in the very osteoporotic, the injuring forces are violent.

2. All patients complain of pain immediately at the moment of injury and are unable to bear weight thereafter.

3. All patients present with a tense hemarthrosis.

4. Some patients present with shortening or an angular deformity.

5. The condylar end of the femur is uniquely tender.

6. Firm palpation of the condylar end of the femur often elicits bony crepitation.

7. Evidence of neurovascular injury may or may not be present.

8. Anteroposterior and lateral x-rays of the knee will identify the fracture

Treatment. The reduction must be precise, as any disturbance of the normal orientation of the condyles to one another will disrupt the joint mechanism and thus decrease the range of motion and increase the wear on the articular surfaces. Neurovascular injury requires immediate repair to avoid paralysis and/or ischemic necrosis below the knee. An orthopaedist and perhaps a vascular surgeon must assume ultimate responsibility for treatment. The primary practitioner should facilitate the treatment goals as follows:

1. Assume every hemarthrosis is a fracture of the condylar end of the femur until proven otherwise.

2. Examine sciatic nerve and arteriovascular function whenever the distal end of the femur is tender or crepitant.

3. Should a neurovascular injury be evident, notify a vascular surgeon and/or an orthopaedist at once, and insure that preparations are begun for surgery within the hour.

4. When neurovascular function is intact, admit the patient to an orthopadist and immobilize the extremity in Buck's traction. Insure that neurovascular function is monitored until arrival of the orthopaedist.

5. Complete the usual anesthesia and surgical clearance.

Epiphyseal Fractures

Children and adolescents may sustain fractures of the distal femoral or proximal

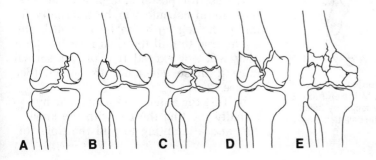

Fig. 12–32. Fractures of the condylar end of the femur. *A,* fracture of the medial condyle. *B,* fracture of the lateral condyle. *C,* "T-shaped" intracondylar fracture. *D,* "Y-shaped" intracondylar fracture. *E,* comminuted fracture.

A   B   C   D   E

tibial epiphyses. These fractures may present as stable or unstable injuries. Their evaluation, prognosis, and management are summarized in Chapter 15.

Methods of Examination

Examination for Sciatic Nerve and Popliteal Artery Malfunction.
Vascular competence may be tested by examining for pedal pulses and capillary return in the toes. Sciatic nerve function may be tested by requiring the patient to dorsiflex the ankle.

Examining for Effusion.
1. Ambulatory patients should be first examined with both knees flexed 90°. Inspect to either side of the patellar ligament. Moderate effusions will cause a bulging in these areas not evident in the normal knee.

2. With the knee fully extended and the extensor apparatus relaxed, compress the knee above and to either side of the patella, and attempt to subject the patella to ballottement with a finger. Sufficient effusion forces the patella away from the femur and allows ballottement. (See Figure 12–33.)

3. If neither of these observations suggests an effusion, attempt to flex the knee fully, unless suspicion of an extensor apparatus injury contraindicates it. A slight effusion is one phenomenon that can interfere with full flexion of the knee. If flexion is not actively resisted, any limitation in full flexion may well be due to an effusion.

4. Arthrocentesis is performed when indicated in the treatment protocols. A method of arthrocentesis is illustrated in Chapter 17.

Examination of the Extensor Apparatus.
1. The quadriceps tendon, the body of the patella, and the patellar ligament are palpated for defects and tenderness. If there is any evidence of a defect over the quadriceps tendon or the patellar ligament, or the body of the patella is tender or palpably fractured, an x-ray must be made. If the x-ray demonstrates a transverse fracture of the body of the patella, or avulsions from either the superior border or the inferior pole, or if the examination by palpation did demonstrate an apparent defect in the quadriceps tendon or patellar ligament, a rupture of the extensor apparatus must be presumed and further examination discontinued until orthopaedic consultation becomes available.

2. When there is no evidence of a rupture of the extensor apparatus, displace the patella laterally and medially to test for a retinacular tear or strain, associated with patellar dislocation or subluxation, and displace the patella proximally while forcing it posteriorly onto its femoral articulation, to test for pain associated with chondromalacia patellae. (See Figure 12–22.)

Examination of the Collateral and Cruciate Ligaments.
1. The area of each collateral ligament is inspected for swelling and palpated for tenderness. If injured, the entire ligament will be tender. (See Figure 12–34.)

2. The ligaments are stressed.

a. Test for posterior cruciate and postero-lateral capsule tear by internally rotating the leg with the knee at 45°, and attempting to pull the tibia forward. Joint play will not exceed that of the normal knee if those ligaments are intact. (See Figure 12–34.)

b. Test for anterior cruciate tear by externally rotating the leg with the knee at 45°, and attempting to pull the tibia for-

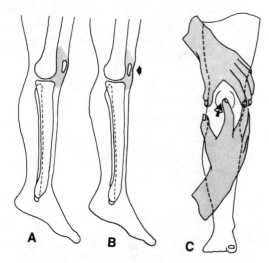

Fig. 12–33. Examination for knee joint effusion. *A*, patella forced away from the femur by the effusion. *B*, patella forced downward onto the femur by ballottement maneuver. *C*, illustration of the ballottement maneuver.

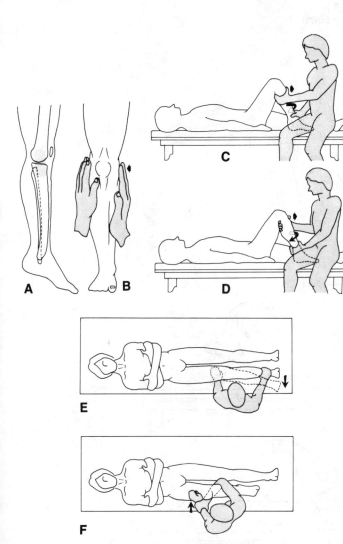

Fig. 12-34. Examination for collateral and cruciate ligament injuries. *A*, area of tenderness. *B*, palpation for tenderness. *C*, manipulation for laxity of posterior cruciate and posterolateral capsule. *D*, manipulation for laxity of anterior cruciate. *E*, manipulation for laxity of anterior cruciate and medial collateral ligament tear. *F*, manipulation for laxity of medial collateral ligament alone.

ward. Joint play will not exceed that of the normal knee, if the anterior cruciate ligament is intact. (See Figure 12-34.)

c. Test for medial collateral and anterior cruciate tear by attempting to open the medial side of the joint with the knee in full extension. If the joint opens, both ligaments are torn. (See Figure 12-34.)

d. Test for medial collateral ligament tear by attempting to open the medial side of the joint with the knee flexed 20°. This maneuver is most easily performed with a half-Nelson. (See Figure 12-34.) If the knee opens slightly more than the normal knee, a partial tear of the medial collateral ligament must be presumed. If the knee opens substantially more than the normal knee, a major or even complete tear of the medial collateral ligament must be presumed, and the possibility of an anterior cruciate tear must be considered. The findings of the previous test should bear on the question of an anterior cruciate tear.

Examination for Meniscus Injury.

1. The joint lines are palpated. Shortly after an acute tear or redisplacement of a chronic tear, the associated joint line will be tender. (See Figure 12-35.)

2. Palpate the joint lines while rotating the leg back and forth. A torn meniscus may cause a palpable click during this maneuver. (See Figure 12-35.)

3. Perform McMurray's maneuver: flex the knee fully, and with the leg externally rotated when testing for medial meniscus tear, and internally rotated when testing

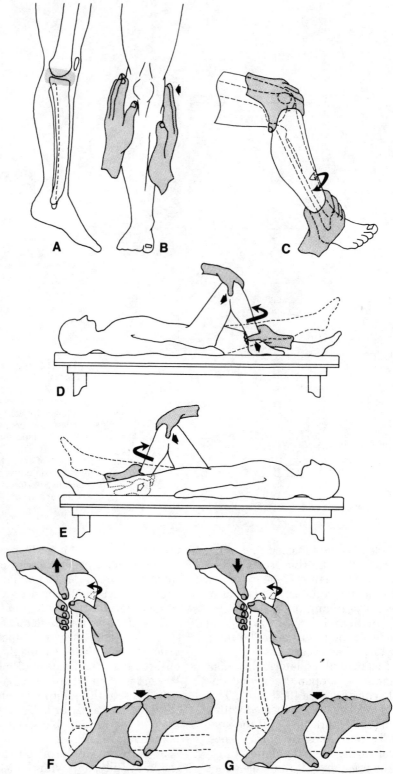

Fig. 12–35. Examination for meniscus injury. *A*, area of tenderness. *B*, palpation for tenderness. *C*, palpation for "click" during alternate internal and external rotation of the leg. *D* and *E*, McMurray's maneuver. *F*, Apley's maneuver; pain is compatible with ligament injury. *G*, Apley's maneuver; pain is compatible with meniscus injury.

for lateral meniscus tear, while maintaining rotation, extend the knee with a firm controlled movement. A painful click in early or mid-extension is very suggestive of a meniscus tear. (See Figure 12–35.)

4. Perform Apley's maneuver: with the patient lying prone, flex the knee to 90°. While applying upward traction on the leg, rotate the leg internally and externally. Pain during this maneuver is more compatible with ligament injury than with meniscus tear. Repeat the rotation while bearing downward on the leg. Pain during this maneuver is more compatible with meniscus injury. (See Figure 12–35.)

Protocols for Evaluation of the Symptomatic Knee

As the reader will have noticed, a variety of knee disorders can present superficially in very similar ways, though nearly every one has its pathognomonic feature. To facilitate recall and avoid errors of inattention, we recommend the following evaluation tables (12–1, 12–2) that should be learned and applied to every symtomatic knee. With experience, a practitioner may find short-cuts to these tables, but we advise the novice to follow them strictly.

Table 12–1
Evaluation of the Non-Traumatic Painful Knee

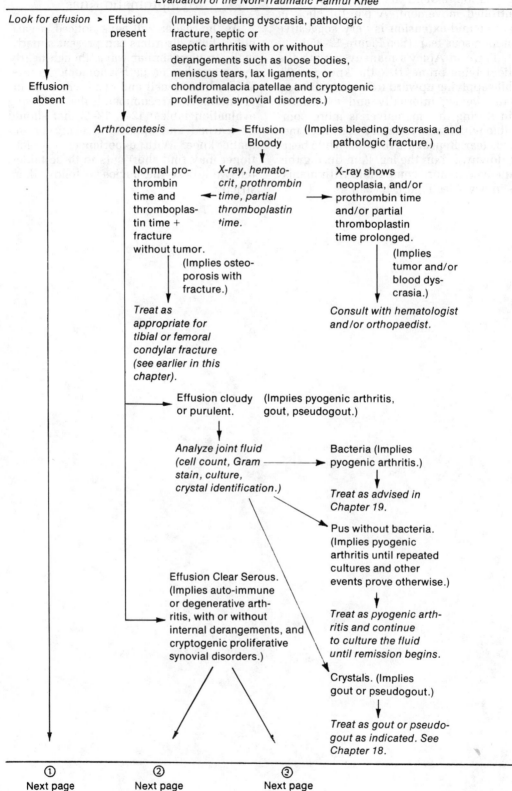

Look for effusion ➤ Effusion present (Implies bleeding dyscrasia, pathologic fracture, septic or aseptic arthritis with or without derangements such as loose bodies, meniscus tears, lax ligaments, or chondromalacia patellae and cryptogenic proliferative synovial disorders.)

Effusion absent

Arthrocentesis ➤ Effusion Bloody (Implies bleeding dyscrasia, and pathologic fracture.)

Normal prothrombin time and thromboplastin time + fracture without tumor.

X-ray, hematocrit, prothrombin time, partial thromboplastin time.

X-ray shows neoplasia, and/or prothrombin time and/or partial thromboplastin time prolonged.

(Implies osteoporosis with fracture.)

(Implies tumor and/or blood dyscrasia.)

Treat as appropriate for tibial or femoral condylar fracture (see earlier in this chapter).

Consult with hematologist and/or orthopaedist.

Effusion cloudy or purulent. (Implies pyogenic arthritis, gout, pseudogout.)

Analyze joint fluid (cell count, Gram stain, culture, crystal identification.)

Bacteria (Implies pyogenic arthritis.)

Treat as advised in Chapter 19.

Pus without bacteria. (Implies pyogenic arthritis until repeated cultures and other events prove otherwise.)

Effusion Clear Serous. (Implies auto-immune or degenerative arthritis, with or without internal derangements, and cryptogenic proliferative synovial disorders.)

Treat as pyogenic arthritis and continue to culture the fluid until remission begins.

Crystals. (Implies gout or pseudogout.)

Treat as gout or pseudogout as indicated. See Chapter 18.

①
Next page

②
Next page

③
Next page

Table 12–1 *Continued*

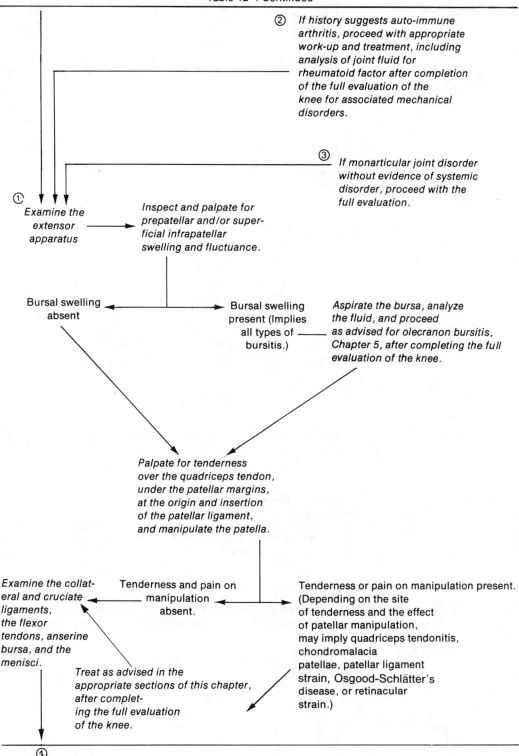

② *If history suggests auto-immune arthritis, proceed with appropriate work-up and treatment, including analysis of joint fluid for rheumatoid factor after completion of the full evaluation of the knee for associated mechanical disorders.*

③ *If monarticular joint disorder without evidence of systemic disorder, proceed with the full evaluation.*

① *Examine the extensor apparatus*

Inspect and palpate for prepatellar and/or super-ficial infrapatellar swelling and fluctuance.

Bursal swelling absent

Bursal swelling present (Implies all types of bursitis.)

Aspirate the bursa, analyze the fluid, and proceed as advised for olecranon bursitis, Chapter 5, after completing the full evaluation of the knee.

Palpate for tenderness over the quadriceps tendon, under the patellar margins, at the origin and insertion of the patellar ligament, and manipulate the patella.

Examine the collat-eral and cruciate ligaments, the flexor tendons, anserine bursa, and the menisci.

Tenderness and pain on manipulation absent.

Tenderness or pain on manipulation present. (Depending on the site of tenderness and the effect of patellar manipulation, may imply quadriceps tendonitis, chondromalacia patellae, patellar ligament strain, Osgood-Schlätter's disease, or retinacular strain.)

Treat as advised in the appropriate sections of this chapter, after complet-ing the full evaluation of the knee.

④
Next page

Table 12–1 *Continued*

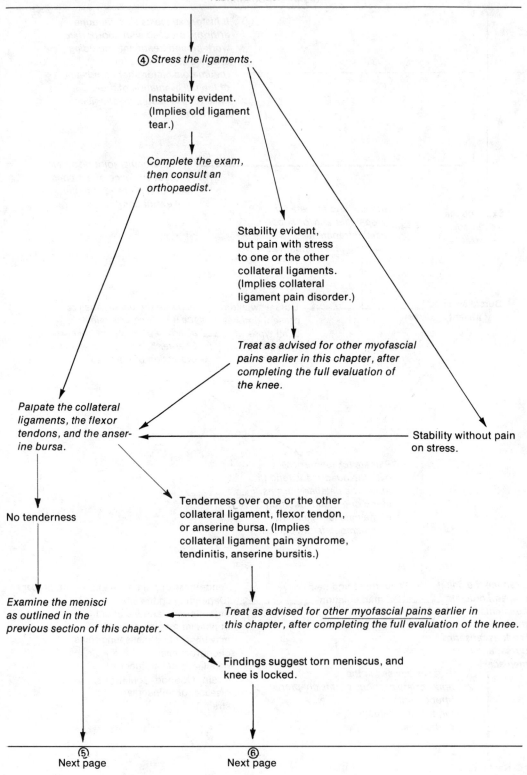

④ *Stress the ligaments.*

Instability evident.
(Implies old ligament
tear.)

*Complete the exam,
then consult an
orthopaedist.*

Stability evident,
but pain with stress
to one or the other
collateral ligaments.
(Implies collateral
ligament pain disorder.)

*Treat as advised for other myofascial
pains earlier in this chapter, after
completing the full evaluation of
the knee.*

Palpate the collateral
ligaments, the flexor
tendons, and the anser-
ine bursa.

Stability without pain
on stress.

No tenderness

Tenderness over one or the other
collateral ligament, flexor tendon,
or anserine bursa. (Implies
collateral ligament pain syndrome,
tendinitis, anserine bursitis.)

*Examine the menisci
as outlined in the
previous section of this chapter.*

*Treat as advised for other myofascial pains earlier in
this chapter, after completing the full evaluation of the knee.*

Findings suggest torn meniscus, and
knee is locked.

⑤
Next page

⑥
Next page

Table 12–1 *Continued*

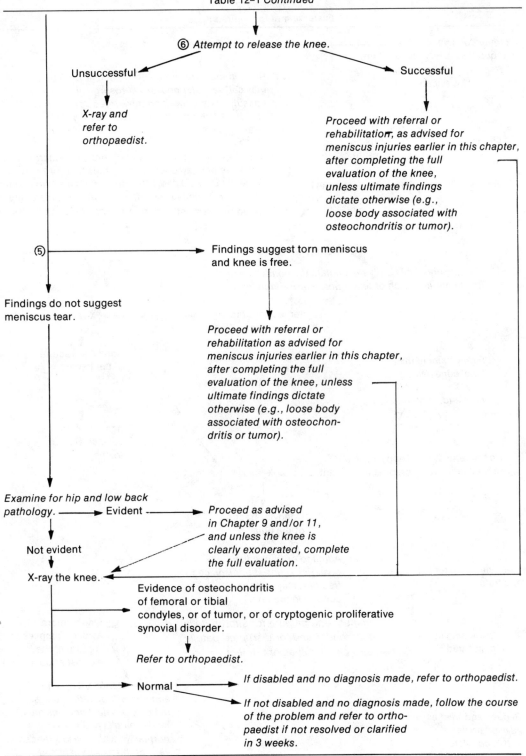

⑥ *Attempt to release the knee.*

Unsuccessful

X-ray and
refer to
orthopaedist.

Successful

*Proceed with referral or
rehabilitation, as advised for
meniscus injuries earlier in this chapter,
after completing the full
evaluation of the knee,
unless ultimate findings
dictate otherwise (e.g.,
loose body associated with
osteochondritis or tumor).*

⑤   Findings suggest torn meniscus
and knee is free.

Findings do not suggest
meniscus tear.

*Proceed with referral or
rehabilitation as advised for
meniscus injuries earlier in this chapter,
after completing the full
evaluation of the knee, unless
ultimate findings dictate
otherwise (e.g., loose body
associated with osteochondritis or tumor).*

*Examine for hip and low back
pathology.* ──────▶ Evident ────────▶ *Proceed as advised
in Chapter 9 and/or 11,
and unless the knee is
clearly exonerated, complete
the full evaluation.*

Not evident

X-ray the knee.

Evidence of osteochondritis
of femoral or tibial
condyles, or of tumor, or of cryptogenic proliferative
synovial disorder.

Refer to orthopaedist.

Normal ──────────▶ *If disabled and no diagnosis made, refer to orthopaedist.*

*If not disabled and no diagnosis made, follow the course
of the problem and refer to ortho-
paedist if not resolved or clarified
in 3 weeks.*

Table 12–2
Evaluation of the Injured Knee

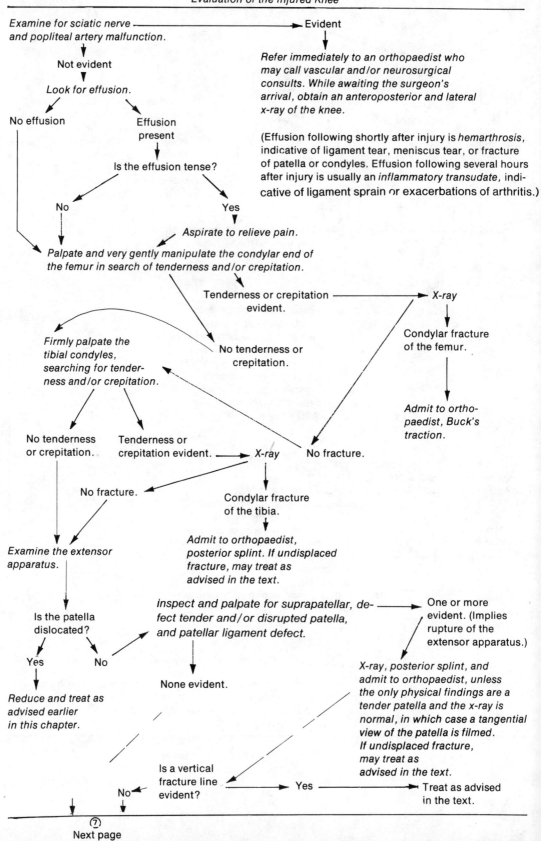

Table 12–2 *Continued*

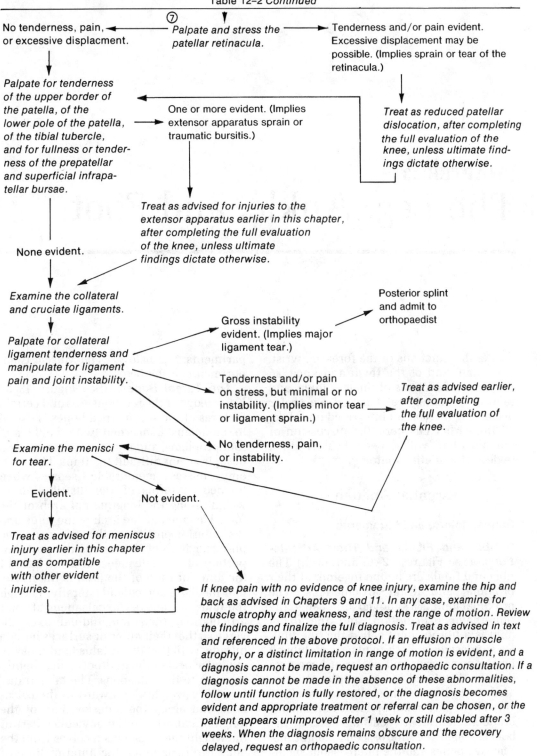

No tenderness, pain, ◄───── ⑦ *Palpate and stress the* ─────► Tenderness and/or pain evident.
or excessive displacment. *patellar retinacula.* Excessive displacement may be
possible. (Implies sprain or tear of the
retinacula.)

Palpate for tenderness
of the upper border of
the patella, of the ◄──── One or more evident. (Implies
lower pole of the patella, ───► extensor apparatus sprain or   Treat as reduced patellar
of the tibial tubercle, traumatic bursitis.) dislocation, after completing
and for fullness or tender- the full evaluation of the
ness of the prepatellar knee, unless ultimate find-
and superficial infrapa- ings dictate otherwise.
tellar bursae.

Treat as advised for injuries to the
extensor apparatus earlier in this chapter,
after completing the full evaluation
None evident. of the knee, unless ultimate
findings dictate otherwise.

Examine the collateral   Posterior splint
and cruciate ligaments.   and admit to
                                                                orthopaedist

Palpate for collateral   Gross instability
ligament tenderness and   evident. (Implies major
manipulate for ligament   ligament tear.)
pain and joint instability.
                             Tenderness and/or pain
                             on stress, but minimal or no   Treat as advised earlier,
                             instability. (Implies minor tear ─── after completing
                             or ligament sprain.) the full evaluation of
                                                                the knee.

Examine the menisci ◄────
for tear. ◄────   No tenderness, pain,
                             or instability.

Evident. Not evident.

Treat as advised for meniscus
injury earlier in this chapter
and as compatible
with other evident
injuries. ─────► If knee pain with no evidence of knee injury, examine the hip and
back as advised in Chapters 9 and 11. In any case, examine for
muscle atrophy and weakness, and test the range of motion. Review
the findings and finalize the full diagnosis. Treat as advised in text
and referenced in the above protocol. If an effusion or muscle
atrophy, or a distinct limitation in range of motion is evident, and a
diagnosis cannot be made, request an orthopaedic consultation. If a
diagnosis cannot be made in the absence of these abnormalities,
follow until function is fully restored, or the diagnosis becomes
evident and appropriate treatment or referral can be chosen, or the
patient appears unimproved after 1 week or still disabled after 3
weeks. When the diagnosis remains obscure and the recovery
delayed, request an orthopaedic consultation.

CHAPTER 13

The Leg, Ankle, and Foot

Like the functions of the forearm, wrist, and hand, and of the thigh and knee, so too are the functions of the leg, ankle, and foot so intimately related that we prefer discussing them as an integrated unit. Like all the earlier chapters, the discussion of the disorders will depend heavily on a review of essential anatomy.

Essential Anatomy

Bones, Joints, and Ligaments

Tibia and Fibula and Their Articulations. (See Figures 12–16 and 13–1.) The tibia and fibula are bound together at their proximal and distal articulations. The proximal joint is a synovial joint called the *tibiofibular articulation,* and the distal joint is a fibrous joint called the *tibiofibular syndesmosis.* Both joints are stabilized by strong anterior and posterior ligaments and the distal end by an additional interosseous ligament. These ligaments allow very slight play at both joints. A thin membrane stretches between the shafts of the bones, called the *interosseous membrane.* The two bones and the interosseous membrane are part of the barrier that separates the leg into anterior and posterior compartments. See below, "*The Muscle Compartments of the Leg.*"

The Tarsal Bones. (See Figure 13–2.) Knowledge of the relationships and certain features of the seven tarsal bones is useful to clinicians concerned with ankle and foot problems, and contrary to the general despair, is not difficult to attain. The anatomy makes memorable sense when learned in terms of the distribution of weight along the longitudinal arch of the foot. The apex of the arch is the *talus* and the anterior portion of the *calcaneus,* the posterior limb of the arch is the posterior portion of the calcaneus, and the base of the anterior limb of the arch is the *navicular* medially and *cuboid* laterally. Though the talus lies above the calcaneus at their articulation, their longitudinal axes diverge so that their anterior surfaces lie side by side, with that of the talus (and thus the medial aspect of the midfoot) lying slightly superior to the calcaneus. The talus transfers body weight downward to the calcaneus and along the anterior limb of the longitudinal arch to the navicular. Part of the weight the calcaneus receives from the talus it directs along the anterior limb of the arch to the cuboid, and part it directs along the posterior limb of the arch into its own posterior extension. The navicular directs its share of the weight further along the anterior limb of the arch to the three cuneiform bones (medial, intermediate, and lateral), and the cuneiforms direct the weight further along to the medial three metatarsals. The cuboid directs its share of the weight along the anterior limb of the arch directly to the 4th and 5th metatarsals.

The hindfoot and midfoot can be viewed as a distorted Y: The posterior portion of the calcaneus forms the base of the Y; the anterior portion of the calcaneus and the cuboid form one limb of the Y; and the anterior portion of the talus, the navicular, and the three cuneiforms, form the other limb of the Y; the articulation between the talus and calcaneus forms the intersection between the base and the two limbs of the Y.

Epiphyses of Clinical Importance. (See Figure 13–3.) *The distal epiphyses of the tibia and fibula* become radiologically visible by the 2nd year of age and unite with their shafts between the 18th and 20th years of age. These epiphyses are vulnerable to injury in childhood and early adolescence. (See below under "Fractures of the Shafts of the Tibia and Fibula," and see Chapter 15.) The calcaneus regularly ossifies from two centers, the large metaphysis and the thin posterior epiphysis. This epiphysis becomes radiologically visible by the 10th year of age and unites with the metaphysis shortly after puberty. It can undergo a painful degeneration, called Sever's disease. (See below, form 8 under "Heel and Ankle Pain.") The posterior process of the talus occasionally ossifies separately from the rest of the talus, and appears on x-ray as a fragment, confused by the novice for a fracture. This anatomic variant is called the os trigonum.

The Ankle Joint (Tibiotalar or Talocrural or Mortice Joint). (See Figure 13–1.) Orthopaedists have been called carpenters, and some of their forebears applied carpenter's terms to their work, when the terms applied. They applied particularly well to the ankle joint which has been called a *mortice joint*. The distal ends of the tibia and fibula form an arch called the *mortice*, into which articulates its *tenon*, the talus. The talus is a dynamic tenon

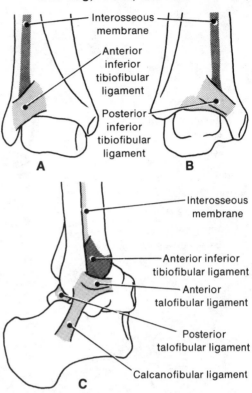

Fig. 13–1. Distal tibiofibular joint and tibiotalar joint. *A*, anterior view. *B*, posterior view. *C*, lateral view.

which fits its mortice variably tightly. As its anterior portion is wider than its posterior portion, it fits most tightly when the ankle is dorsiflexed and rather loosely when plantarflexed. The ankle is clearly more stable when dorsiflexed and more mobile when plantarflexed. The joint is surrounded by a thin, fibrous, and synovial capsule. Its articulating surfaces are cartilagenous. Seven ligaments maintain the stability of the ankle joint. The *interosseous and the anterior and posterior tibiofibular ligaments* maintain the width of the mortice. When they are torn, the mortice widens, and it no longer fits is tenon, the talus. The *deltoid ligament*, a strong fan-shaped ligament medially, and the three lateral ligaments, the *anterior and posterior talofibular*, and the *calcaneofibular ligaments*, hold the talar tenon within its mortice. To the degree that they are torn, the talus rocks unstably in the mortice.

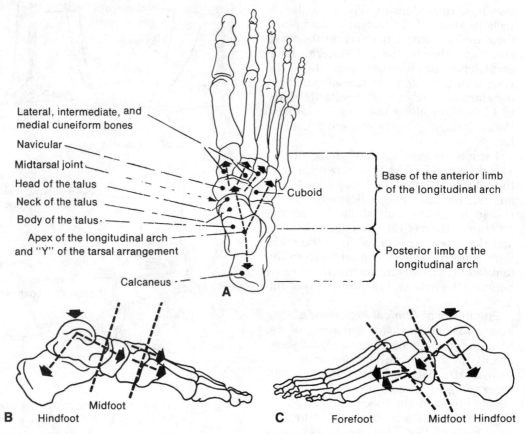

Lateral, intermediate, and
medial cuneiform bones

Navicular

Midtarsal joint

Head of the talus

Neck of the talus

Body of the talus

Apex of the longitudinal arch
and "Y" of the tarsal arrangement

Calcaneus

Cuboid

Base of the anterior limb
of the longitudinal arch

Posterior limb of the
longitudinal arch

A

B Hindfoot Midfoot

C Forefoot Midfoot Hindfoot

Fig. 13–2. The tarsal bones and the dispersion of weight throughout the foot. *A,* superior view. *B,* medial view. *C,* lateral view.

The Talocalcaneal Articulations. (See Figure 13–4.) The talus and calcaneus articulate through two joints, the posterior *subtalar joint* and the anterior *talocalcaneonavicular joint.* The two joints are separated from one another by a thickened interarticular fusion of their capsules, called the *interosseous talocalcaneal ligament,* which extends vertically between the bones in the tarsal canal. The sinus tarsi is a funnel-shaped lateral depression between the bones, which provides direct access to the tarsal canal. The sinus tarsi is palpable just anterior and inferior to the tip of the fibula, particularly when the heel is inverted.

The *subtalar joint* inclines anteriorly and inferiorly. The talocalcaneal portion of the talocalcaneonavicular joint inclines anteriorly, inferiorly, and medially. These inclinations tend to guide the weighted talus toward an anteromedial slip which is opposed only by the talocalcaneal liga-

ments. Much of the current understanding of chronic foot strain is based on the fact of this "talar slip." (See Figure 13–25.)

The Talonavicular Articulation. (See Figure 13–5.) The convex anterior pole of the talus articulates with the concave posterior surface of the navicular to form a shallow ball-and-socket joint, the talonavicular portion of the talocalcaneonavicular joint. This joint is the highest point on the medial side of the anterior limb of the longitudinal arch of the foot. As such, it is subject to severe shearing stress, particularly severe when weight applies through a dorsiflexed ankle and a pronated foot. Such directed forces tend to dislodge the talus plantarly out of articulation with the navicular. Two structures oppose this disaster:

1. The *plantar calcaneonavicular ligament,* also called the spring ligament (another carpenter's term), which cradles the talus and forms a portion of the articular

surface, which receives the anterior pole of the talus;

2. The tendon of the tibialis posterior, a supinator, which passes beneath (superficial to) the plantar calcaneonavicular ligament.

As will be emphasized again in the clinical sections, strong supinator forces protect against chronic foot strain in two ways:

1. Supinating forces also invert the heel, which decreases the medial inclination of the talocalcaneal articulation, and the tendency to talar slip.

2. Supination forces oppose the strain on the talonavicular joint.

The Calcaneocuboid Articulation. (See Figure 13–5.) The concavoconvex surfaces of the anterior pole of the calcaneus and posterior surface of the cuboid form a shallow saddle joint. This joint is the highest point on the lateral side of the anterior limb of the longitudinal arch of the foot. As such, like the talonavicular joint, it is subject to shearing forces, which would dislocate the joint were it not strongly stabilized by several dorsal and plantar ligaments.

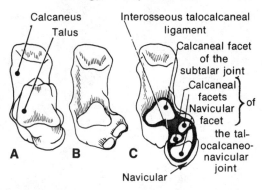

Fig. 13–4. Talocalcaneal articulation. *A,* superior view of the talus on the calcaneus. *B,* superior view of the calcaneus. *C,* superior view of the calcaneus, navicular, and talocalcaneonavicular ligaments.

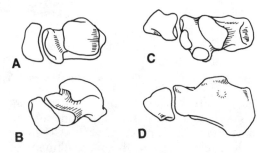

Fig. 13–5. *A* and *B,* talonavicular articulation. *A,* superior view. *B,* medial view. *C* and *D,* calcaneocuboid articulation. *C,* superior view. *D,* lateral view.

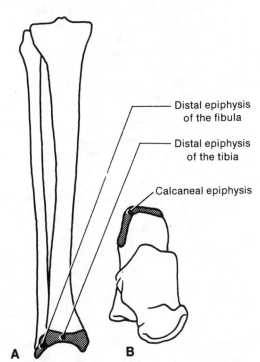

Fig. 13–3. Epiphyses of clinical importance at the ankle and hindfoot. *A,* anterior view of the ankle. *B,* superior view of the hindfoot.

Distal epiphysis of the fibula

Distal epiphysis of the tibia

Calcaneal epiphysis

The Midtarsal Joint. (See Figure 13–2.) The talonavicular and calcaneocuboid joints form together this articular plane, which is the nominal separation between the midfoot and the hindfoot. The reader will recall that the talonavicular joint is a ball-and-socket joint, and the calcaneocuboid joint a saddle joint. Both kinds of joints allow circular motion. Thus, the movement of the midfoot and forefoot on the hindfoot, though small, can be circular. The following terms are applied to this movement: plantarflexion, dorsiflexion, supination (inversion and adduction), and pronation (eversion and abduction).

The Midfoot. (See Figure 13–2.) The *cuneonavicular, cubonavicular, cuneocuboid,* and *intercuneiform* joints are much less mobile than the transverse tarsal joint, and are rarely of clinical importance. The *navicular bone,* however, is not so immune: (See below under "Midfoot Pain.")

1. The point of attachment of the posterior tibialis tendon to its medial surface

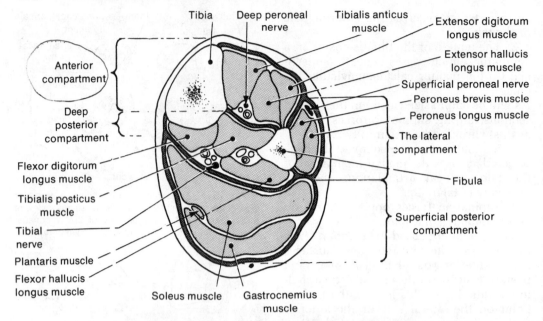

Fig. 13–6. Muscle compartments of the leg in cross section.

may ossify separately and stand as a sesamoid bone medial to the body of the navicular. This anatomic variant is more vulnerable to strain at the attachment of the posterior tibialis tendon.

2. In childhood, the navicular may undergo aseptic necrosis.

The Tarsometatarsal Articulation. (See Figure 13–2.) The metatarsals articulate with the tarsal bones by three joints: the joint between the 1st metatarsal and the medial cuneiform, the joint between the 2nd and 3rd metatarsals and the intermediate and lateral cuneiforms, and the joint between the 4th and 5th metatarsals and the cuboid. The medial two joints allow for very little motion and are rarely of clinical significance. The lateralmost joint allows for modest range of motion in eversion and in dorsal and plantar flexion. This joint is often sprained.

The Metatarsophalangeal (MP) and Interphalangeal (IP) Articulations. The structure and the relationships of these joints to supporting ligaments and controlling tendons are very similar to those of the hand. The differences are clinically unimportant.

The Neuromuscular Organization

Muscle Compartments of the Leg. The bones and muscles of the leg are surrounded by a strong fascial sheath called the *crural fascia.* This fascial sheath is densely adherent to muscles and tibia anteriorly, and loosely adherent to muscles posteriorly. Three fibrous septa which extend inward from the crural fascia, with the interosseous membrane, divide the leg into four compartments: the anterior compartment, the lateral compartment, the deep posterior compartment, and the superficial posterior compartment. (See Figure 13–6.)

The Nerves of the Leg. (See Figure 13–7.) The sciatic nerve divides into the *common peroneal* and *tibial nerves* on the popliteal surface of the femur, superficial to the popliteal artery and vein. The *common peroneal nerve* passes laterally to divide into the *superficial and deep peroneal nerves,* either anterior or posterior to the head of the fibula. When the division occurs posterior to the fibula, the superficial peroneal nerve passes directly distally in the lateral compartment, and the deep peroneal nerve rounds the fibula from posterior to anterior, to pass distally in the anterior compartment. When the division occurs anterior to the fibula, both branches pass directly distally in their respective compartments. The deep peroneal nerve, when the division is posterior, or the common peroneal nerve when the division is anterior, is palpable and vulnerably superficial as it rounds the neck of the fibula. The tibial nerve passes medially between the two femoral attachments of the gastrocnemius muscle to continue distally in the deep posterior compartment. These nerves share the cutaneous innervation of the leg and foot, as illustrated in Figure 13–8.

The Muscles of the Leg and Their Innervations. The muscles of the *anterior compartment* are the dorsiflexors of the

ankle and toes. (See Figure 13–9A.) They are all innervated by the deep peroneal nerve. The *tibialis anterior* is the most medial of the muscles. It takes long origin from the tibia and intermuscular septum, and ends in a tendon that crosses the anteromedial aspect of the ankle to insert on the plantar surface of the medial cuneiform and base of the 1st metatarsal. The *extensor hallucis longus* takes origin from the fibula and intermuscular septum and crosses medially to lie posterior to the belly

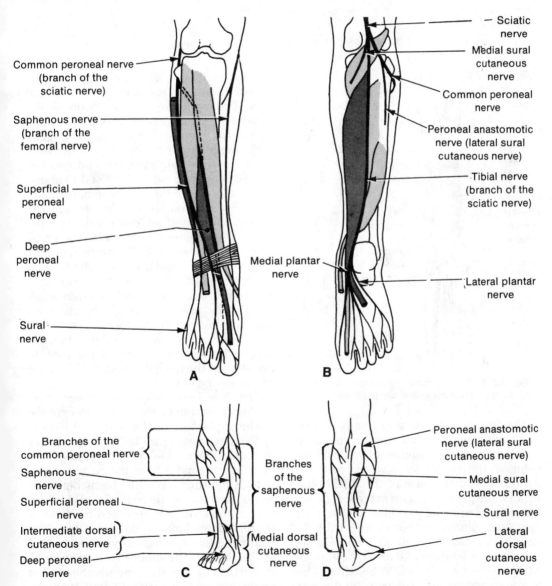

Fig. 13–7. Nerves of the leg. *A* and *B*, major divisions. *A*, anterior view. *B*, posterior view. *C* and *D*, cutaneous nerves of the leg. *C*, anterior view. *D*, posterior view.

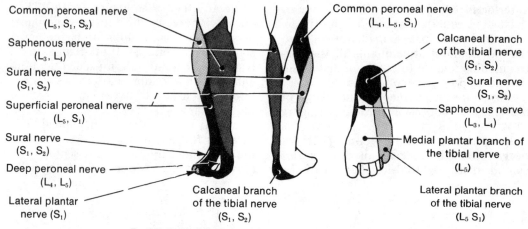

Common peroneal nerve
(L_5, S_1, S_2)

Saphenous nerve
(L_3, L_4)

Sural nerve
(S_1, S_2)

Superficial peroneal nerve
(L_5, S_1)

Sural nerve
(S_1, S_2)

Deep peroneal nerve
(L_4, L_5)

Lateral plantar
nerve (S_1)

Calcaneal branch
of the tibial nerve
(S_1, S_2)

Common peroneal nerve
(L_4, L_5, S_1)

Calcaneal branch
of the tibial nerve
(S_1, S_2)

Sural nerve
(S_1, S_2)

Saphenous nerve
(L_3, L_4)

Medial plantar branch of
the tibial nerve
(L_5)

Lateral plantar branch
of the tibial nerve
(L_5 S_1)

Fig. 13–8. Distribution of the cutaneous nerves of the leg.

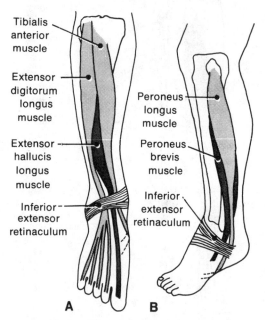

Tibialis
anterior
muscle

Extensor
digitorum
longus
muscle

Extensor
hallucis
longus
muscle

Inferior
extensor
retinaculum

Peroneus
longus
muscle

Peroneus
brevis
muscle

Inferior
extensor
retinaculum

A   **B**

Fig. 13–9. *A*, muscles of the anterior compartment. *B*, muscles of the lateral compartment.

of the tibialis anterior, and finally to end in a long tendon which crosses the ankle just lateral to the tendon of the tibialis anterior and passes distally to insert on the dorsum of the base of the distal phalanx of the great toe. The *extensor digitorum longus* and the *peroneus tertius* take long and common origin from the fibula and intermuscular septum, separate as they become tendons and cross the anterolateral aspect of the ankle together. The peroneus tertius inserts upon the dorsum of the base of the 4th and 5th metatarsals,

and the extensor digitorum longus divides into four tendons, one to each of the lateral toes. The structure and insertion of the extensor tendons at the toes is very like that of the extensor tendons to the fingers: they divide into a central slip to the base of the intermediate phalanx, and two lateral slips to the base of the distal phalanx.

The muscles of the *lateral compartment*, the *peroneus longus* and *brevis*, are the pronators of the foot and everters of the ankle. (See Figure 13–9*B*.) Both are innervated by the superficial peroneal nerve. Both originate (usually separately) from the lateral surface of the fibula, and pass as separate tendons around the lateral malleolus. The peroneus brevis inserts upon the base of the 5th metatarsal. The peroneus longus rounds the cuboid to pass across the plantar surface of the foot, to insert upon the medial cuneiform and base of the 1st metatarsal.

The three long muscles of the *deep posterior compartment* are the inverters of the ankle, supinators of the foot, and flexors of the toes. (See Figure 13–10*A*.) The *flexor hallucis longus*, the most lateral of the muscles, originates from the posterior surface of the fibula, rounds the medial malleolus, and passes through the plantar aspect of the foot, to insert upon the base of the distal phalanx of the great toe. The *flexor digitorum longus*, the most medial of the muscles, originates from the posterior aspect of the tibia, rounds the medial malleolus, and divides into four tendons, which pass through the plantar aspect of the foot to insert upon the bases of the distal phalanges of the four lateral toes. The *tibialis posterior* originates between the two flexor muscles from the tibia, fibula, and interosseous membrane, rounds the medial malleolus, and inserts upon the plantar medial surface of the navicular, the plantar surfaces of the cuneiform bones and the bases of the 2nd, 3rd, and 4th metatarsals. A fourth muscle is the short *popliteus* which originates between the fibrous and synovial capsules of the knee joint from the lateral femoral condyle and the lateral meniscus, and crosses medially to insert into the posterior surface of the upper end of the tibia. Its rotating action and its traction on the lateral meniscus facilitate knee motion in the last few degrees of extension.

The large muscles of the *superficial posterior compartment* are the strong plantar flexors of the ankle. They are the *gastrocnemius* and *soleus*. (See Figure 13–10B.) The more superficial of the two, the *gastrocnemius*, originates by two attachments, one from each femoral condyle, and the deeper *soleus* originates from a broad attachment to the upper third of the tibia and fibula. Both merge to form the *achilles* tendon which inserts upon the calcaneus. Crossing between the soleus and gastrocnemius from its origin upon

the lateral femoral condyle to its insertion with the fibers of the achilles tendon is the vestigeal *plantaris* muscle and its long narrow tendon.

The muscles of the deep and superficial posterior compartments are all innervated by branches of the tibial nerve.

The Retinacula of the Ankle. Four transverse thickenings of the crural fascia hold the long tendons to the foot in positions of mechanical advantage as they cross the angles of the ankle (see Figure 13–11):

1. The *inferior extensor retinaculum* binds the tendons of the anterior compartment and the *deep peroneal nerve.*

2. The *flexor retinaculum* binds the tendons of the deep posterior compartment and the *tibial nerves.*

3 and 4. The *superior and inferior peroneal retinacula* bind the tendons of the lateral compartment.

The long tendons of the ankle are sheathed as they pass through the retinacula. The relationship of the tendons to each other at the ankle is illustrated in Figure 13–11.

The Fascia, Intrinsic Muscles, and Nerves of the Foot. The *plantar aponeurosis and its deeper septa* are clinically important in two respects (see Figure 13–12):

1. It shares with the strong plantar lig-

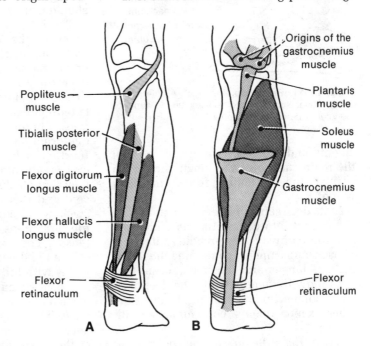

Fig. 13–10. *A,* muscles of the deep posterior compartment. *B,* muscles of the superficial posterior compartment.

Popliteus muscle
Tibialis posterior muscle
Flexor digitorum longus muscle
Flexor hallucis longus muscle
Flexor retinaculum
Origins of the gastrocnemius muscle
Plantaris muscle
Soleus muscle
Gastrocnemius muscle
Flexor retinaculum

A　B

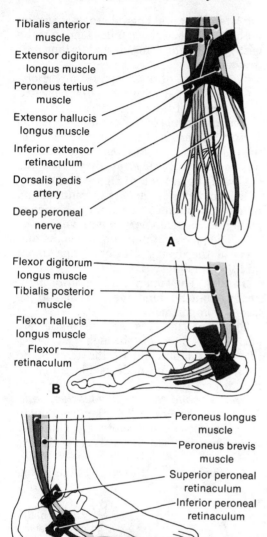

Tibialis anterior muscle

Extensor digitorum longus muscle

Peroneus tertius muscle

Extensor hallucis longus muscle

Inferior extensor retinaculum

Dorsalis pedis artery

Deep peroneal nerve

A

Flexor digitorum longus muscle

Tibialis posterior muscle

Flexor hallucis longus muscle

Flexor retinaculum

B

Peroneus longus muscle

Peroneus brevis muscle

Superior peroneal retinaculum

Inferior peroneal retinaculum

C

Fig. 13–11. Retinacula of the foot. *A,* inferior extensor retinaculum. *B,* flexor retinaculum. *C,* superior and inferior peroneal retinacula.

aments and intrinsic muscles of the foot the maintenance of the longitudinal arch against the flattening forces of body weight.

2. Its deep septa divide the plantar space of the foot into compartments which define the pathways of spreading infection. Those compartments containing the flexor hallucis longus and flexor digitorum longus follow the tendons into the deep posterior compartment of the leg. None of the other compartments communicate with the leg.

The *intrinsic flexors of the foot* are of

great clinical significance. If strong, they oppose tendencies to three kinds of painful degenerative foot disorders:

1. Metatarsalgia and plantar fasciitis, both manifestations of chronic foot strain;
2. hallux valgus;
3. hammer toes.

A brief review of the anatomy and actions of these muscles will demonstrate how they oppose these degenerations. The muscles lie in four layers:

1. The most superficial layer with the tendon of the flexor hallucis longus flexes the toes and abducts the great toe and least toe. (Abduction of toes is movement in the frontal plane of the foot away from the middle toe.)

2. The second layer takes origin from the flexor digitorum longus tendons and acts as do the lumbricals of the hand.

3. The third layer flexes the great and least toes and adducts the great toe. (Adduction of the toes is movement in the frontal plane of the foot toward the middle toe.)

4. The fourth layer acts very like the interosseous muscles of the hand.

The anatomy of each layer and its potential contribution to the prevention or development of degenerative foot disorders have been illustrated in Figures 13–13 through 13–16. A few minutes' study should clarify the pertinent details.

The *intrinsic extensors of the foot* take origin in the lateral hindfoot. From this common origin the *extensor hallucis brevis* passes as a single muscle to join over the first metatarsal head with the extensor hallucis longus tendon, and the extensor digitorum brevis passes as three muscle to join the tendons of the extensor digitorum longus to the second, third, and fourth toes. In some individuals these muscles create quite a mass anterior to the lateral maleolus. Novice clinicians have confused this muscle mass for traumatic swelling of a ganglion. These erroneous interpretations constitute the intrinsic extensors' greatest clinical significance.

The tibial nerve rounds the medial malleolus with the tendons of the deep posterior compartment, passes deep to the superficial layer of intrinsic flexors, and divides into the *medial and lateral plantar nerves.* These nerves emerge to either side of the flexor digitorum brevis at the midfoot, and form an arch superficial to the flexor digitorum brevis and deep to the plantar aponeurosis. From this arch, branch the plantar digital nerves. As the tibial nerve rounds the medial malleolus, it gives rise to the medial calcaneal branches. The plantar nerves and the medial calcaneal branches share the sensory innervation to the sole of the foot as illustrated in Figure 13–17. The plantar nerves innervate the intrinsic flexors of the foot as follows: The *medial plantar nerve*—abductor hallucis, flexor hallucis brevis, flexor digitorum brevis, 1st lumbrical; *lateral plantar nerve*—quadratus planti, the lateral 3 lumbricals, the abductor digiti minimi, the flexor digiti minimi, the two heads of the adductor hallucis, and all the interossei.

The dorsum of the foot is innervated by four nerves (See Figure 13–7): the superficial peroneal nerve divides terminally into two dorsal cutaneous nerves in the lower third of the leg, the *medial dorsal cutaneous nerve* (1) and the *intermediate dorsal cutaneous nerve* (2). In the popliteal fossa, the tibial nerve gives rise to the *medial sural cutaneous nerve*. With a branch from the common peroneal nerve, it forms the *sural nerve*, which terminates as the *lateral dorsal cutaneous nerve* (3). The *deep peroneal nerve* (4) terminates as

dorsal digital nerves to the web between the great toe and the second toe. These four nerves share the cutaneous sensory innervation to the dorsum of the foot as illustrated in Figure 13–8. The *deep peroneal nerve* innervates the intrinsic extensors of the foot as it passes deep to them over the midfoot.

The Work of Weightbearing in the Normal Foot

During normal stance, the plantar ligaments and the plantar aponeurosis resist the entire tension on the longitudinal arch. The balance between the tone of the soleus muscle and the gravitational forces tending to dorsiflex the ankle distribute the total body weight about equally between the forefoot and the hind foot, and the balance of tone between the pronators and supinators distributes two-sixths of the weight on the forefoot to the head of the 1st metatarsal, and one-sixth of the weight on the forefoot to the heads of the other 4 metatarsals.

During normal walking (See Figure 13–17), the tibialis anterior and the extensors hallucis and digtorum longus resist the moment arm at heel strike, preventing foot slap, and coordinating a smooth transfer of weight from the hindfoot to the

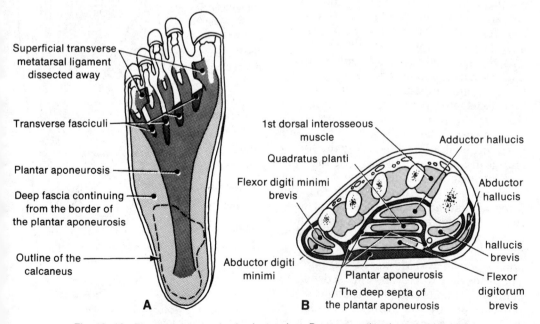

Fig. 13–12. Plantar aponeurosis. *A,* plantar view. *B,* cross section through the midfoot.

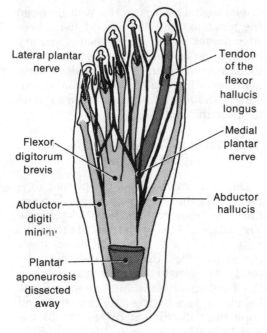

Fig. 13–13. First layer of muscles, tendons, and nerves in the foot.

the greater the relief they can afford to the plantar ligaments and aponeurosis. During recovery, the dorsiflexors of the ankle again increase their tone to allow the foot to clear the ground and to prepare for heel strike. During barefoot walking, the intrinsic toe flexors invariably participate during push-off. Try to walk barefooted without toe gripping, particularly through sand or over gravelly surfaces. Progress through sand will be tedious and, over a gravelly surface, painful. Full employment of toe gripping facilitates both tasks. During shoe walking, on the other hand, these provocations to toe gripping are blocked. Hence, the use of shoes will, for most people, decrease the participation by the intrinsic muscles of the foot. However, it will not decrease participation by the long dorsiflexors of the ankles and toes as recovery and heel strike demand their participation, whether in or out of shoes. As the intrinsic muscles weaken, the strain on the plantar ligaments and aponeurosis increases, and

forefoot. During weight transfer from the hindfoot to the forefoot, the tibialis posterior adds its supinating force to that of the tibialis anterior and extensor hallucis to cause the initial weight transfer to occur along the outer border of the foot. During these initial stages of weight transfer, the peroneal muscles are relatively quiescent, and supinator tone dominates. As weight transfers to the lateralmost heads of the metatarsals and the phase of push-off begins, the peroneal muscles rapidly increase their tone as the tibialis anterior, extensor hallucis, and tibialis posterior decrease their tone, and the foot pronates, transferring weight from the lateralmost metatarsal heads to the 1st metatarsal head and great toe. Push-off is effected by the soleus and gastrocnemius muscles and the long and intrinsic flexors of the toes. The moment arms of the foot are such that the force of plantar flexion must be at least twice body weight to effect push-off. Thus, at the moment of push-off, the tension forces on the longitudinal arch of a 150-pound person would exceed 300 pounds. These tension forces are opposed by the plantar ligaments and plantar aponeurosis and variably by the intrinsic muscles to the toes. The stronger these muscles are,

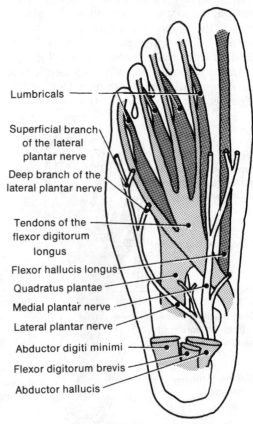

Fig. 13–14. Second layer of muscles, tendons, and nerves in the foot.

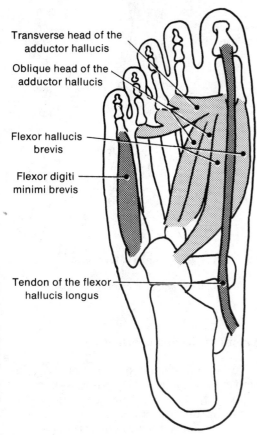

Fig. 13–15. Third layer of muscles, tendons, and nerves in the foot.

Transverse head of the adductor hallucis

Oblique head of the adductor hallucis

Flexor hallucis brevis

Flexor digiti minimi brevis

Tendon of the flexor hallucis longus

the tendency of the long extensors and flexors to flex the IP joints while extending the MP joints will be unopposed by the lumbricals and interossei. If, in addition, the heel of the shoe be elevated, the tendency toward talar slip will increase, and if the toe of the shoe be pointed, the adduction forces on the great toe will exceed abduction forces much of the time. Thus, as normal function is prevented, and abnormal postures are forced, painful distortions in the anatomy will begin to emerge. (See below under "Foot Pain.")

Congenital Disorders of the Leg and Foot

Feet and legs can and have been developmentally distorted in every direction. Most of the possibilities are rare, and the primary practitioner cannot hope to keep them all in mind. If the primary practitioner knows the normal, the abnormal

can be defined through careful examination. Because they are so prevalent or so generally known to lay people, five distortions should be fairly well understood by the primary practitioner. The definitions of foot posture, the limits of normal, and the anatomy and treatment of the five prevalent or generally known distortions will be described in the next several paragraphs.

Definitions of Posture (See Figure 13–18)

Normal, spontaneous posture varies from that which causes the toes to point directly forward parallel to the midsagittal plane, to that which causes the toe to point slightly away from the midsagittal plane.

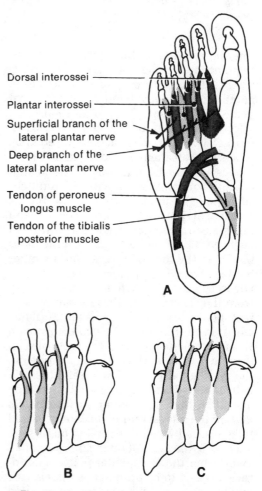

Dorsal interossei

Plantar interossei

Superficial branch of the lateral plantar nerve

Deep branch of the lateral plantar nerve

Tendon of peroneus longus muscle

Tendon of the tibialis posterior muscle

A

B   C

Fig. 13–16. Fourth layer of muscles, tendons, and nerves in the foot. *A,* plantar view of all the structures. *B,* plantar interossei alone. *C,* dorsal interossei alone.

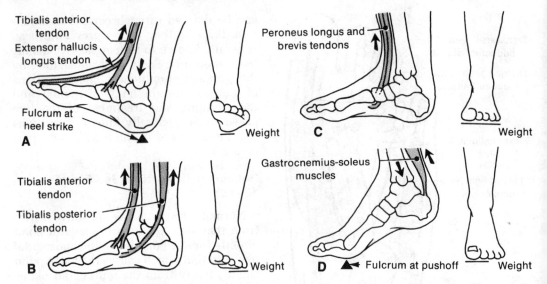

Tibialis anterior tendon

Extensor hallucis longus tendon

Fulcrum at heel strike

A

Weight

Peroneus longus and brevis tendons

C

Weight

Tibialis anterior tendon

Tibialis posterior tendon

B

Weight

Gastrocnemius-soleus muscles

D Fulcrum at pushoff

Weight

Fig. 13–17. *A* through *D*, the sequential distribution of weight and the action of extrinsic controllers of the foot during the phases of stepping.

Internal rotation of the leg causes the toes to point toward the midsagittal plane. *External rotation* of the leg causes the toes to point farther away from the midsagittal plane than the outer limit of normal.

The *foot* is said to be in *calcaneus* when the calcaneus is vertical and in *equinus* when the calcaneus is horizontal. A *forefoot* is said to be in *varus* or *adduction* when it forms an angle with the hindfoot such that the inner border of the foot is concave and the outer border convex, and in *valgus* or *abduction* when it forms an angle with the hindfoot such that the inner border of the foot is convex and the outer border concave. The *heel* is said to be in *varus* or *inversion* when it angles away from the vertical such that its plantar surface points toward the midsagittal plane, and it is said to be in *valgus* or *eversion* when it angles away from the vertical such that its plantar surface points away from the midsagittal plane. The forefoot is said to be *inverted* when it is rotated on its long axis such that the plantar surface points toward the midsagittal plane, and it is said to be *everted* when it is rotated on its long axis such that the plantar surface points away from the midsagittal plane. The forefoot is said to be *pronated* when everted and in valgus, and it is said to be *supinated* when inverted and in varus.

Limits of Normal in Infancy

1. The plantar fat pad causes every infant's foot to be "flat." However, every infant's foot is not *pronated,* and that is the important question.

2. The foot with straight borders is normal. When borders are not straight, rule No. 3 must be applied before the foot is called abnormal.

3. For the normal foot, the passive range of motion of the tibiotalar, subtalar, midtarsal, and tarsometatarsal joints is full. During the first few months of life, the child's foot may be held in calcaneovalgus or equinovarus and still be normal, as the passive range of motion of its joints is full. Note that range of motion is "full" only when it includes an arc to either side of neutral.

4. The normal tibia may be slightly rotated internally or externally. The internal rotation is more common than external rotation. Two tests for tibial rotation are useful (see Figure 13–19):

a. While the child lies supine, the foot is held at right angles to the leg and neither inverted nor everted. In such a position, a line projected from the anterosuperior iliac spine through the middle of the patella will intersect the second toe. This test may be employed when the foot is normal.

b. With the child prone, the knees are flexed at 90°. A line drawn through the two malleoli will create an angle of about 75° with a line extending from the axis of the thigh. This test should be employed when the foot is distorted.

Tibial Torsion

Most children are born with a moderate degree of internal tibial torsion as indicated in the previous section. Fewer children are born with a marked degree of internal tibial torsion. Rarely is a child born with any degree of external tibial torsion. Internal tibial torsion is one of the causes of "the inturning foot," or the "pi-geon-toed stance." Almost invariably, it can and should be ignored. As the otherwise normal, active child grows, the torsion corrects without exception. Indeed, a homologous developmental process occurs with the growth of those children whose femurs are anteverted. The femoral anteversion does not correct, but the tibia compensates by rotating externally.

Pronated Foot (Flat Foot) (See Figure 13–20)

An infant's feet may be pronated for one of four reasons:

1. The foot is *hypermobile*. Some children are constitutionally lax in some or all

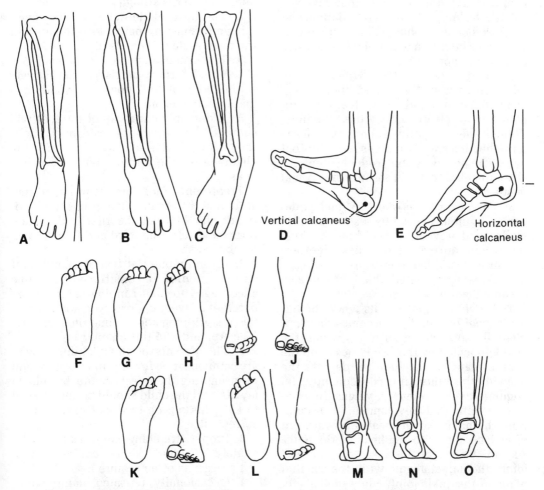

Vertical calcaneus

Horizontal calcaneus

Fig. 13–18. Definitions of posture of the leg and foot. *A* through *C*, rotations of the leg. *A*, normal—0–15° external rotation. *B*, abnormal internal rotation—greater than 0°. *C*, abnormal external rotation—greater than 15°. *D* and *E*, postures of the ankle. *D*, calcaneus. *E*, equinus. *F* through *L*, postures of the forefoot. *F*, normal. *G*, varus. *H*, valgus. *I*, eversion. *J*, inversion. *K*, supination. *L*, pronation. *M* through *O*, postures of the heel. *M*, normal. *N*, valgus. *O*, varus.

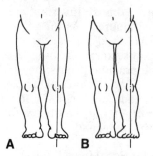
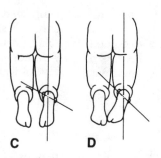

Fig. 13-19. Examining for tibial torsion. *A* and *B*, child supine. *A*, normal. *B*, internal tibial torsion. *C* and *D*, child prone, knees flexed 90°. *C*, normal. *D*, internal tibial torsion.

of their joints, and when stressed, their joints move easily and painlessly beyond the limits of normal. The orientation of the talocalcaneal-talonavicular joints are such that a laxity of ligaments will cause the heel of a hypermobile foot to angulate to valgus, the longitudinal arch to flatten, and the forefoot to pronate. The non-weight-bearing or intentionally supinated foot will assume the normal posture.

2. Children with *internal tibial torsion* who are continually chided about being pigeon-toed may force their feet into pronation in an effort to obey their mentors. Though they may thus silence their mentors, they may well be punished with foot pain. The non-weightbearing or intentionally supinated foot will assume the normal posture.

3. The *heel cord is short.* A modest degree of equinus caused by a short achilles tendon will prevent the heel from touching the ground during stance unless the forefoot pronates. When non-weightbearing or intentionally supinated, this foot will also assume the normal posture.

4. A *rigid flat foot* results when the *talocalcaneal articulation* becomes developmentally so oriented as to (a) widen the angle projected by the two bones upon the frontal plane of the foot, (b) depress the head of the talus and, consequently, (c) angulate the calcaneus in valgus. In association with that developmental orientation, the navicular dislocates upward out of articulation with the head of the talus. As the "tenon" of the ankle or "mortise" joint, the talus aligns with the sagittal plane of the ankle joint, while the cuboid, cuneiforms, and metatarsals remain in alignment with the calcaneus. Shortened ligaments hold this deformation fairly rigidly.

In consequence of these developmental distortions and alignments, the disorder presents the following clinical characteristics:

1. The medial plantar border of the foot is convex rather than concave, and the lateral border is straight.

2. The head of the talus and the overlying navicular are palpable at the apex of the medial plantar convexity.

3. The heel is angulated in valgus.

4. The deformity persists in the actively supinated foot and does not yield to a manipulative exam.

5. A dorsoplantar x-ray of the foot will show the abnormal talocalcaneal angle, the talonavicular dislocation, and the alignment of the forefoot with the calcaneus.

Treatment. Each form of pronated foot is treated differently. The primary practitioner should treat the first and second forms and refer the third and fourth to an orthopaedist.

1. Hypermobile flat feet are painless if strong. Children so constructed should be encouraged to play running sports, to go barefoot at every opportunity, and to practice toe-gripping and supination exercises. (See Appendix to this chapter.)

2. The parents of those children who are compensating for internal tibial torsion by pronating their feet should be told to lay off, and the child should be encouraged to keep his pigeon-toed gait until growth corrects it.

3. Proper stretching exercises may adequately lengthen a short achilles tendon, but surgery is often required.

4. Occasionally, repeated manipulation and casting will correct the talocalcaneal alignment and relocate the navicular in articulation with the talus and cuneiforms, but usually surgery is necessary. Results of either method are poor, and arthrodesis

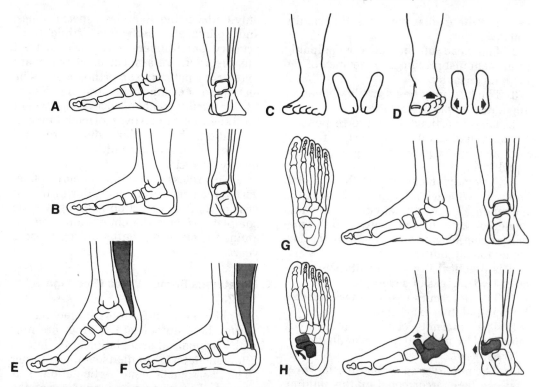

Fig. 13-20. Pronated foot. *A* and *B*, hypermobile flatfoot. *A*, non-weightbearing. *B*, weightbearing. *C* and *D*, correction of internal tibial torsion by intentional pronation. *C*, pigeon-toed stance of internal tibial torsion. *D*, straight stance at expense of pronation. *E* and *F*, adaptation to short heel cord by intentional pronation. *E*, non-weightbearing. *F*, weightbearing. *G* and *H*, a form of rigid flatfoot. The talus is angulated medially and plantarward. The navicular is dislocated and lies dorsal to the head of the talus. *G*, normal. *H*, the rigid flatfoot.

to relieve pain is often required in adult life.

Metatarsus Varus. (See Figure 13-21)

Like the rigid flat foot, *metatarsus varus* is partially characterized by a *widened talocalcaneal angle.* Unlike the rigid flat foot, however, the head of the talus is not depressed, and the talonavicular joint remains in articulation. Like the rigid flat foot, the midfoot remains in alignment with the calcaneus, causing the navicular to angulate laterally at its articulation with the head of the talus. Unlike the rigid flat-foot, the forefoot angulates medially at the tarsometatarsal joints, aligning with or radial to the axis of the talus. The calcaneus may rotate into valgus or into varus or remain in alignment with the axis of the leg. The ligaments are not markedly shortened and the involved joints retain a variable degree of play.

In consequence of these developmental

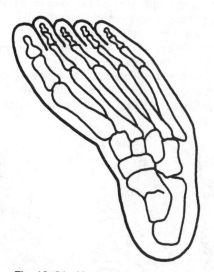

Fig. 13-21. Metatarsus varus, superior view.

distortions and alignments, the disorder presents the following clinical characteristics:

1. The lateral border of the foot is con-

vex, and the medial border is abnormally concave.

2. The head of the talus is palpably prominent just proximal to the apex of the medial concavity.

3. The heel may be normally aligned or angulated in valgus or varus.

4. The distortions are more responsive to manipulation than are the rigid flatfoot and the talipes equinovarus, but not all are equally so.

5. A dorsoplantar x-ray of the foot will show the widened talocalcaneal angle, the alignment of the cuboid, cuneiforms, and navicular with the calcaneus, and the medial angulation of the forefoot at the tarsometatarsal joints.

It is practical to view metatarsus varus as of two degrees of severity:

1. The deformity can be *overcorrected* by manipulative examination.

2. The deformity can, at best, be only *corrected* by manipulative examination.

Treatment.

1. The *mild degree of metatarsus varus* that can be *overcorrected* by the manipulative examination can well be treated by the primary practitioner. The child should wear outflare shoes during sleeping hours until the foot corrects (6–12 months is usual). The child should be examined as often as necessary to reinforce compliance and avoid a missed progression of the deformity. We find it adequate to follow most of our patients bimonthly.

2. The *severe degree of metatarsus varus* that cannot be overcorrected by the manipulative examination will correct only with casting. Exercises, special shoes, and splints are ineffective. While some primary practitioners may learn to treat this disorder, we suspect most will want to refer the patient to an orthopaedist. The technique of casting is illustrated in Figure 13–22. Casts are changed every 2 weeks until the foot can be overcorrected by manipulation, then outflare shoes are used during sleeping hours until the foot completely corrects.

3. Regardless of the initial degree of severity, recurrences are likely during the 1st year or 2 after correction is thought to be complete. Hence, the child should be examined every 4–6 months during those 2 years.

Metatarsus Primus Varus (See Figure 13–23)

Unlike the rigid flatfoot and metatarsus varus, the hindfoot and midfoot are normal. The plane of articulation of the lateral 2 tarsometatarsal joints (see above under "The Tarsometatarsal Articulation.") is normal. The plane of articulation of the medialmost tarsometatarsal joint faces medially, causing the 1st metatarsal to lie in varus relative to the rest of the forefoot.

In consequence of this developmental distortion and alignment, the disorder presents the following clinical characteristics:

1. The lateral border of the foot is straight in alignment with the calcaneocuboid axis.

2. The medial border of the foot is abnormally concave with the apex of the concavity at the medial tarso-metatarsal joint.

3. The heads of the 1st and 2nd metatarsals are palpably more separate, and the great and second toes are splayed apart.

4. A dorsoplantar x-ray of the foot will show the medial angulation of the medial tarsometatarsal joint and the 1st metatarsal.

Treatment. This deformity is generally not treated unless by osteotomy later in life. Unless shoes are chosen to accommodate the deformity, *hallux valgus* will result.

Talipes Equinovarus (See Figure 13–24)

This deformity is the more common form of "clubfoot" (talipes calcaneovalgus

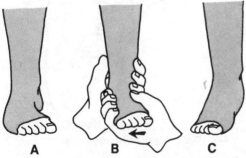

Fig. 13–22. Correction of metatarsus varus by casting (3-month child). *A,* plaster is molded to the deformed foot. *B,* the forefoot and midfoot are maximally abducted, and the position is held until the plaster sets. *C,* appearance of the foot and cast after the plaster sets.

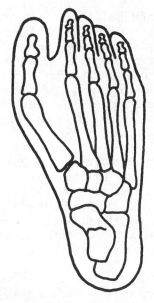

Fig. 13–23. Metatarsus primus varus.

being the less common). It is the result of four developmental distortions:

1. The tibiotalar joint is in marked plantar flexion, and the posterior compartment muscles of the leg are commensurately shortened and atrophied.

2. The talocalcaneal articulation is so oriented as to narrow the angle projected by the two bones upon the frontal plane of the foot, elevate the head of the talus, and consequently angle the calcaneus in varus.

3. The midfoot and forefoot are supinated with the medial angulation (varus) and internal rotation (inversion) occurring equally in the midtarsal, naviculocuneiform, and tarsometatarsal joints.

4. Ligaments and tendons on the concave side of the deformity are commensurately shortened.

In consequence of these developmental distortions and alignments, the deformity presents the following clinical characteristics:

1. The calf muscles are atrophic and the heel cord very tight with the ankle thus held in marked plantar flexion (equinus).

2. The heel is angulated in varus.

3. The mid- and forefoot are markedly supinated, such that the lateral dorsal border of the foot becomes the weightbearing surface.

4. The distortions are rigidly held by

shortened muscles, tendons, and ligaments and do not yield to manipulative examination.

5. A dorsoplantar x-ray of the foot will show the narrow talocalcaneal angle and the medial angulation and internal rotation at the junction of the midfoot and forefoot.

Treatment. Results of treatment are always less than ideal, and surgery is often required. The primary practitioner should refer these children promptly to an orthopaedist. *The younger the infant when treatment begins,* the better the final result. Treatment usually starts with a trial of casting. The equinus is initially overlooked, and the supination deformity manipulated and casted, much as is the metatarsus varus deformity. Casts are changed weekly. If correction has not occurred within 4 months of casting, surgery must be considered. Once correction occurs, it is maintained during early growth by applying outflare shoes, so attached to a Denis-Browne bar as to hold the heels in valgus. Once the supination deformity is corrected, the equinus is treated by heel cord stretching and/or by tendon-lengthening surgical procedures.

Non-Traumatic Disorders of the Leg, Ankle, and Foot

Leg and Ankle Pain

Stress Myalgia. Muscle-working and/or -stretching activity, to which an individual is unaccustomed, is likely to result in muscle pain of varying severity and persistence. *Shin splints* is a term common among runners, used to refer to pains along the tibia that result when the muscles of the

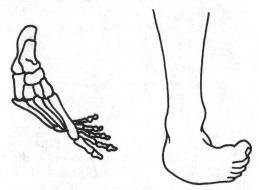

Fig. 13–24. Talipes equinovarus.

anterior or deep posterior compartments are overstressed. Heel-toe running, particularly downhill, if practiced too vigorously early in a season, will often overstress the muscles of the anterior compartment, and use of spiked track shoes too early in a season will often overstress the muscles of the deep as well as superficial posterior compartments. Visible evidence of inflammation suggests that the pain syndrome represents myositis and periostitis.

Characteristic clinical features are the following:

1. The patient complains of pain over a muscle compartment near to the tibia. Pain may refer into the foot and up into the knee.

2. Movements that stretch or work the affected muscles increase the pain.

·3. Palpation over the affected muscle group and the adjacent tibia will reveal tenderness.

4. Slight swelling and redness may be visible over the affected muscle and its tibial origin.

Treatment. Minor stress myalgias can be ignored and the provoking activity continued.

When pain is quite intense and/or inflammation visibly evident, the provoking activity should be avoided until recovery is well advanced. Ice is the safest applied analgesic during the first 2 or 3 days. Thereafter, heat or ice may be used, whichever is most comforting. Stretching and mild working exercise may begin as soon as visible evidence of inflammation has subsided. The provoking activity should be resumed quite gradually.

Tenosynovitis. The long tendons to the foot and their synovial sheaths are vulnerable to irritation where they pass under the retinacula at the ankle. Activity that requires prolonged repetitive movement of a tendon is most likely to provoke its inflammation. The tibialis anterior and posterior, and the peronei longus and brevis are most commonly involved.

Characteristic clinical features are the following:

1. Pain is felt over the affected tendon and may refer into that portion of the foot distal to it: tibialis anterior—anteromedial aspect of the ankle and dorsum of the foot; tibialis posterior—posteromedial aspect of

the ankle and medial plantar aspect of the foot; peronei—posterolateral aspect of the ankle and lateral aspect of the foot.

2. Tenderness, visible fullness, and often a creaky crepitation are evident over the tendon where it passes beneath the retinaculum.

3. Any movement of the tendon usually increases the pain.

Treatment.

1. When mild, ambulation may continue, but activities requiring prolonged repetitive movements should be avoided. When severe, ambulation should also be curtailed. When remission is delayed beyond 2 weeks and the individual must be ambulating, a walking cast should be considered.

2. Ice is the safest applied analgesic until visible evidence of inflammation has disappeared. Thereafter, either heat or ice may be used, whichever the patient finds most comforting.

3. Anti-inflammatory agents, either oral drugs or local corticosteroid injections, can be helpful. (See Chapter 18.)

Foot Pain

Congenital and acquired disorders of the feet can lead directly to foot pain: a short heel cord, either singly or as part of the talipes equinovarus syndrome, can lead to heel pain syndromes; rigid flat feet can lead to subtalar, midtarsal, and cuneonavicular joint arthritis; residual contracture of supinators and of ligaments on the medial aspect of the equinovarus foot can lead to painful calluses and chronic contusion on the outer border of the foot, and chronic strain of the plantar ligaments; the cavus foot can lead to metatarsalgia and hammer toes. Most foot pain, however, represents a manifestation of *chronic foot strain*. While congenital pronated feet of the hypermobile or adaptive form (adaptive to a short achilles tendon or to an internal tibial torsion) predispose to chronic foot strain, the sedative effect of shoes alone is responsible for chronic foot strain in the large majority of those who consult a primary practitioner. The compressive effect of cosmetic shoes increases the shoe-related foot pains by another sizeable increment: hallux valgus, hammer toes, onychocryptosis, interdigital corns, and corns over the outer border of the 5th metatarsal head.

The following discussion will summarize the pathogenesis of chronic foot strain and its relationship to foot pain, and then will review the forms of foot pain regionally, whether resulting from chronic foot strain or not. It will be noted that those forms resulting from chronic foot strain are all treated essentially alike, as effective treatment must neutralize the forces provoking the chronic foot strain.

Pathogenesis of Chronic Foot Strain.
The entire process of chronic foot strain illustrated in Figure 13–25 begins with talar slip (see above under "The Talonavicular Articulation.") which moves the head of the talus and the articulating navicular medially downward and distally. Medial movement increases the medial moment arm, acting on the calcaneus, and causes the calcaneus to evert (valgus heel). Downward and distal movement will lower the apex of the longitudinal arch and, with the medial movement, will broaden and evert

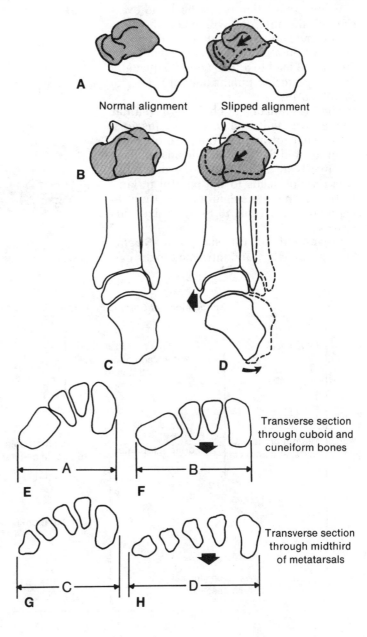

Fig. 13-25. Talar slip and the dynamics of chronic foot strain. A and B, the talar slip. A, medial view. B, superior view. C and D, eversion of the calcaneus in consequence of talar slip. C, normal. D, eversion after slippage. E through H, widening and eversion of the midfoot (E and F), and forefoot (G and H). E, normal midfoot. F, widened midfoot. G, normal forefoot. H, widened forefoot.

the transverse arch of the midfoot. The forefoot will correspondingly broaden and shift into pronation. As the forefoot pronates and the apex of the longitudinal arch descends, the plantar aponeurosis will be stretched and the normal curving line of the weight transfer from heel strike along the lateral border of the foot across the metatarsal heads to a push-off point from the first metatarsal head and the great toe will shift to a straight line of weight transfer from heel strike to a push-off point from the middle metatarsal heads.

Valgus angulation of the heel and eversion of the midfoot will place the long flexor and supinator tendons, and the tibial nerve on stretch. The consequent irritation will lead to a *tenosynovitis* (usually of the posterior tibialis tendon), and, to *tibial neuritis.*

The irritation of stretch upon the plantar aponeurosis will lead to *plantar fasciitis.*

The concentration of the push-off point upon the middle metatarsal heads subjects the overlying soft tissue to a degree of stress which leads to the painful inflammation of *metatarsalgia* and, in time, to *digital neuritis.* Table 13.1 summarizes this process.

Prevention of Chronic Foot Strain. Strong supinators and intrinsic flexors can oppose the process of chronic foot strain, as illustrated in Figure 13-26. Circumstances that increase the talocalcaneal incline plane and inhibit supinator and intrinsic flexor tone will facilitate the process of chronic foot strain. As suggested in a previous paragraph, most standard shoes can inhibit supinator and intrinsic flexor tone, and high heels will increase the talocalcaneal incline plane. Barefoot walking is healthiest for the feet, but in urban society and in winter climates shoes should be chosen that have been made with a flexible last that most closely approxi-

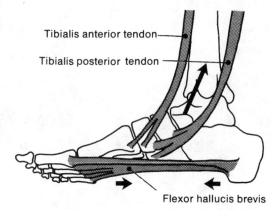

Tibialis anterior tendon

Tibialis posterior tendon

Flexor hallucis brevis

Fig. 13–26. Actions of the supinators and intrinsic flexors oppose the process of chronic foot strain.

Table 13.1

Pathogenesis of Chronic Foot Strain Summarized

Talar Slip →	Valgus heel	→	Long flexor and supinator tendons and tibial nerve are stretched	→	Tibial Neuritis
					Tenosynovitis (usually of posterior tibialis)
	Midfoot broadens, everts, and abducts		Forefoot pronates	→	Push-off point shifts to middle metatarsal heads	→	Metatarsalgia
							Digital neuritis
					→ Plantar aponeurosis stretches → Plantar fasciitis
	Apex of longitudinal arch descends				

mates the shape of the foot, with close-fitting counter, ample toe room (regular shoes should extend two fingerbreadths beyond the longest toe, and pointed toe shoes should extend three fingerbreadths beyond the longest toe), and low heel. Wearers should consciously practice toe gripping and supination when walking.

Basic Treatment Regimen. When chronic foot strain emerges, particular treatments are applied for particular manifestations, but a basic treatment regimen is employed as well for all manifestations:

1. Shoes must be corrected as discussed in the paragraph concerning prevention.

2. Supination should be supported by certain shoe modifications. (See Figure 13–27.)

a. A ⅛″ to ¼″ inner heel wedge should be placed in a shoe with a firm, well-fitting counter.

b. A supinator longitudinal arch support should also be fitted into the shoe.

3. Active supination and toe-gripping exercises must be practiced several times daily, and toe gripping during walking should be intended until it becomes habitual. (See Figure 13–28.)

4. When pain is disabling, weightbearing should be minimized until remission is well advanced.

5. Hot baths can be comforting when the feet ache at rest. We recommend they be used prior to exercise.

Acute Foot Strain. Any foot can be acutely strained by stress to which it is unaccustomed. The manifestations of acute strain emerge either during the uncustomary activity or within 24 hours thereafter. Any or all of the three regions of the foot can be affected. Nearly all acute strains are muscle strains, fatigue fractures, or both. Its form will be identified in the regional discussions immediately following.

Heel and Ankle Pain. The primary practitioner encounters eight forms of heel pain with sufficient regularity to warrant a summary. The first four of the eight forms are manifestations of chronic foot strain.

1. Plantar Fascitis. When strain of the plantar aponeurosis leads to inflammation at its attachment to the calcaneus, heel pain results. The patient complains of heel

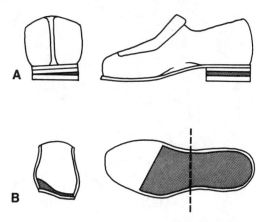

Fig. 13–27. Shoe modifications which support supination. *A,* inner heel wedge. *B,* supinator longitudinal arch support.

pain when standing or walking, and occasionally when at rest. Point tenderness is evident, usually over the medial plantar aspect of the midsection of the heel.

Treatment. In addition to the basic treatment regimen for chronic foot strain, injections of corticosteroids into the tender focus occasionally speed the remission.

2. Tenosynovitis beneath the Flexor Retinaculum. See the discussion above of tenosinovitis under "Leg and Ankle Pain." The syndrome may emerge from acute or chronic foot strain. Treatment of tenosynovitis when a manifestation of acute foot strain has been summarized above under "Tenosynovitis." When tenosynovitis is a manifestation of chronic foot strain, treatment must employ the basic treatment regimen for chronic foot strain. Oral anti-inflammatory drugs or local corticosteroid injections may be employed as well. (See Chapter 18.)

3. Tibial Neuritis. When the tibial nerve is irritated beneath the flexor retinaculum, painful paresthesias and eventual intrinsic muscle weakness follow. Usually, the medial calcaneal branch of the tibial nerve is first involved. Hence, initial symptoms are usually felt in the medial aspect of the heel. In addition to the basic treatment regimen for chronic foot strain, a corticosteroid injection around the tibial nerve beneath the flexor retinaculum will sometimes speed remission.

4. Subtalar Arthritis. Following from the degenerative effects of talar slip, sub-

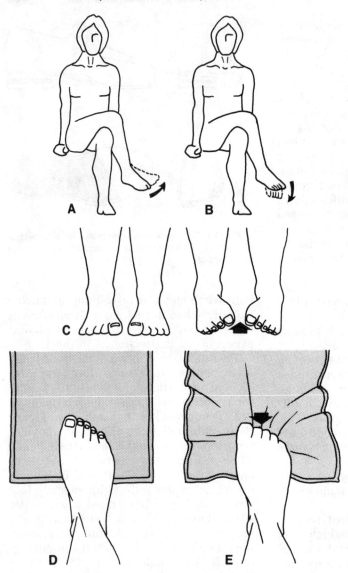

Fig. 13-28. Active supination and toe-gripping exercises. *A,* supination. *B,* toe gripping. *C,* standing supination. *D,* grasping with the toes.

talar arthritis emerges as a late manifestation of chronic foot strain. It may also follow several years after a calcaneal fracture has damaged the posterior talocalcaneal articulation.

The patient complains of heel and ankle pain, worsened by weightbearing. The joint line is tender—tenderness is particularly evident in the sinus tarsi. Manipulation of the subtalar joint produces pain. Lateral x-ray of the ankle and heel may show the bony changes of degenerative arthritis about the subtalar joint.

Treatment. When subtalar arthritis is a late manifestation of chronic foot strain,

the basic treatment regimen for chronic foot strain must be employed. Whether a late complication of a calcaneal fracture, or a late manifestation of chronic foot strain, the heel of the shoe should be cushioned and weightbearing should be minimized permanently. Corticosteroid injections into the joint through the sinus tarsi may induce temporary remissions which will last the longer the more compliantly the basic regimen is followed.

When these conservative methods prove inadequate, the patient should be referred to an orthopaedist for consideration of an arthrodesis.

5. Posterior Calcaneal Bursitis. A posterior calcaneal bursa can be irritated by friction of the upper border of a heel counter that is too firm and too convex. Ladies' cosmetic shoes are most capable of irritating the posterior calcaneal bursa. The patient complains of posterior heel pain and a tender bump on the back of the heel. Examination reveals the tender firm bump on the back of the heel, at the insertion of the achilles tendon.

Treatment. Ideally, open-heel shoes or sandals should be used until the inflammation subsides. Local injections of a corticosteroid may speed remission. When shoes with heel counters are again worn, the counter should be less convex, and its upper border should be soft. A posterior wedge can be cut away from the posterior counters of cosmetic heels and soft leather sewn across the defect. (See Figure 13–29.)

6. Retrocalcaneal Bursitis. Activity requiring repetitive dorsiflexion of the ankle can irritate the retrocalcaneal bursa. The patient complains of heel pain, worsened by dorsiflexion of the ankle. Tenderness is evident to palpation just anterior to the insertion of the achilles tendon upon the calcaneus. When inflammation is intense, swelling and redness may be evident above the insertion of the achilles tendon.

Treatment. Weightbearing is minimized and, when necessary for extended periods, is performed with a ½″ elevation of the heel. (See Figure 13–30.) Hot or cold compresses may afford some relief of pain. Oral anti-inflammatory drugs or corticosteroid injections may speed the remission. (See Chapter 18.)

7. Paratendinitis Achilles. The reticular fascia surrounding the achilles tendon can become irritated whenever the achilles tendon is subjected to uncustomary repet-

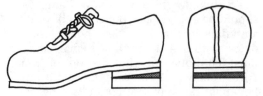

Fig. 13–30.   A ½″ heel lift.

itive stress, such as a long hike or jog. The patient complains of pain in the back of the heel and leg which worsens when the achilles tendon is stretched or worked. The space just anterior to the achilles tendon is always tender and may be swollen.

Treatment is essentially the same as that for retrocalcaneal bursitis.

8. Calcaneus Apophysitis (Sever's Disease). Prepubertal children may suffer a painful necrosis of the calcaneal epiphysis. The cause is not known and is probably like that of Osgood-Schlatter's disease. The child may limp and will complain of heel pain, worsened by heel strike on hard surfaces and by running. The sides of the calcaneus posteriorly are tender.

Treatment. Running should be curtailed, and a ½″ elevated heel should be used when walking. (See Figure 13–30.) Full remission generally occurs within 3–6 months.

Midfoot Pain. Three forms of midfoot pain are of importance to the primary practitioner. The first two forms are unique to older children and adolescents, and the last form is a manifestation of chronic foot strain.

1. Aseptic Necrosis of the Navicular (Köhler's Disease). This occurs for unknown reasons (perhaps akin to those of Legg-Perthes' disease) in prepubertal schoolchildren. The child limps and complains of pain along the inner aspect of the foot. Physical examination will demonstrate tenderness over the medial aspect of the midfoot and pain during active or passive supination of the foot. X-ray will confirm the diagnosis eventually but may be normal if the child is first seen early in the course of the illness. Any child who complains of midfoot pain should be followed at biweekly intervals with this diagnosis in mind until pain remits or the x-ray confirms necrosis or is normal 6 weeks after the first consultation.

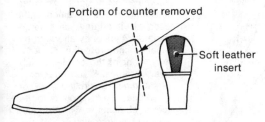

Portion of counter removed

Soft leather insert

Fig. 13–29. Insertion of soft leather into the back of the heel counter.

Treatment. A short-leg walking cast should be applied and the child allowed to ambulate in the cast. New bone consolidates within 4–6 months, hence casting must continue for that period of time. After removal of the cast, the child must be taught range of motion and strengthening exercises of the ankle and foot. (See Figure 13–31.) Ambulation should begin with partial weightbearing and should advance as range of motion and strength return.

2. Chronic Strain of the Navicular Insertion of the Tibialis Posterior Tendon. This is likely to occur when the point of insertion stands as a separate bone with only fibrous attachment between it and the navicular proper. The problem typically appears in adolescence and young adulthood, and women are more likely to suffer the problem than are men. The young person complains of midfoot pain, worsened by weightbearing. Examination demonstrates a tender prominence over

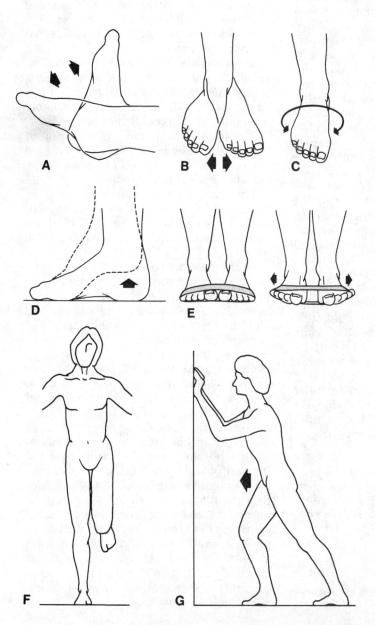

Fig. 13–31. Range of motion and strengthening exercises of the foot and ankle. *A,* active movement of the tibiotalar joint by alternate dorsiflexion and plantarflexion. *B,* active movement of the subtalar, intertarsal, and tarsometatarsal joints by alternate supination and pronation. *C,* active movement of the tibiotalar, subtalar, intertarsal, and tarsometatarsal joints by circling the foot. *D,* repeated elevation onto the toes, standing. *E,* pronation against elastic resistance. *F,* balancing on one foot. *G,* heel cord stretching.

the medial aspect of the navicular. Strong passive pronation and resisted active supination may provoke the pain. X-ray will confirm the separated point of insertion. This entire clinical picture and an otherwise normal examination are necessary for a valid diagnosis.

Treatment. The patient should be referred to an orthopaedist as excision of the fragment and reattachment of the tendon to the plantar surface of the navicular are commonly required.

3. Plantar Fasciitis. Chronic stretch may irritate the plantar aponeurosis in the midfoot region, in which case the patient will complain of pain in the midfoot, worsened by weightbearing. Examination will demonstrate a uniquely tender point in the midfoot segment of the plantar aponeurosis. Other stigmata of chronic foot strain may be evident.

Treatment is essentially that of plantar fasciitis in the hindfoot.

Forefoot Pain. Seven forms of forefoot pain are important to the primary practitioner: the first three are forms of acute foot strain, the fourth and fifth, are manifestations of chronic foot strain, the sixth is a bony aseptic necrosis that afflicts adolescents, and the last a cryptogenic degeneration of the plantar aponeurosis.

1. Acute Intrinsic Flexor Strain. When a person walks or runs more vigorously or longer than he or she is accustomed to doing, the intrinsic flexor muscles are likely to be strained. Pain will begin late in the activity or several hours thereafter. The patient complains of forefoot pain, worsened by weightbearing. Examination demonstrates tenderness deep within one or more spaces between the metatarsal bones, pain with passive dorsiflexion of the toes, and pain with resisted active flexion of the toes.

Treatment. When the condition is mild, the person may continue usual activity and apply no treatment as such. Gentle extension and flexion exercises while the feet are in a hot bath can be quite relieving.

When ambulation is very painful, it should be limited to that most essential. Transverse strapping of the forefoot and the use of a longitudinal arch support may allow more comfort during ambulation. (See Figure 13–32.) When quiescent, the

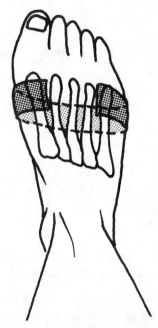

Fig. 13–32. Transverse strapping for acute foot strain.

feet should be elevated and the toes frequently gently exercised in flexion and extension. Warm foot baths may be used as desired for comfort. Full remission is rarely delayed more than 2 weeks.

2. March Fracture. When a person walks longer than he or she is accustomed to doing, a fatigue fracture of a metatarsal shaft may result. Pain begins while walking and in time becomes hardly bearable. Examination reveals tenderness and often swelling over a metatarsal shaft and pain when that metatarsal is stressed. (See Figure 13–33.) X-ray may show a hairline fracture or nothing early after the onset, but after 2 weeks will show typical callus. When acute-onset forefoot pain does not remit within 2 weeks, a repeat x-ray is indicated to exclude the possibility of March fracture.

Treatment. The foot is immobilized in a short leg walking cast. Ambulation is allowed as desired within the cast. The cast may be removed after 6 weeks. Though bony union is not complete at that time, it will progress normally in spite of unprotected weightbearing. When the cast is removed, the patient must be taught range of motion and strengthening exercises of the ankle and foot. (See Figure 13–31.)

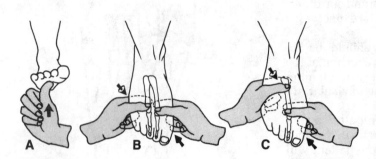

Fig. 13–33. Manipulative examination of the forefoot. *A,* upward pressure on the head of the metatarsal will cause pain when the attached intrinsic muscles are strained, when the tarsometatarsal joint is sprained, and when the metatarsal is fractured. *B,* manipulation of one metatarsal on the other will cause pain under similar circumstances without also stressing the midfoot, hindfoot, and ankle. *C,* manipulation of one metatarsal by stabilizing its base with one hand, while attempting to move its distal end with the other, will cause pain only when the metatarsal is fractured.

Weightbearing is partial at first and is advanced as range of motion and strength return.

3. Tendinitis of the Flexor Pollicis Longus. When a person walks or runs more vigorously or longer than he or she is accustomed to doing, the flexor pollicis longus tendon may be strained. It may be strained alone or along with the intrinsic flexors. The patient complains of forefoot pain worsened by walking. Examination reveals tenderness over the medial plantar aspect of the foot. Four features distinguish the condition from plantar fasciitis.

a. Tendinitis is typically a form of acute strain, while plantar fasciitis is typically a manifestation of chronic strain.

b. Dorsiflexion of the ankle and foot does not increase pain as long as the great toe is allowed to flex.

c. Dorsiflexion of the great toe as such, after the ankle is dorsiflexed, increases the pain.

d. Palpation of the tendon, after it is made to stand out by dorsiflexion of the great toe, reveals it to be uniquely tender along most of its plantar course.

Treatment. The basic treatment is identical to that employed for acute intrinsic flexor strain. Oral anti-inflammatory agents in addition may speed the recovery. (See Chapter 18.)

4. Metatarsalgia. Chronic foot strain is thought to product this syndrome through three mechanisms: (a) The transverse metatarsal arch of the pronated foot is splayed, and the transverse metatarsal ligaments are thus subject to undue strain;

(b) the transfer of weight from the heel to the push-off point is not shared by the outer border of the foot and all the metatarsal heads, but is directed immediately to the middle metatarsal heads; (c) because the intrinsic flexors are weak, the push-off is made from the metatarsal heads without assistance from the toes—thus the subcutaneous fascia is subject to chronic irritation. Examination may reveal a reverse transverse metatarsal arch with callus formation over the midmetatarsal heads; the hammer-toe deformity is usually evident; and the middle metatarsal heads are uniquely tender. X-ray is normal.

Treatment. The basic treatment for chronic foot strain must be applied. In addition, the middle metatarsal heads may be protected in one of two ways (see Figure 13–34): (a) When the problem is of recent onset and the stigmata of chronic foot strain are not advanced, a metatarsal pad may be placed in the shoe. (b) When the problem is of long standing, and stigmata of chronic foot strain are advanced, a metatarsal bar should be fitted to the shoe by a shoemaker.

When symptoms persist in spite of efforts to encourage compliance with the conservative regimen, the patient should be referred to an orthopaedist or podiatrist. One of a variety of surgical modifications of the distal end of the metatarsal may be performed.

5. Interdigital Neuritis (Morton's Neuroma). The irritations described above to which the transverse metatarsal arch of the chronically pronated foot are vulnerable can so irritate an interdigital nerve as to lead to a mechanical neuritis and, in time, to the fibrous reaction called a neuroma. The patient typically complains of burning and aching pain in the plantar aspect of the forefoot and into the third and fourth toes. Examination reveals the stigmata of metatarsalgia and a unique tenderness between the heads of the 3rd and 4th metatarsals: deep palpation in that interspace produces sudden, intense burning pain in the third and fourth toes.

Treatment. Conservative treatment is as advised for metatarsalgia. When this treatment proves inadequate, the patient should be referred to an orthopaedist or podiatrist. Excision of the neuroma will relieve the pain at the expense of a permanent numbness of the third and fourth toes, and a small risk of a transection neuroma and a resulting chronic pain problem.

6. Aseptic Necrosis of the 2nd Metatarsal Head (Freiberg's Disease). For unknown reasons (perhaps akin to Legg-Perthes' and Köhler's diseases), the head of the 2nd metatarsal may undergo aseptic necrosis in adolescence. The young person will complain of forefoot pain, worsened by weightbearing and extreme movements of the second metatarsophalangeal joint. Examination reveals tenderness of the 2nd metatarsal head and often a visible and tender swelling over the dorsum of the metatarsal head. X-ray confirms the necrotic process within 2–3 weeks of the onset of symptoms.

Treatment. The foot may be immobilized in a short leg walking cast, the plantar surface of which extends beyond the toes. New bone will consolidate within 4–6 months, hence the cast must be maintained for that period of time. When the cast is removed, the patient must be taught range of motion and strengthening exercises for the ankle and foot. (See Figure 13–31.)

Some orthopaedists and podiatrists recommend immediate excision of the metatarsal head, on grounds that relief is quick, and that degenerative arthritis is a common late complication after conservative treatment. Unfortunately, a lasting pain can follow the surgery itself.

7. Dupuytren's Contracture. Dupuytren's contracture can occur in the plantar aponeurosis as well as in the palmar aponeurosis. Initially, its manifestations are indistinguishable from plantar fasciitis. In time, the nodular degeneration of Dupuytren's contracture becomes palpably evident.

Treatment. The treatment is as advised for Dupuytren's contracture of the palmar aponeurosis.

Painful Toes. Except for relatively rare tumors and rheumatoid arthritis, all toe pain results from short narrow shoes, short stockings, and/or weak intrinsic flexors. Even the hammer toes inevitably associated with the cavus foot would not be painful if shoes were roomy, and intrinsic flexors remained strong. Seven forms of painful toe syndromes are of particular importance to the primary practitioner. The first form is associated with metatarsalgia, the second with hammer toes and

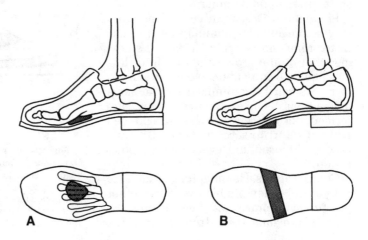

Fig. 13-34. Shoe modifications employed when treating metatarsalgia. *A*, metatarsal pad. *B*, metatarsal bar.

A   B

shoe pressure, the third with shoe pressure alone, the fourth with shoe pressure and developmental predisposition, the fifth with an inflammation of the 1st metatarsophalangeal joint and/or its medial overlying bursa, and the sixth and seventh with a constitutional or acquired distortion of nail plates.

1. Interdigital Neuroma. This may accompany metatarsalgia. Both of these disorders were discussed in the previous section regarding the forefoot.

2. Hammer Toes. These may be developmental. They always accompany the cavus foot, but also may appear in late childhood, in children whose feet are otherwise normal. Hammer toes may also be degenerative: They will emerge when intrinsic flexors become weaker than extrinsic extensors, or when persons wear shoes and/or stockings that are too short and crowd the toes into flexion. Most people who wear shoes have relatively weak intrinsic flexors, but not all have hammer toes. Most people whose feet are degeneratively pronated have hammer toes, but not all. These facts suggest that hammer toes develop in those with weak intrinsic flexors, who are constitutionally predisposed to the development of hammer toes. However, it may be that the harmfully short shoe or stocking is another critical difference between those with weak flexors who develop hammer toes and those who do not. Figure 13–35 illustrates hammer toes and the degenerative mechanisms that facilitate their development.

Corns over the interphalangeal joints and over the ends of the toes result when shoes press upon hammer toes.

Prevention. Degenerative hammer toes may be prevented by maintaining intrinsic flexor tone and wearing shoes and stockings that do not crowd the toes into flexion. The deformity of developmental hammer toes can be minimized by the same precautions. Once hammer toes are formed, they rarely can be straightened without resort to surgery, as the IP joints become fibrosed and even undergo bony fusion.

Complications. Hammer toes as such are not painful. They predispose to two other painful syndromes: (a) The flexion deformity prevents them from sharing the stresses of push-off with the metatarsal heads. Thus, they predispose to the development of metatarsalgia; (b) the dorsal prominence of the proximal interphalangeal (PIP) joints and the plantar prominence of the ends of the toes predispose to corns if toe pieces of shoes are insufficiently roomy. These corns are always painful.

Treatment. Conservative treatment of the complications should be attempted initially. Treatment of metatarsalgia was reviewed in the previous section dealing with the forefoot. Corns are treated as follows: (a) Only shoes with roomy toe pieces are worn, or no shoes are worn. (b) Corns are pared thin and kept so. We do not favor corn plasters; rather, we recommend paring the corns when necessary after a foot bath. (c) Corticosteroids are injected beneath the corns, as they are usually associated with a painful inflammation of subcutaneous fascia.

When conservative measures prove inadequate, the patient should be referred to

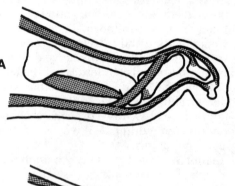

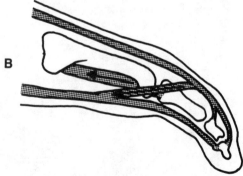

Fig. 13–35. Hammer toes. *A,* weak interosseous and lumbrical muscles allow the long extensor and flexor muscles to produce the hammer toe deformity. *B,* when strong, the interosseous and lumbrical muscles oppose the hammer toe deformity by flexing the metatarsophalangeal joint and extending the proximal interphalangeal joint.

an orthopaedist or podiatrist who may consider excision of the prominent PIP joints.

3. Corns on the Sides of the Toes. Tight shoes press the IP joints of one toe against the phalanges or IP joints of its neighbors, and press directly against the MP and IP joints of the fifth toe. If the joints be prominent, as they will become with degenerative change, the pressure will be great enough to cause the development of corns on each of the toes at their points of contact. These corns are always painful. Interdigital corns tend to ulcerate and become infected.

Treatment. (a) Only shoes with roomy toe pieces are worn, or no shoes are worn. (b) Corns are pared thin and kept thin by paring when necessary after a foot bath. (c) Corticosteroids are injected beneath the corn as they are usually associated with a painful inflammation of the subcutaneous fascia. (d) Lamb's wool placed between the toes or just proximal to the lateral aspect of the 5th MP joint may divert pressure away from the corns. (e) Should infection and/or ulceration supervene, the patient should be advised to rest the feet out of shoes, elevate them to waist level, block the affected toes apart with small blocks of cork or wood, and to bathe the feet several times daily. A culture should be made and appropriate antibiotics given when infection is manifest by cellulitis and/or lymphangitis.

When conservative measures prove inadequate, the patient may be referred to an orthopaedist or podiatrist who may consider removal of bony prominences from the pressing joint margins.

4. Hallux Valgus. Persons who chronically wear shoes with pointed toe pieces develop some degree of hallux valgus in time. Three developmental anomalies predispose to hallux valgus: metatarsus primus varus, metatarsus varus, and a malformed first metatarsal head. Metatarsus primus varus and metatarsus varus can predispose to hallux valgus only when shoes with narrow toe pieces are worn, while a malformation of the 1st metatarsal head may predispose to hallux valgus, even among the barefooted. Figure 13–36 illustrates the manner by which the malformed metatarsal head does this.

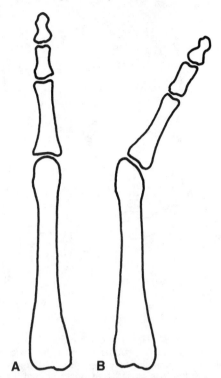

Fig. 13–36. Hallux valgus resulting from a malformed metatarsal head. *A*, normal. *B*, abnormal.

Prevention and Early Correction. If the abductor hallucis is intentionally strengthened, its tone can prevent progression of hallux valgus. Most people, particularly those who chronically wear shoes and give their feet next to no thought, are unable selectively to contract the abductor hallucis. However, unless atrophy is advanced and/or the MP joint bound into abduction by shortened ligaments and a shortened adductor pollicis, they can learn to abduct the great toe. Figure 13–37 illustrates exercises designed to facilitate the learning of abduction. When manipulative examination shows passive abduction to be limited to an angle short of the longitudinal axis of the foot, a night abduction splint should be worn. (See Figure 13–38.) Roomy, straight-toe shoes, open sandals, or no footwear are mandatory. When hallux valgus results from a malformed metatarsal head, non-surgical correction is unlikely. However, maintenance of abductor tone and full MP range of motion may protect the MP joint from subluxation and the consequent increased wear which will hasten its degeneration.

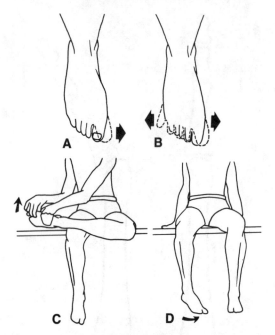

Fig. 13–37. Hallux abduction exercises. *A,* push against a finger, a rubber band, or the side of the shoe. *B,* keep the feet and toes on the floor and spread the toes apart. *C,* manually abduct the great toe to stretch the adductor hallucis, and the lateral aspect of the first metacarpophalangeal joint capsule. *D,* keeping the heel stationary, slide the forefoot internally toward the other foot.

Late Treatment. Once the toe is bound in adduction by shortened ligaments and a shortened adductor pollicis, exercises and splints become useless. Also, by this time, shoe pressure over the prominent 1st MP joint has nearly always produced a *bunion,* which is a painful prominence consisting of reactive bony overgrowth and thickened subcutaneous fascia. Patients hurting with this advanced hallux valgus and its associated bunion must be referred to an orthopaedist or podiatrist for consideration of a variety of surgical procedures.

5. Bursitis and Arthritis of the 1st MP Joint. Gout and degeneration can predispose to acute exacerbation of arthritis in the 1st MP joint, and hallux valgus predisposes to an acute degenerative bursitis over its medial aspect. A phlegmonous cellulitis or pyogenic arthritis can mimic all three. The clinician differentiates among these five disorders by attending to the following:

a. Premorbid state of the joint. Gout often emerges in a previously normal joint. Exacerbations of degenerative arthritis always emerge in a previously degenerative joint. Degeneration of an MP joint is suggested when the range of motion is limited and attended by crepitation. X-ray will confirm the degeneration. An exacerbation of bursitis is more likely to occur when the great toe is in valgus. A phlegmonous cellulitis or pyogenic arthritis can emerge about or in a normal or degenerated joint.

b. Onset. Gout develops very rapidly, often without any history of stress by pressure or by movement. An exacerbation of degenerative arthritis or of bursitis may emerge rapidly, but usually some history of uncustomary usage prior to onset is elicited. Cellulitis or pyogenic arthritis can emerge rapidly, without recognized predisposing events, or they may follow any superficial injury to the overlying skin.

c. Physical findings. Gouty, degenerative, and pyogenic arthritis show redness and swelling about a tender MP joint which is tender on all sides. Bursitis shows a redness and swelling over a tender me-

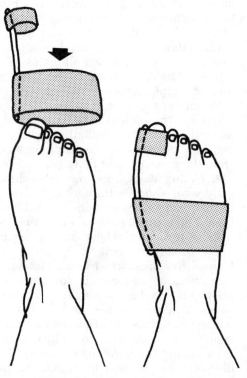

Fig. 13–38. Hallux abduction splint.

dial aspect only. Cellulitis shows a generalized redness and swelling of a tender great toe and adjacent forefoot, with tenderness not limited to the joint line or bursa. Lymphangitis and/or inguinal and femoral lymphadenitis, fever, and leukocytosis are more likely to be associated with pyogenic arthritis and phlegmonous cellulitis than with the other disorders. Although pyogenic arthritis cannot be certainly excluded without aspiration of the joint, we find it rarely necessary to aspirate these joints. Prior history of gout or degenerative arthritis and the absence of fever, lymphadenopathy, and leukocytosis allow us a presumptive exclusion of pyogenic arthritis. We follow our patients closely, and should toxic signs or regional evidence of infection appear, or 2 days' treatment with anti-inflammatory agents pass with no improvement, we attempt an arthrocentesis and start antibiotics.

Treatment.

1. At the outset, bursitis, gouty arthritis, and degenerative arthritis are all treated with indomethacin or phenylbutazone, ice applications, and rest. (See Chapter 18.)

2. X-ray is made, and serum uric acid is determined.

3. When bursitis or degenerative arthritis appears to have been the problem, efforts are begun to correct any hallux valgus, to strengthen the intrinsic flexors and extensors of the great toe, and to increase the painless range of motion of the great toe. Pressure diversion away from a bursa is effected with bunion pads and/or lamb's wool.

4. When gouty arthritis appears to have been the problem, we switch to maintenance gout therapy as soon as remission is well advanced. (See Chapter 18.)

Hallux rigidis is a late complication of degenerative arthritis of the 1st MP joint. The range of motion is initially painfully restricted by capsular congestion and fibrosis. In time, the joint may undergo bony fusion. A rocker-bottom shoe or a regular shoe with a rigid shank, or surgery are the only treatments available.

6. Embedded Nail Margins ("Ingrown Toenail," Onychocryptosis). All nail plates are dorsally convex from side to side. The convexity of some nail plates is rather shallow, and of others quite deep. The

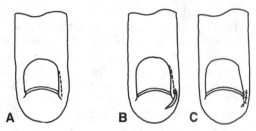

Fig. 13–39. *A*, embedded nail margin (ingrown toenail). *B* and *C*, surgical delivery of the embedded nail margin by retraction of the nail fold.

lateral borders of nails with deep convexities are likely to become embedded beneath the distal verge of their nail grooves. (See Figure 13–39.) Nail margins so embedded cannot continue to grow without cutting into the distal verge of the nail groove. This wound becomes inflamed, as would any wound containing a foreign body, and becomes secondarily infected with saprophytes and occasionally with aggressive parasites, particularly the coagulase-positive Staphylococcus. The resultant chronic paronychia is annoyingly painful at best, and can become disablingly so when infected by an aggressive parasite.

The deep lateral margins may become embedded in one of two ways: (a) Shoe pressure either forces the nail plate downward or the nail fold upward, such that one of the margins of the nail plate cuts into the nail groove. As this injury becomes inflamed, the nail fold and the distal verge of the nail groove swell upward over the nail margin. As the nail plate continues to grow forward, the distal angle of the embedded nail margin begins to cut into the verge of the nail groove. At this point, the chronic paronychia is established. (b) If the distal angle of a nail margin is trimmed or broken back, the verge of the nail groove may swell over the new distal angle in response to the inevitable congestion of hot dependent feet. With growth of the nail plate, the new distal angle will cut into the swollen verge of the nail groove. At that point, the chronic paronychia is established.

Efforts to trim the corners of embedded nail plates inevitably create a deep spicule which hooks into the verge of the nail groove in a manner which prevents the nail margin from being delivered except by surgery.

For deep convexity (not my office tech)

Treatment.

1. At the first appearance of a parony-chia, antibiotics, ice packs, and elevation for several days may be rewarded by a remission of the paronychia and a subsid-ence of the nail fold. At that point, the potentially embedded nail margin may sometimes be wedged over the verge of the nail groove with cotton packing.

2. When the paronychia has been pre-sent for several weeks, medical treatment is ineffective, as the foreign body effect of the angle of the nail plate in the verge of the nail groove is established, and the in-flammation will not subside until it is re-moved.

3. Occasionally, the angle of the nail plate can be thoroughly removed under local anesthesia, following which the par-onychia will remit. When the paronychia has remitted, and the nail fold and nail groove are no longer tender, and the nail fold is no longer swollen, the new angle of the nail plate may sometimes be wedged over the verge of the nail groove by re-peated cotton packings. This technique has been successful in our hands only for nail plates of rather shallow convexity.

See previous page

4. When the nail plate is of shallow convexity and the superficial treatments of the nail plate described above are un-successful, the verge of the nail fold can be surgically retracted, thus delivering the embedded nail margin. (See Figure 13–39, B and C.) This method and the superficial treatments of the nail plate are usually unsuccessful when the nail plate is of deep convexity.

5. For nail plates of deep convexity, the embedded margin of the nail plate, its nail bed, and its matrix must all be removed or destroyed if the distal angle of the growing nail plate is to remain liberated from the nail groove. Figure 13–40 illustrates the sharp surgical method of removal. This is the method we have used. When care is taken to remove nail bed and matrix down to the periosteum of the distal phalanx, permanent cures can be expected. The pro-cedure disables the patient about 3 days. We examine and clean the wound after 2 or 3 days, and apply a simple band-aid dressing. Any sutures are removed in 7 days. The patient is instructed to soak the toe in soapy water for 20 minutes at least

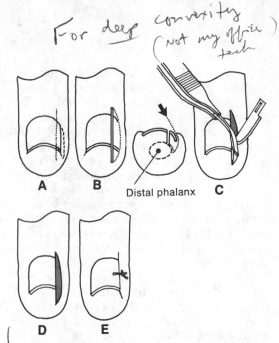

A   **B**   Distal phalanx   **C**

D   **E**

Fig. 13:40. *A* through *E*, excision of the embedded margin of the "ingrown toenail" with its nail bed and matrix. Excision extends to the periosteum of the distal phalanx.

daily, and to rinse thoroughly afterward. A new band-aid is applied after each soak-ing. The toe is gratifyingly comfortable after 1 week, and usually painless after 2–3 months.

6. Some physicians remove only the nail plate and cauterize the bed and matrix with saturated carbolic acid. Phenol crys-tals to which a few drops of water have been added create a saturated solution of carbolic acid. The carbolic acid treatment is asserted to be less painful than and equally effective as sharp surgical re-moval, provided the carbolic acid is al-lowed to remain in contact with the tissue for sufficient time. The advocates of the method advise that a cotton applicator, soaked in carbolic acid, be rubbed vigor-ously over the nail bed and matrix for 2 minutes. (See W. R. Ross and D. S. Wolf, The Foot-Podiatry, page 818, in George J. Hill II, *Outpatient Surgery,* W. B. Saunders and Company, 1973.)

7. **Onychomycosis.** Fungus infection of the nail bed usually begins in one or an-other lateral margin and very slowly pro-gresses across the distal margin and back toward the matrix. The nail bed produces a thick keratin debris which elevates the nail plate, and in time the nail plate be-comes thickened, yellow, and fibrous. The

distortion proves to be a cosmetic problem for some, and as the nail plate thickens, one or two pain problems may emerge as well: (a) The thick nail plate may be pressed downward by a tight-fitting toe piece, and the resultant pressure may irritate the subungual fascia; (b) as the thickened nail plate assumes a deep transverse convexity, one of its lateral margins may injure its nail groove and thus become embedded, leading to the chronic perionychia of the "ingrown toenail."

Treatment. In our experience, there is no sure cure. Fulvicin 500 mg. twice daily for 12 months can produce a regression and even an apparent cure in most patients who can take the drug that long. Unfortunately, a number of these suffer a relapse after the drug is withdrawn.

When this treatment is impossible due to drug reaction or is ineffective, and the pain syndrome complicates the problem, we treat the pain syndrome as follows:

1. Contused subungual fascia. The nail plate is thinned with an emory wheel. Various hand-held motor-powered emory wheels are available from medical supply houses. This treatment is repeated whenever growth of the nail plate necessitates.

2. "Ingrown toenail." We remove the entire nail plate and that portion of the nail bed and matrix which lies in the affected nail groove.

3. Occasionally, patients request permanent removal of the nail. We remove the entire nail plate, bed, and matrix, rongeur the distal phalanx as necessary to allow the flap of distal skin to be sutured to the epinychial wound margin, then remove all dog ears and complete the closure. Other physicians remove the nail plate only and cauterize the matrix with carbolic acid, and await keratinization of the nail plate. (See W. R. Ross and D. S. Wolf, page 820, in George J. Hill II, *Outpatient Surgery*, W. B. Saunders and Company, 1973.)

Injuries of the Leg, Ankle, and Foot

The prognosis of lower extremity injuries depends heavily upon the circulation. This obvious contingency bears emphasis because the lower extremity is uniquely vulnerable to arterial and venous disease, and because novice clinicians tend to ignore this fact in their preoccupation with the details of the injury. In contrast, an initial concern of the clinician must be the vascular competence of the injured extremity. In our opinion, in the face of venous or arterial insufficiency, the following injuries should be referred immediately to an orthopaedist or general surgeon when at all possible:

1. Extensive muscle contusion.

2. Fractures of tubular bone (shafts of tibia and fibula).

3. Unstable sprains and dislocations.

4. Compound injuries and avulsions of the integument.

This general rule will not be stated again, but we urge the reader to keep its injunctions in mind when interpreting the remainder of this chapter, as the treatments recommended assume an extremity with competent arterial and venous systems.

Contusion of the Leg

Because the *crural fascia* is tough and tense over the anterior compartment, contusions to the anterior compartment can be of grave import. Modest bleeding and effusion into the confined anterior compartment can so increase the tissue pressure as to lead to ischemic necrosis of the muscle. Because the skin over the anterior aspect of the leg is tightly bound to the crural fascia, it too tolerates swelling poorly, and contusions of the anterior skin almost invariably lead to necrosis of the central zone of the contused skin. We have never seen a large hematoma between the anterior crural fascia and the overlying skin that was not complicated by necrosis of the central zone of overlying skin.

Therefore, contusions of the anterior compartment of the leg must be respected. The clinician must do what can be done to minimize swelling, and must watch closely for signs of anterior compartment muscle ischemia.

Treatment. The primary practitioner should proceed as follows:

1. Any associated abrasions must be scrubbed as free of ground dirt as possible. We use a brush gently, after applying 2% Xylocaine topically.

2. The extremity must be elevated above heart level, and toe-gripping exercise be performed repeatedly every few minutes to encourage venous and lymphatic return.

3. Ice packs may be applied over the injury for the first 24 hours.

4. The leg should not be bound.

5. <u>Dorsiflexion of the ankle and extension</u> of the toes should be attempted every 30 minutes for the first 12 hours, and several times daily thereafter. Any decline in apparent strength or increase in pain with the effort suggests muscle ischemia. Of course, pain alone can inhibit extensor tone, but many patients who are made aware of the importance of the test will generate a stronger movement with a well-nourished muscle than with an ischemic muscle. If at any point muscle ischemia is suspected, an orthopaedist or general surgeon must be asked to consider fasciotomy.

6. As swelling and pain subside, active stretching and working exercises of the anterior compartment muscles are begun.

7. The patient should avoid ambulation during the first 48 hours, except for bathroom needs only, and then ambulation should be non-weightbearing with crutches. Partial weightbearing may begin when active stretching and working exercises have been performed for 1 day without increase in pain or swelling.

Contusions to the posterior compartment are practically never subject to the danger of muscle ischemia, so restorative treatment can proceed more rapidly. Active working and stretching exercises and weightbearing as tolerated can begin after 24 hours elevation and ice.

Vigorous running and exposure to further contusion should be avoided until healing is complete, as repeated intramuscular bleeding can lead to myositis ossificans.

Tennis Leg

A violent push-off, as occurs when a tennis player makes a desperate dash for the net may be rewarded by a sudden pain in the calf, which feels to the afflicted as though the calf had been kicked or hit by a stone. Indeed, a middle-aged gentleman who suffered the injury while playing badminton next to a yard that was being trimmed by a rotary mower was initially convinced that the mower had thrown a stone into his calf. Classically, a rupture of the plantaris muscle has been blamed for this injury. A current view denies our ability clinically to distinguish such an injury from a partial tear of the gastrocnemius or soleus muscles, and abstains from judging the matter. Some clinicians suspect that a suddenly activated discoordinate contraction can subject a group of motor units to a rupturing force. The calf becomes tender and tense within a few hours of the injury, and the distal posterior aspect of the leg becomes ecchymotic, usually by the next day. Any stress to the gastrocnemius-soleus muscles increases the pain.

Treatment. The primary practitioner should proceed as suggested for a contusion of the posterior aspect of the leg, with one additional measure: An elevated heel allows more comfortable walking during the first 1–2 weeks after injury. Patients are often troubled by the prolonged convalescence. The injury often takes 6–8 weeks for complete resolution. But the bark is worse than the bite, and full recovery always occurs. When pain is disabling for too long, a walking cast with the ankle in slight plantar flexion can be very comforting. We leave such a cast in place for 4 weeks.

Rupture of the Achilles Tendon

Like the tennis leg, this injury occurs during sudden stress to the posterior compartment muscles. However, the force is much greater and is usually applied when passive dorsiflexion is strongly resisted, as can occur when an individual slips off a high curb or the tailgate of a truck and takes full weight on the ball of the plantar-flexed foot. The impact is heralded by sudden pain and a sense of snapping. Patients often believe they have fractured or severely sprained an ankle. They sometimes do not notice the weakness of plantar flexion that follows. Swelling and ecchymosis appear about the lower leg and ankle within 12 hours.

Diagnosis. Achilles tendon rupture must be suspected of every "ankle injury" until examination proves otherwise. When the patient attempts to plantar flex against

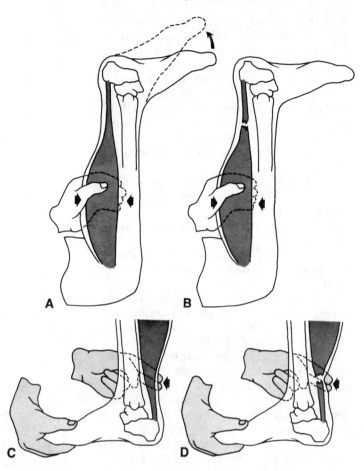

Fig. 13–41. Diagnosis of the ruptured achilles tendon. *A,* normal. *B,* ruptured. *C,* normal. *D,* ruptured.

resistance, the movement is noted to be weak. Two observations confirm the diagnosis (See Figure 13–41):

1. When the calf of the injured extremity is gripped, the ankle and foot will not plantar flex, whereas when this maneuver is applied to the normal extremity, the ankle will plantar flex.

2. When the ankle is gently dorsiflexed, instead of the firm achilles tendon, a tender soft depression is palpable at the musculotendinous junction.

Treatment. Many surgeons prefer open repair of the tendon, but we have had uniformly satisfying results with casting. Thus, in our opinion, the injury can fall within the competence and responsibility of the primary practitioner. To be effective, a cast must accomplish two ends:

1. The ends of the tendon must be held in contact.

2. The gastrocnemius and soleus muscles must be protected from stretch.

Full plantar flexion will accomplish the first end, and, as the soleus originates from the tibia and fibula, will prevent the soleus from stretching. However, the gastrocnemius originates from the femoral condyles and will be stretched by knee extension. The gastrocnemius is ideally free of tension when the knee is flexed to or beyond 90°. For the knee to be immobilized at 90° for the requisite 2–3 months would be very awkward at best, and would add the need of knee mobilization and strengthening to the rehabilitation task. Some clinicians have recommended that the knee be immobilized at 135–150° as a compromise. We prefer a different compromise, which keeps the knee nearer to 90° most of the time—the short leg cast. We believe this method works for three reasons:

1. While the patient could intentionally extend the knee at every opportunity, none of our patients have done so when told

why they should not. Or, if they have done so, and kept their activities secret from us, it has at least not prevented a satisfactory result.

2. With the ankle fully plantar flexed, whether non-weightbearing or weight-bearing, the knee must be carried at 135° or less for the foot to clear the ground. When sitting, the knee is at 90°

Hence, in summary, we recommend the following treatment:

1. Immobilize the extremity in a short leg cast with the ankle in full plantar flexion. (See Figure 13–42).

2. Keep the patient non-weightbearing for 6 weeks.

3. Add a walking surface to the toe of the cast and allow weightbearing for the next 4 weeks.

4. Remove the cast after the full 10 weeks and instruct the patient to return to partial weightbearing—initially resting only the weight of the leg on the ground.

5. Begin gastrocnemius-soleus stretching and strengthening exercises. These exercises must be advanced very gradually. Full rehabilitation is not expected before 6 months. A physical therapist's services are mandatory.

6. The patient must not engage in activity that would abruptly stress the achilles tendon until that 6-month rehabilitation program is complete.

Dislocation of the Peronei Tendons.

Some persons' peroneal retinacula are relatively weakly bound to the underlying fascia and will, in time, tear loose, allowing the tendons to dislocate anteriorly over the lateral malleolus during a full dorsiflexion of the ankle. (See Figure 13–43). The initial episode may be painful, and may be followed by the appearance of swelling and ecchymosis. Usually, the tendons spontaneously relocate when the ankle is plantar flexed. Thus, the tendons may come repeatedly to dislocate and relocate, producing an unpleasant snapping sensation at each occurrence. Patients often complain that their ankle keeps "popping out." When the tendons remain dislocated, pronation is weak or impossible, and the lateral ligaments of the ankle are therefore unusually vulnerable to injury.

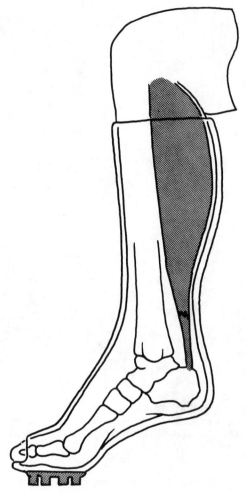

Fig. 13–42. Cast treatment of achilles tendon rupture.

Diagnosis. When patients give the history summarized above, the peroneal tendons must be examined. If dislocated, the diagnosis is made. If not dislocated, they can usually be made to dislocate if the patient actively rotates the ankle in full range of motion.

Treatment. The primary practitioner should proceed as follows:

1. If dislocated, the tendon must be relocated. This may occur spontaneously when the patient actively plantar flexes the ankle. Posteriorly directed pressure on the tendon will facilitate the relocation, if necessary.

2. The ankle should be casted in slight plantar flexion and pronation. The plaster should be carefully molded to apply firmly

to the contour of the lateral malleolus. A walking heel may be applied for full weight bearing.

3. The cast is removed after 8 weeks, and partial weightbearing is begun.

4. Active range of motion and ankle-strengthening exercises are begun and gradually advanced over a 2-month period. (See Figure 13–31). A physical therapist's services are recommended.

Should the problem recur, the patient should be referred to an orthopaedist who must consider a surgical modification of the peroneal retinacula.

Fractures of the Shafts of the Tibia and Fibula

The nature of these bones and their relationships dictate 11 principles upon which secure diagnosis and effective treatment are founded.

1. As in the case of the radius and ulna, a single fracture of the tibia or fibula cannot displace grossly unless one of the tibiofibular joints dislocates.

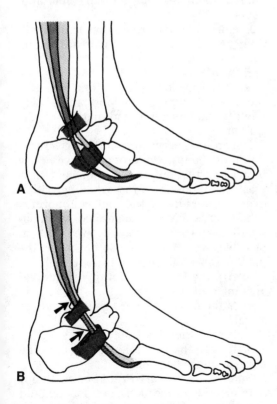

Fig. 13–43. Subluxation of the peroneal tendons. *A*, normal. *B*, subluxed.

2. Correlatively, a dislocation of one of the tibiofibular joints necessitates a dislocation of the other joint or a displaced fracture of one of the bones.

3. An intact fibula can prevent firm apposition of the fragments of the tibial fracture, thus delaying and even preventing healing. (See Figure 13–44).

4. Only the lower end of the fibula, which enters into formation of the ankle mortice, is clinically important, and its proper function does not depend on its proximal shaft, but upon the tibiofibular ligaments and the collateral ligaments of the ankle. (See Figure 13–44B.) The shaft of the fibula is important only as an origin for the muscles of the lateral, anterior, and deep posterior compartments of the leg. It can serve this function without being an entirely intact bone.

5. Fractures of the upper end of the fibula may injure the common or the deep peroneal nerve.

6. Healing of fibular fractures is practically never a problem; indeed, a single fracture of the fibula will heal without immobilization.

7. On the other hand, the shaft of the tibia is distinctly vulnerable to delayed union and non-union, though contemporary treatment has greatly diminished the incidence of these misfortunes.

8. Because the tibia is a superficial bone, and the forces that fracture it are violent, its fractures are more likely to compound than are any other fractures in the body.

9. The forces that fracture the shaft of the tibia and fibula are direct impact forces, angulating forces, twisting forces, and axial compressive forces.

Direct impact forces to the lateral aspect of the leg rarely produce injury more serious than a simple fracture of the fibula, which may or may not be complicated by a peroneal nerve injury.

Direct impact forces to the anterior and medial aspects of the leg are likely to produce compound fractures of the tibia.

Angulating forces are likely to produce transverse or shallow oblique fractures of the tibia, or fracture separations of the tibial epiphysis in childhood and adolescence. When the force is sufficiently prolonged, a transverse or shallow oblique fracture of the fibula will also occur. When

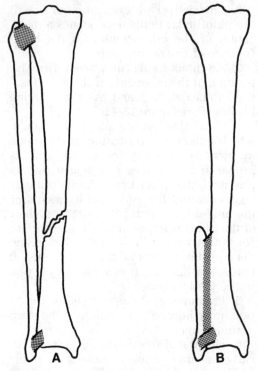

Fig. 13–44. *A*, distraction of a tibial fracture by an intact fibula. *B*, portion of fibula necessary to the structure of the ankle mortice.

may produce injuries at either the knee or ankle. Why one injury will occur and not another is a matter of speculation. A reasonable notion consistent with some clinical experiences presumes that the spiral fracture will occur when both knee and ankle are strongly splinted by posture and muscle action, and by boots. Rarely, spiral fractures will enter the ankle or knee joints.

Axial compressive forces produce injuries which are reviewed below under "Injuries of the Ankle."

10. Impacting forces favor healing. Distracting forces impede it.

11. Spiral fractures are least amenable to weightbearing treatment, as they do not impact.

Diagnosis. The following symptoms and signs suggest fracture of the shaft of the fibula and/or tibia.

1. The patient may report abrupt pain and sometimes a snapping sensation at the moment of violence to the leg.

2. Tenderness and swelling are usually evident about the shafts of the tibia and fibula.

3. Pain and often crepitation are evident when gentle shearing forces are applied to the bones.

Evaluation.

1. Anteroposterior and lateral x-rays of the leg, including knee and ankle, will identify the location and nature of the fracture.

2. Peroneal nerve and tibial nerve function must be tested: Peroneal nerve injury is suggested when pronation of the foot is weak or impossible, and when sensation over the dorsum of the foot is abnormal. Tibial nerve injury is suggested when supination and toe flexion are weak or impossible, and when sensation over the plantar aspect of the foot is abnormal.

3. Are the fragments in apposition and alignment or nearly so?

4. Is the fracture transverse, oblique, or spiral?

5. Is only the tibia fractured?

6. If only the fibula is fractured, is the mortice injured or not?

Role of the Primary Practitioner. In our opinion, the primary practitioner should complete the above evaluation and proceed as follows:

both bones fracture, they fracture at the same level (See Figure 13–45*A*.) When angulating forces disrupt the ankle mortice, they may fracture out the lower third of the fibula. (See below under "Pronation," under "Injuries of the Ankle.") Transverse and shallow oblique fractures occur most commonly in the lower third of the leg. These fractures usually occur when a sudden decelerating force is applied at the foot. The following are typical examples: (a) A skier drives a ski tip into a mogul, is catapulted over his boottops, and the forward release jams. (b) A baseball player catches a cleat on the edge of home plate at the beginning of a late violent slide. (c) A downhill runner steps into a hole.

Twisting forces are likely to produce spiral fractures of both tibia and fibula. The tibial fracture is typically in the lower third of the leg, and the fibular fracture in the upper third (See Figure 13–45*B*.) These fractures occur when the body rotates violently on a fixed leg, or a leg rotates violently on a fixed body. Similar forces

1. Treat the following fractures definitively:

a. Transverse fractures of both tibia and fibula in or near apposition and alignment.

b. Single fractures of the fibula, without injury to the mortice and without peroneal nerve injury.

2. Treat the following fractures with orthopaedic consultation:

a. Undisplaced fractures of the tibia alone, whether spiral, oblique, or transverse. If the fibula is tending to distract the tibial fracture, an orthopaedist may elect to excise a small segment of the fibula.

b. Undisplaced spiral and oblique fractures of the tibia and fibula. If these fractures should tend to displace with time, an orthopaedist may elect to immobilize the fractures internally.

c. Salter I and II fractures of the distal tibial epiphysis. (See Chapter 15.)

3. Provide emergency immobilization of the following fractures and refer the patient to an orthopaedist:

a. Grossly displaced or compound fractures of any form.

b. Fractures accompanied by disruption of the mortice.

c. Fractures that have entered the ankle or knee joint.

d. Salter III, IV, and V fractures of the distal tibial epiphysis. (See Chapter 15.)

Treatment.

1. Transverse fractures of both tibia and fibula, in or near apposition and alignment. Alignment must be anatomic, while apposition need be only so much as to allow impaction during weightbearing and to avoid an unacceptable cosmetic result. Only the tibia need be in apposition. The ankle should be at 90°, and efforts to place it there will tend to angulate the fracture anteriorly. We grapple with this paradox as follows (see Figure 13–46):

a. The patient is placed supine with the leg dependent over the side of the treatment table.

b. In addition to the usual padding, an additional several layers are placed around the fracture site.

c. Plaster is applied from the tibial tubercle to 1″ above the fracture site.

d. Plaster is applied over the foot and ankle to a point 1″ below the fracture site. As the plaster sets, the ankle is held at 90°, and the plaster is molded firmly about the ankle and distal portion of the leg.

e. When the plaster is firmly set, the angulation at the fracture site is corrected, and the cast is completed and extended above the knee.

The patient must be placed at bed rest with the leg elevated to heart level for 48 hours. During this time, careful watch must be kept for symptoms and signs of circulatory impairment: increased pain, paresthesias, pallor or cyanosis of the toes, and sluggish capillary return in the toes. The cast must be split and levered open should any evidence of circulatory impairment appear. The clinician should not leave the patient until normal circulation has been restored. If splitting and levering the cast are insufficient, the padding under the cast must be cut. If that is insufficient, the cast must be split on the opposite side as well. If that is insufficient, the cast must be removed and an orthopaedist's services requested.

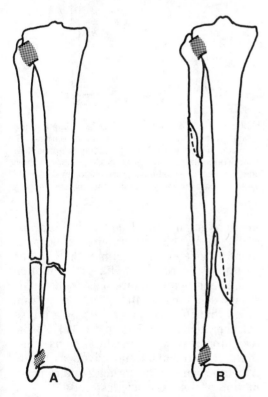

Fig. 13–45. *A*, transverse or shallow oblique fracture through the distal third of the tibia and fibula. *B*, spiral fracture of the tibia and fibula.

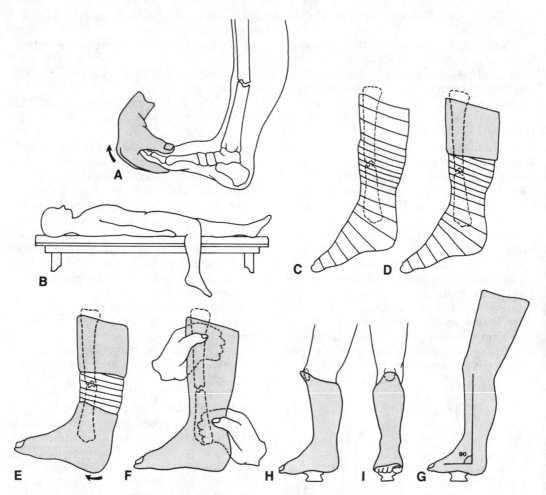

Fig. 13–46. Immobilization of transverse and shallow oblique fractures of the tibia and fibula. *A,* the fracture will angulate anteriorly when the ankle is placed at 90°. *B* through *G,* one way to avoid producing a deformity. *B,* patient is positioned supined with the leg dependent over the side of the table. *C,* cast padding is applied. *D,* plaster is applied around the proximal fragment. *E,* plaster is applied to the foot and ankle while the ankle is held at 90°. *F,* plaster is applied to bridge the gap, the angulation is corrected, and the desired position is held while the bridging plaster sets. *G,* a long leg cast is completed. *H* and *I,* patellar weightbearing cast. *H,* side view. *I,* front view.

After 48 hours, if the patient is comfortable in a proper cast, and circulation to the toes is brisk, non-weightbearing ambulation is begun. The leg must be elevated whenever the patient is not moving about. After 2 weeks, a walking heel can be applied and gradually increasing weightbearing begun. By the end of 3 weeks, most patients are fully weightbearing and will continue so for the entire period of immobilization. At 6 weeks, the long leg cast can be changed to a patellar weightbearing cast. (See Figure 13–46, *H* and *I*.) This cast allows early rehabilitation of the knee and still prevents rotation of the fracture fragments. Usually the fracture is clinically stable, and abundant bridging callus is evident on x-ray by the 4th month. If so, the cast may be removed. Range of motion and strengthening exercises for the ankle must begin immediately, and we recommend that they be supervised by a physical therapist (See Figure 13–31.) Partial weightbearing with crutches begins when the cast is removed and advances to full weightbearing as the strength and range of motion of the ankle are restored.

Radiographic examinations are made as advised in Chapter 17.

Delayed union. If callus is minimal or

the fracture not clinically stable after 4 months, an orthopaedist's consultation should be obtained. Most of these fractures go on to heal by 6 months without other treatment, but the potential gravity of the situation warrants the early participation of a specialist.

2. Single fractures of the fibula without injury to the mortice or peroneal nerve. A short leg walking cast is applied for comfort. If the fracture is in the distal half, a regular short leg cast is adequate. If the fracture is in the proximal half, a patellar weightbearing cast may be necessary. Once again, the practitioner and the patient must realize that the cast is for comfort only. The fracture will heal, though nothing be done. The cast can be removed after 4–6 weeks. At this time, range of motion and strengthening exercises of the ankle should begin (See Figure 13–31.) Full weightbearing, if cautious, can begin when the cast is removed. Vigorous walking and athletic activities must not resume until the ankle is fully rehabilitated. The patient who rejects immobilization and continues to walk about, albeit with crutches or a cane, will rehabilitate more quickly than will the patient who accepts immobilization. Follow-up radiographic examinations are not necessary.

3. Undisplaced fractures of the tibia alone are immobilized in long leg plaster and followed as recommended for transverse fractures of the tibia and fibula. Occasionally, the orthopaedic consultant may elect surgically to excise a fragment of fibula when it appears that the tibia is being distracted. Radiographic examinations are made as advised in Chapter 17.

4. Undisplaced spiral and oblique fractures of the tibia and fibula are immobilized in long leg plaster. Weightbearing is not allowed until adequate callus bridges the fracture lines. Therefore, external immobilization of spiral and oblique fractures may require 4 months of non-weightbearing ambulation. As soon as any bridging callus is evident, usually by 2 months, the long leg cast may be exchanged for a patellar weightbearing cast, and quadriceps strengthening and range of motion exercises of the knee may be started. Radiographic examinations are made as advised in Chapter 17.

5. Emergency immobilization of injuries that require referral to an orthopaedist is often satisfactorily accomplished in a long leg posterior splint, or in a Thomas splint. These patients are generally admitted to hospital.

Injuries of the Ankle

The effect of an injury upon the articular surfaces and the stability of the talar tendon in its tibiofibular mortice determine the choice of treatment and the prognosis of the injury.

The following forces injure these regions:

Supination. (See Figure 13–47.) These forces produce the majority of sprains. They result when the extremity rotates externally upon a fixed foot, or when a weight acting on the forepart of a plantar-flexed foot and ankle causes the foot and ankle to supinate under the extremity. The structures injured depend partially upon the degree of plantar flexion at the moment of injury and partially upon the duration and/or magnitude of the force.

When plantar flexion at the moment of injury is marked, the lateral talocalcaneal ligament is likely to be injured first. When plantar flexion is less, the anterior talofibular ligament is likely to be injured first. As the duration of the force increases, the fibulocalcaneal ligament will be injured as well. The severity of injury depends largely upon the magnitude of the forces. The talocalcaneal and anterior talofibular, and calcaneofibular ligaments are sprained by lesser forces and torn by greater forces. These greater forces, rather than tear the ligaments, may either avulse the attachment of the calcaneofibular ligament from the tip of the fibula, or with the anterior and posterior talofibular ligaments, avulse the entire end of the lateral malleolus. Having avulsed the end of the lateral malleolus, these forces can then fracture out the medial malleolus and shift the talus and attached malleoli medially out of articulation with the tibial articular surface.

Pronation. (See Figure 13–48.) These forces produce the majority of fractures. They result when the extremity rotates internally upon a fixed foot, or when body

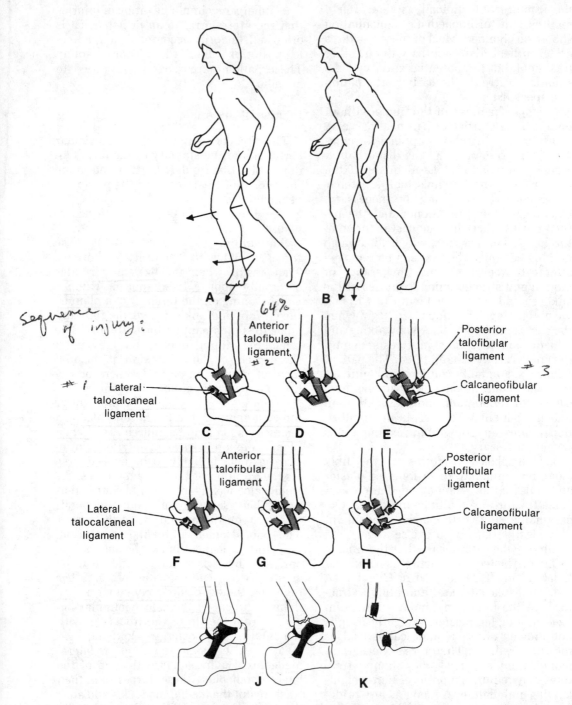

sequence of injury:

64%

Anterior
talofibular
ligament.
 # 2

Posterior
talofibular
ligament

 # 3

 # 1   Lateral
talocalcaneal
ligament

Calcaneofibular
ligament

C   D   E

Anterior
talofibular
ligament

Posterior
talofibular
ligament

Lateral
talocalcaneal
ligament

Calcaneofibular
ligament

F   G   H

I   J   K

Fig. 13–47. Supination injuries to the ankle. *A* and *B*, modes of injury. *A*, extremity rotates externally on the fixed foot. *B*, plantar-flexed foot is forced into supination. *C* through *E*, sequence of injuries. Lateral talocalcaneal ligament (*C*) is injured before the anterior talofibular (*D*), which is injured before the calcaneofibular (*E*). *F* through *H*, when the injuring force is sufficient, the ligaments will tear completely and in the same sequence. *I* through *K*, rather than tear the lateral ligaments, the injuring force may avulse a flake of fibula (*I*), or fracture off the end of the fibula (*J*), or fracture off both the end of the fibula and the medial condyle (*K*).

weight—acting on the lateral aspect of the forepart of the foot—forces it into extreme pronation. The structures injured depend partially upon the duration and magnitude of the force.

The weaker and briefer pronating forces will either fracture out the lateral malleolus or avulse the medial malleolus, leaving the talotibial joint unstable but still in articulation.

The stronger pronating forces can produce one of three injuries:

1. They may fracture out the lateral malleolus and tear the deltoid ligament.

2. They may fracture out the lateral malleolus and avulse the medial malleolus.

3. They may tear the deltoid ligament and the tibiofibular ligament, and fracture out the lower third of the fibula.

All three injuries destroy the mortice and displace the talus laterally out of articulation with the tibia.

When the injuring forces cause forward displacement of the tibia as well as pronation of the foot and ankle, the posterior margin of the tibia (sometimes called the posterior malleolus) may be fractured out as well. This fracture may accompany any

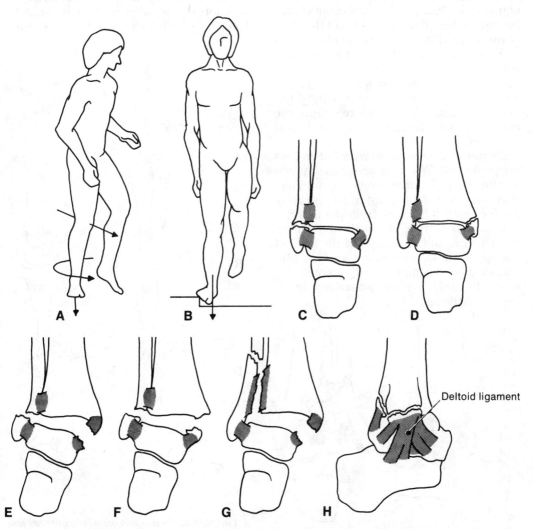

Fig. 13–48. Pronation injuries of the ankle. *A* and *B*, modes of injury. *A*, extremity rotates internally on the fixed foot. *B*, the foot is forced into pronation by weight taken on the lateral aspect of the forefoot. *C* and *D*, brief forces of lesser severity may fracture a malleolus without tearing a ligament. *E* through *G*, forces of greater severity will destroy the mortice in one of three ways. *H*, when forward displacement of the tibia accompanies severe pronation forces, the posterior margin of the tibial articular surface may be fractured as well.

of the injuries described in the previous paragraph.

Axial Compression. (See Figure 13–49.) These forces are encountered less often than supination and pronation forces. They usually result when individuals fall from a height and land on their feet. When the impact creates some dorsiflexion as well as compression vectors, the anterior margin of the tibia is fractured out, and the talus is displaced anteriorly out of articulation with the tibia. When the impact creates pure compression forces, the talus is driven upward through the tibial articular surface, thus producing a comminuted fracture of the articular surface of the tibia, a tear of the tibiofibular ligaments, and an outward fracture of the lower third of the fibula.

When children sustain such an injury, a Salter V epiphyseal fracture is almost unavoidable. See Chapter 15 regarding the prognosis and treatment of epiphyseal fractures.

Flexion and Anteroposterior Shear. (See Figure 13–50.) When of lesser magnitude and/or when shearing forces are minimal, dorsiflexion and/or plantar flexion may produce a chip fracture from the anterior or posterior margin of the tibial articular surface or from the dorsum of the head of the talus. These injuries are very painful and may be accompanied by a contusion of the tibiotalar and/or posterior talocalcaneal cartilages.

When of greater magnitude, the following injuries may result:

1. Dorsiflexion may produce a fracture through the neck of the talus. This fracture is frequently complicated by aseptic necrosis of the head of the talus.

2. When associated with posterior shear, dorsiflexion may produce a posterior dislocation of the talus with or without the fracture of the neck of the talus. More rarely, a posterior oblique fracture of the distal end of the tibia may occur.

3. When associated with anterior shear, dorsiflexion may produce an anterior dislocation of the talus with or without the fracture of the neck of the talus. More

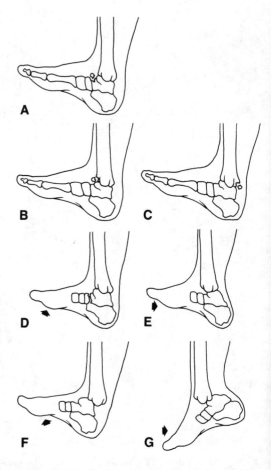

Fig. 13–50. Flexion and anteroposterior shearing forces. *A* through *C*, forces of lesser severity may produce a chip fracture of: *A*, the dorsum of the talus. *B*, the anterior margin of the tibia, or *C*, the posterior margin of the tibia. *D* through *G*, forces of greater severity may fracture the neck of the talus and/or dislocate the tibiotalar joint.

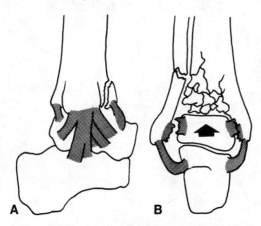

Fig. 13–49. Axial compression injuries of the ankle. *A*, when dorsiflexion accompanies compression, an oblique fracture of the anterior margin of the tibial articular surface may result. *B*, direct axial compression of sufficient force will destroy the mortice.

rarely, an anterior oblique fracture of the distal end of the tibia may occur.

4. Plantar flexion, which except in the rarest of circumstances is accompanied by posterior shear, may produce a posterior dislocation of the talus.

These dislocations occur independently of any disruption of the mortice itself. They are the rarest of ankle injuries, and the posterior dislocation is the more common of the two. The dislocations that do occur are often compounded.

Whether all these forces tear ligaments or fracture malleoli may depend upon structural differences among individuals that make their bones more or less resilient than their ligaments. However, subtle differences in direction of the vectors may also make their contribution.

Evaluation of the Injured Ankle. A harmfully simplistic notion presumes that the evaluation of ankle injuries seeks simply to determine whether an injury be a fracture or not. The reader who has understood the previous paragraphs will appreciate the final irrelevance of that question.

The proper evaluation will categorize an ankle injury into one of three groups:

1. Stable injuries.

2. Unstable injuries with an intact mortice or a mortice only one side of which has been distorted.

3. Unstable injuries with a completely distorted mortice (either by tibiofibular distraction or by fracture of both lateral and medial malleoli).

We recommend the following examination protocol. The significance of each finding is indicated in context. *Both ankles and feet must be examined together, as all is relative, and only a contrast is meaningful.* Each observation should be made on the normal side and that finding compared with the finding on the injured side.

Inspection.

1. Does the ankle appear dislocated?

2. Is the ankle swollen and/or ecchymotic? Early after an injury, swelling is indicative of bleeding.

3. Is the joint space distended? With the ankle at 90°, note the scaphoid depression to either side of the extensor tendons. A joint effusion will cause the depressions to bulge in comparison to the normal.

Palpation.

1. Are the malleoli tender or crepitant? Tenderness without crepitation suggests an undisplaced fracture. Tenderness with crepitation suggests a displaced fracture. Tenderness over the body of the malleolus suggests a fracture line through the body of the malleolus. Tenderness over the tip of the malleolus suggests an avulsion of the attachment of the ligament from the malleolus.

2. Does compression of the fibula on the tibia in the midleg produce pain? When this maneuver produces pain, it suggests a fracture of the fibula above the tibiofibular ligaments which, when associated with evidence of an ankle injury, suggests a distraction of the mortice. (See Figure 13-51.)

3. Which ligaments are tender? (See Figures 13-1 and 13-52.)

Manipulation. (See Figure 13-53.)

1. If the ankle does not appear to be dislocated, if the malleoli are not crepitant, and if compression of the fibula on the tibia in the midleg does not produce pain, the mortice may be tested for stability. The sooner after injury this manipulation is performed, the more likely is the manipulation to yield useful information. Holding the ankle at 90°, grasp the heel and attempt alternately to evert and invert the hindfoot. After noting the effect of the same maneuver on the normal side, some sense of stability or instability on the abnormal side may be achieved.

2. If the ankle seems stable, gently move the ankle between dorsiflexion and plantar flexion, and with the ankle at 90°, gently apply rhythmic traction to the ankle. If these maneuvers can be effected with little increase in pain, an effusion into the joint and/or an unstable disruption of collateral ligaments is unlikely. (Painful stretch to the commonly injured lateral talocalcaneal and anterior talofibular ligaments is less likely to occur if plantar flexion is performed with the foot everted and traction performed with the ankle at 90°.)

Note. The effect of any grip should be observed before performing a manipulation. The grip may touch a tender spot, and the unwary examiner may incorrectly interpret the patient's increased pain to have been produced by the manipulation.

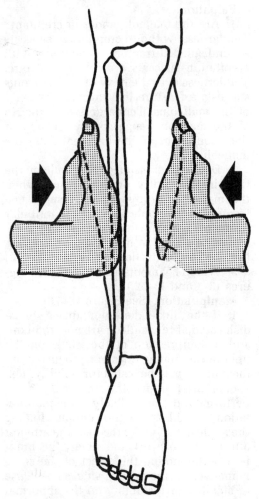

Fig. 13–51. Examination of the ankle—compression of the fibula on the tibia.

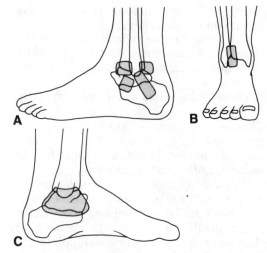

Fig. 13–52. Examination of the ankle—zones oɪ tenderness of the individual ligaments. *A,* the lateral ligaments. *B,* the anterior-inferior tibiofibular ligament. *C,* the deltoid ligament.

The evidence of physical examination is interpreted before ordering x-rays. The following are the physical characteristics of the three groups of injuries:

1. Stable injuries.

a. "Sprain." Early after the injury, swelling is confined to one side of the ankle and may be slight or marked. Early after the injury, the opposite scaphoid depression is the same as that of the normal ankle. After many hours with the ankle dependent, generalized edema may obscure this sign. The malleoli are not tender or crepitant, and compression of the fibula on the tibia in the midleg does not produce pain. Only one group of ligaments is tender—the *lateral talocalcaneal, anterior talofibular,* and *fibulocalcaneal ligaments,* on the one

hand, or the *deltoid ligament* on the other—not both. The ankle seems stable to manipulation in inversion and eversion, and gentle manipulation in plantar and dorsiflexion and in traction does not increase the pain.

b. Chip fractures from the anterior or posterior borders of the tibial articular surface or from the dorsum of the head of the talus. Early after injury, the scaphoid depressions may bulge as compared to the normal ankle. Compression of the fibula on the tibia in the midleg does not produce pain. The malleoli are not tender. Both collateral ligaments may be tender posteriorly or anteriorly. The ankle is stable to inversion and eversion, but gentle manipulation in plantar and dorsiflexion and in traction does increase the pain.

2. Unstable injuries with an intact mortice, or a mortice only one side of which has been distorted.

a. Pronation and supination injuries. Early after the injury, swelling is confined to one side of the ankle and is usually marked. The opposite scaphoid depression often bulges in comparison to the normal ankle when examined early after injury, before generalized edema has obscured the sign. One of the malleoli is tender, and may or may not be crepitant. Compression of the fibula or the tibia in the midleg does not produce pain. The ankle seems unsta-

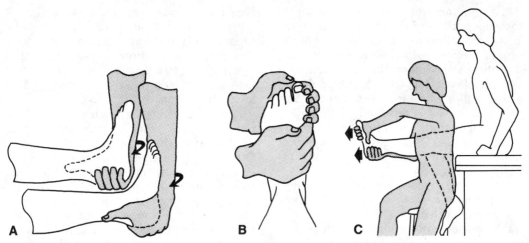

Fig. 13–53. Examination of the ankle—manipulation of the ankle. *A,* manipulation for instability of the tibiotalar joint. The injured ankle may be compared to the normal ankle by simultaneous manipulation. *B,* gentle manipulation in dorsal and plantar flexion. *C,* application of rhythmic traction to the ankle.

ble to manipulation in inversion or eversion, and gentle manipulation in dorsiflexion, plantar flexion, and/or traction does increase the pain. Only one group of ligaments is tender, those either on the same side or on the opposite side of the tender malleolus. (See examples in Figure 13–47 and 13–48.)

b. Anterior or posterior dislocation of the ankle, and fractures of the neck of the talus (See Figure 13–50.) The dislocation and any compounding are obvious. Fractures of the neck of the talus and, after reduction, simple dislocations both present a bulging of the scaphoid depressions as compared to the normal ankle. Compression of the fibula on the tibia does not produce pain. Neither malleolus is tender. Both collateral ligaments are tender. The ankle may not be stable to inversion and eversion, and gentle manipulation in plantar and dorsiflexion and in traction does increase the pain.

3. Unstable injury, with a completely distorted mortice. Swelling is bilateral early after the injury and is marked. The scaphoid depressions, if not hidden beneath the subcutaneous blood, bulge in comparison to the normal. One or both malleoli are tender and crepitant, either over the outer surface of the body or over the tip. Compression of the fibula on the tibia in the midleg may or may not produce

pain. One or both groups of ligaments may be tender. In the face of these findings, manipulation is not done. (See examples in Figures 13–47 through 13–49.)

All injuries that are not clearly in Group 1a injuries are x-rayed.

Treatment.

1. Stable injuries.

a. "Sprain." The stable ligament injuries of the ankle are taped as illustrated in Figure 13–54. When swelling is marked, a compression dressing is applied over the tape, and the tape and dressing are removed and reapplied every 3 or 4 days.

Ice compresses are applied many times throughout the day for the 1st several days after injury. These compresses help to prevent further swelling, and may hasten the resolution of swelling.

Weightbearing may be performed as tolerated. Tolerance in this sense is defined as comfortable walking without limping. If limping is necessary, crutches and partial weightbearing are requisite.

Mobilizing exercises in full range of motion are begun immediately. (See Figure 13–31.) Once full weightbearing is comfortable, pronation strengthening exercises are added to the regimen. (See Figure 13–31.)

Full weightbearing is usually tolerable after 1–2 weeks. Full recovery is usually complete within 3 months.

b. Chip fractures from the anterior or posterior borders of the tibial articular surface or from the dorsum of the head of the talus. To relieve pain and facilitate healing of cartilage, the injury should be immobilized in plaster for 4 weeks. Ambulation with a walking heel may begin at the outset. Once the cast is removed, mobilization and strengthening exercises of the ankle must begin (See Figure 13-31.) The patient must be warned of the possibility of traumatic arthritis.

2. Unstable injuries with an intact mortice or a mortice only one side of which has been distorted.

a. Pronation and supination injuries and reduced, simple dislocations. Contemporary teaching in orthopaedics seems increasingly to favor open surgical repair of all these injuries. We remain skeptical of this global approach and reserve open surgery for only those injuries that appear grossly unstable to very modest stress. When the talus can be rocked out of the mortice 45° or more, by only modest stress, we consider the joint to be grossly "unsta-

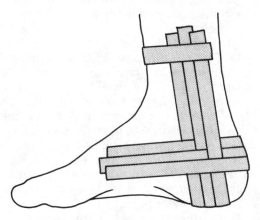

Fig. 13-54. Taping of a stable sprain.

ble." Injuries characterized by lesser instability, in our opinion, can be treated quite satisfactorily by closed methods of reduction and imobilization. These latter injuries may be quite properly managed by the primary clinician. We recommend the following protocol:

(1) If the injury is a dislocation, it is reduced. The primary practitioner can usually effect this reduction fairly readily. Often no pharmacologic analgesia is necessary and then, unless contraindicated, intravenous narcotics are usually quite adequate. Rarely, sciatic and femoral nerve blocks at the hip may be necessary. (See Chapter 16.) The dislocation is reduced by straight traction on the foot in line with the axis of the leg. Figure 13-55 illustrates the grip used.

(2) Any distortion of the mortice is then corrected. Figure 13-56 illustrates manipulations to reduce the three varieties of distortion.

(3) The extremity is then immobilized in a short leg walking cast. Supination injuries are casted in slight pronation. Pronation injuries are casted in slight supination. During the first 2-5 days after casting, the extremity is elevated continuously, except when attending the bathroom. After the first 2-5 days, swelling has usually stabilized, and full weightbearing can usually safely be allowed. Patients are instructed to elevate the foot any time that they are sitting down for any length of time. Follow-up radiographic examinations are made as indicated in Chapter 17.

(4) Plaster is retained for 8 weeks.

(5) Toe-gripping exercises are begun at the outset, and continued many times daily throughout the period of immobilization.

(6) When the cast is removed, partial

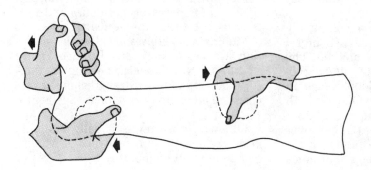

Fig. 13-55. Reduction of a dislocated ankle by straight traction. Both anterior and posterior dislocations can be reduced by this maneuver unless soft tissue interposition blocks closed reduction.

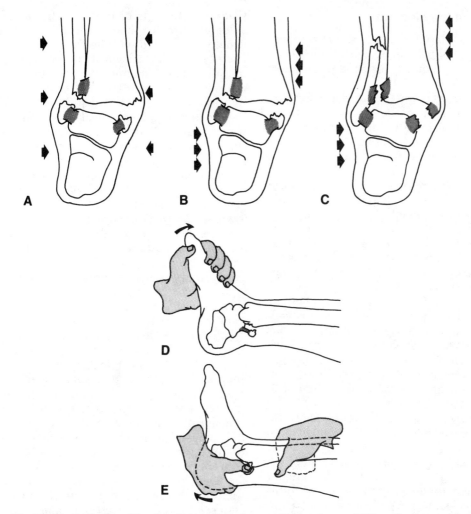

Fig. 13–56. Reduction of the distorted mortice—incorrect (*A*) and correct (*B*) application of reducing forces. *A* and *B*, fractured lateral malleolus and torn deltoid ligament, or avulsed medial malleolus. *C*, torn tibiofibular ligament, deltoid ligament, and fractured lower third of fibula. *D* (incorrect) and *E* (correct) reduction of fractured posterior margin of the articular surface of the tibia.

weightbearing is begun and mobilizing and strengthening exercises of the ankle are begun and continued until function is fully restored—usually after 1-2 months. (See Figure 13-31.) Weightbearing is increased as increasing mobility and strength allow.

b. Grossly unstable injuries, compound dislocations, fractures of the neck of the talus and oblique anterior or posterior fractures of the distal end of the tibia. The primary practitioner should apply a posterior splint and refer the patient to an orthopaedist in hospital. When an interval of hours is expected before the orthopae-

dist can arrive, the primary practitioner should attempt to reduce a compound dislocation before splintage and admission.

3. Unstable injuries with a completely distorted mortice. The great majority of these injuries will require open reduction and immobilization. The primary practitioner should correct any obvious dislocation, apply a posterior splint, and refer the patient to an orthopaedist in hospital.

Patients who have suffered axial compression fractures of the ankle and/or heel (see below) must be examined physically and by x-ray for a fracture of the spine.

Injuries of the Hindfoot.

These are contusions of the bursae and tendons about the heel, contusions of the plantar aspect of the heel, and fractures of the calcaneus.

Contusions of the Bursae and Tendons. These are treated as are non-traumatic bursitis tenosinovitis, and paratendinitis achilles. (See the discussion of these entities in the earler section dealing with "Heal and Ankle Pain.")

Contusions of the Plantar Aspect of the Heel. These result when the heel (usually barefoot) takes weight heavily on a prominence like a stone. Indeed, these injuries are often called "stone bruises." The injuring forces rupture the subcutaneous fibrous septae and bruise the attachment of the plantar aponeurosis.

Treatment. Ice packs are applied as many times daily as possible, until swelling and pain have begun to diminish—3–7 days is usual. A shoe with an elastic heel, like the ripple sole, is fitted with a supination longitudinal arch support, and weightbearing is allowed from the outset as tolerated.

Fractures of the Calcaneus. These result when people fall from a height onto their heels. (See Figure 13–57.) The lesser forces may produce crack fractures of the tuberosity of the calcaneus, the greater forces may produce compression fractures of the calcaneus. While any axial compression force applied through the heel can contuse the posterior talocalcaneal articulation, thus predisposing to traumatic subtalar arthritis, this complication is not usually associated with undisplaced crack fractures of the calcaneal tuberosity. On the other hand, compression fractures of the calcaneus are characterized by impaction of the calcaneal articular surface of the posterior talocalcaneal joint downward into the body of the calcaneus. Its surface is thus shattered into numerous fragments.

Treatment. The undisplaced crack fracture of the calcaneal tuberosity should be protected in a short leg walking plaster for 6 weeks. The ankle is immobilized at 90° and the plaster is molded firmly to the heel. Rehabilitation is as discussed for group 2 injuries of the ankle. (See above.) The primary practitioner can manage this injury from the outset. The patient must be warned of the possible development of traumatic subtalar arthritis.

Following a compression fracture, the anatomic reduction of the calcaneal surface of the posterior talocalcaneal joint is impossible and traumatic subtalar arthritis is an inevitable complication. Two forms of treatment are employed: (a) Full active range of motion exercises of the tibiotalar and talocalcaneal joints, non-weightbearing for 6 weeks, or (b) Immediate subtalar arthrodesis. We believe an orthopaedist should make the choice unless the primary practitioner knows the patient very well, shares a candid respectful rapport with the patient, and the patient categorically declines surgery. In this case, primary practitioners should monitor the non-weightbearing active range of motion regimen themselves. Hospital support for the 1st few days is humane and will provide optimal opportunity for exercise training.

All other patients should be referred to an orthopaedist in hospital.

Injuries of the Midfoot.

Fractures of other tarsal bones are rare. Many are simply treated by 4 weeks' immobilization in a short leg walking cast. It is perhaps wisest that a primary practitioner consult an orthopaedist before assuming responsibility for one of these rare and necessarily unfamiliar fractures.

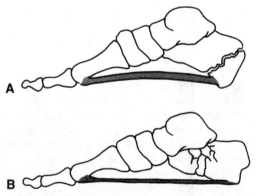

Fig. 13–57. Fracture of the calcaneus. *A,* crack fracture of the tuberosity of the calcaneus. *B,* compression fracture of the body of the calcaneus.

The midtarsal joint may dislocate. (See Figure 13-58.) Often these dislocations are compounded. We recommend the primary practitioner refer all these injuries to an orthopaedist. Any compound injuries should be cleaned of debris and thoroughly irrigated while awaiting arrival of an orthopaedist. When a delay of hours is expected before an orthopaedist's services will be available, we recommended that the primary practitioner attempt the reduction to decrease the pain and the danger of vascular and cartilage injury.

A tibial nerve block posterior to the medial malleolus and a peroneal nerve block, between the tibialis anterior and the common extensor tendons, and lateral to the common extensor tendons, usually provides adequate anesthesia. (See Chapter 16.) The dislocation can usually be reduced very readily by straight traction on the forefoot with one hand while resisting at the ankle with the other. Occasionally, forward pressure by the thumb of the resisting hand on the protruding shelf of the distal tarsal row will help to guide the distal portion toward rearticulation. (See Figure 13-58B.)

Injuries of the Forefoot and Toes.

These injuries commonly result from crushing, grinding, lacerating, and levering forces. Crushing and grinding forces typically lead to compound injury. Levering forces rarely do so.

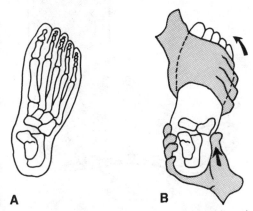

A   **B**

Fig. 13-58. *A,* dislocation of the midtarsal joint—forefoot angulated in valgus. *B,* reduction of midtarsal dislocation.

Crushing Forces. Heavy weights falling on the forefoot or toes burst the soft tissues while fracturing the bones.

Injuries to the toes can be definitively managed by a primary practitioner. Ruptures of the skin are thoroughly irrigated and closed with suture. Injuries to nail plates and nail beds are treated as summarized in Chapter 6 under "Fingertip Injuries." Dislocations are reduced, and fractures are reduced as possible. Often, fractures are comminuted and thus irreducible. A walking cast with a toe platform gives the greatest comfort and protection to these injuries. Two to three weeks cast protection is usually sufficient.

Persons who have suffered a crush injury to the forefoot are generally in severe pain. If and as soon as contraindications can be excluded and any necessary life support provided, the primary practitioner should administer an intravenous narcotic slowly until the patient experiences relief. The wound should then be cleansed as best can be done with no debridement and little manipulation. A bulky gauze dressing should then be applied, leaving the tips of the toes exposed to allow capillary return to be assessed, and the patient should be admitted to a hospital for an orthopaedist's prompt services. Surgical and anesthesia risks at the time of admission should be assessed and documented in the chart.

Grinding Injuries. In motorcycle accidents, a foot may be trapped between the motorcycle and the road as the momentum of the cycle and rider spends itself in a slide along the road. The rough road surface will grind through the integument and eventually through ligament or tendon and bone.

When confined to digits, these compound injuries can be definitively treated by primary practitioners. All loose debris must be removed. Debris that is ground into tissue should be left to slough with the devascularized tissue. No attempt is made to close these wounds. They are dressed with gauze over antibiotic ointment, and the dressings are changed at least daily. At the time of dressing change, the injury is soaked in warm soapy water for 20-30 minutes, then thoroughly rinsed before applying the new dressing. This procedure continues until the wound is clean and granulating well. Then the decision can be made whether to graft, to otherwise revise the wound, or to await full healing by secondary intention. Details of these procedures have been presented in Chapter 6 in the discussion of "Fingertip Injuries."

Grinding injuries to the forefoot, if extensive and deep, are treated as are crush injuries to the forefoot. Shallow injuries to small areas that do not cross the ankle should be treated definitively by the primary practitioner as are grinding injuries to the toes.

Lacerating Forces. The principles of laceration repair were reviewed in Chapter 6 under "Lacerations in the Hand and Wrist." These apply equally to the foot. Extensor and flexor tendons to the great toe must be repaired. Single extensor or flexor tendon injuries to the other toes need not be repaired. Laceration of the common extensor or flexor tendon and of the tibialis posterior, tibialis anterior, and peroneal tendons must be repaired. When both ends of the tendon are easily accessible, it is proper for the primary practitioner to repair the tendon by methods outlined in Chapter 6 under "Repair of Tendons, Ligaments and Nerves." When the ends are not easily accessible, or have been badly frayed, the injury should be repaired by an orthopaedist.

Laceration of the tibial nerve posterior to the medial malleolus or of either plantar nerve just forward of the heel will paralyze the intrinsic flexors of the foot and deprive the plantar surface of cutaneous sensation. A foot so impaired is seriously disabled. These nerves must be repaired if at all possible. Otherwise, the skin wound should be treated as appropriate, and the patient should be referred for secondary repair after 3 weeks. (See "Repair of Tendons, Ligaments, and Nerves" in Chapter 6.)

Levering Forces. Simple metatarsal fractures heal kindly in every case. A short leg walking cast may be applied for comfort for 3 weeks. The fracture of the base of the 5th metatarsal may be associated with ligament injuries that prolong the pain. Because the fracture line is not radiologically healed for 2–3 months, it has been blamed for the persistent pain, in our view incorrectly. Too many patients with these fractures are pain free after 3 weeks and those who are not are usually more tender proximal and dorsal to the base of the metatarsal than over the fracture site itself.

A small bone, called the os vesalianum, is occasionally present proximal to the base of the 5th metatarsal. It can be confused for an avulsion fracture until the clinician notes its smooth borders and evidence of the same structure on the uninjured foot.

Fractures of the digits result from angulating forces that are produced when the bare foot kicks an object. The fifth toe can be fractured at the base of the proximal phalanx and angulated laterally. The prox-

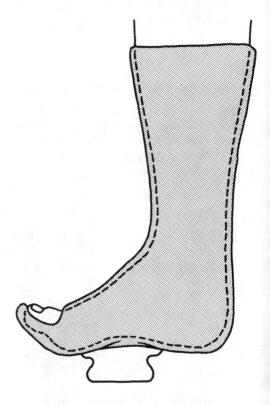

Fig. 13–59. Modification of the short leg cast for immobilization of an avulsed extensor pollicis longus tendon.

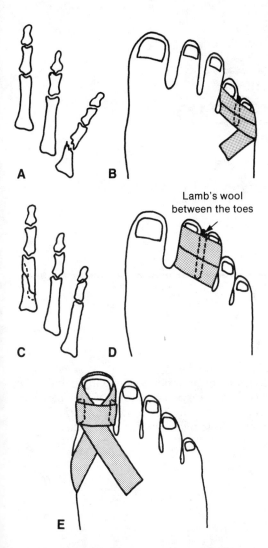

Lamb's wool
between the toes

Fig. 13-60. Immobilization of phalangeal fractures. *A* and *B*, fracture of the proximal phalanx of the fifth toe. *C* and *D*, fracture of the proximal phalanx of the second, third, or fourth toes. The protective and splinting effects of a roomy shoe are usually adequate, but some patients are more comfortable if the toe is taped as diagrammed. *E*, fracture of the proximal phalanx of the great toe.

imal phalanx of the great toe is often obliquely fractured when stubbing forces flex it abruptly under the foot. Occasionally stubbing forces will avulse the attachment of the extensor tendon from the base of the distal phalanx. Fractures of the proximal phalanx of the great toe that enter the MP or IP joints must be anatomically reduced. Reduction of all other digital fractures need merely restore normal appearance.

Fractures of the great toe are best protected on a toeplate in a short leg walking cast for 6 weeks. The avulsion fracture at the extensor tendon insertion requires that the toe be held in dorsiflexion by the toe plate. (See Figure 13-59.) All other angular force digital fractures can be ignored unless grossly unstable. (Fractures that require reduction—most commonly fractures of the base of the fifth toe—are usually unstable.) For comfort, a roomy shoe is best. When a fracture is grossly unstable or patients are uneasy and request more protection, we tape the injured toe to its neighbor after placing lamb's wool between the toes. (See Figure 13-60.) When used to immobilize the grossly unstable fracture, this dressing should remain untouched for 2 weeks. When used for comfort or security, we teach our patients to remove the dressing and wash and dry carefully between the toes every 2 days. They may retape the toes as they desire.

Dislocations of the MP and IP joints are reduced by maneuvers similar to those advised for the homologous dislocations in the hand. Once reduced, nothing further is done except to protect the toe in a roomy shoe for 2 weeks. As for fractures, taping may be required for comfort.

Sprains of the MP and IP joints are treated as reduced dislocations.

CHAPTER 14

Non-Traumatic Pain Syndromes of the Lower Extremity Summarized

The lumbosacral neuropathies and the painful disorders of the pelvis, hips, and knees all produce lower extremity pain, and the differentiation among them is not always obvious. This chapter presents a tabliform summary intended to help the student grasp the extent of the problem and to provide the practicing clinician an accessible overview for office use.

Table 14–1

The Disorder	Distribution of Pain	Usual Presentation	Distinctive Physical Findings	X-ray Findings	Prodromes and/or Predisposing Circumstances
L₅ nerve root irritation, secondary to L₄–L₅ disc herniation.	Ipsilateral buttock, posterior thigh, anterolateral leg, and dorsum of foot.	Dysesthesia in the area of pain distribution. Weak hallux extension.	Occasional lumbosacral lordosis and/or kyphosis. Variable restriction in low back movement. Increased pain with straight leg raising. Symmetrical deep tendon reflexes.	Lumbosacral spine may be normal or show early degenerative changes. Myelogram shows an indentation of the spinal canal anterolaterally at the L₄–L₅ disc.	Repeated episodes of acute low back pain over the previous 5–10 years. Unilateral spondylolysis and rotational facet malformation may predispose to disc degeneration.
L₅ nerve root irritation, secondary to L₅–S₁ facet degeneration.	Same as disc.	Same as disc.	Same as disc.	Advanced degenerative changes. Myelogram may show variable degrees of spinal stenosis.	Repeated episodes of acute low back pain over the previous 10+ years.
S₁ nerve root irritation, secondary to L₅–S₁ disc herniation.	Ipsilateral buttock, posterior thigh, posterolateral leg, and outer aspect of the heel.	Dysesthesia in the area of pain distribution. Variable weakness of plantar flexion.	Same as L₄–L₅ disc, except achilles deep tendon reflex is diminished or absent.	Same as L₄–L₅ disc, except the myelogram shows the indentation of the spinal canal anterolaterally at the L₅–S₁ disc.	Same as the L₄–L₅ disc.
Narrow spinal canal syndrome.	Both buttocks and legs.	Pain intensified by walking, secondary to the associated lumbosacral lordosis. Bladder and bowel function may be impaired. Sensation and strength in the lower extremities is variably impaired.	Accentuation of the lumbosacral lordosis will increase pain. Variable restriction in low back motion.	Advanced degenerative changes. Myelogram shows narrow spinal canal.	Repeated episodes of acute low back pain over the previous 10+ years.
Sacroiliac strain or arthritis.	Ipsilateral low back and buttock.	Walking and other postural changes may increase the pain.	Tenderness over the affected sacroiliac joint. Pain increased by axial compression of the trunk, especially while sitting on the ipsilateral buttock.	Lumbosacral spine may be normal or show variably severe degenerative or Paget changes at the affected sacroiliac joint.	Pregnancy in the third trimester. Generalized psoriasis, active ulcerative colitis or regional enteritis, family or personal history of ankylosing spondylitis, or Paget's disease.
Acute and chronic septic arthritis of the hip.	Groin and anteromedial aspect of the thigh and knee.	Cannot bear weight. Infants and young children will manifest a flaccid extremity. Hectic fe-	The slightest manipulation of the hip provokes pain behavior.	No findings early. If untreated, cystic subchondral bone resorption, signs of degener-	The greatest incidence occurs among children prior to 3 years of age. Premature newborns

TABLE 14-1—Continued

The Disorder	Distribution of Pain	Usual Presentation	Distinctive Physical Findings	X-ray Findings	Prodromes and/or Predisposing Circumstances
		ver and various degrees of toxicity: Newborns and infants may be prostrate, and even unresponsive; older children and adults are miserably ill but alert and somewhat active.		ative joint disease, and often signs of chronic osteomyelitis will emerge.	are particularly vulnerable.
Transient synovitis of the hip in early childhood.	The articulate child may describe pain in the groin and anteromedial aspect of the thigh and knee. Some children will complain of knee pain only.	The child is reluctant to bear weight on or to move the affected hip. The child appears otherwise well.	Internal rotation, extension, and abduction are limited by pain.	Normal x-ray throughout the course of the illness.	Typically occurs in children between 3 and 5 years of age.
Aseptic necrosis of the femoral head (Legg-Perthes disease).	Groin and anteromedial aspect of the thigh and knee.	The child limps without recognized antecedent injury, particularly after some hours of weight-bearing. The child appears otherwise well.	Internal rotation, extension, and abduction are limited by pain.	Normal x-ray at the onset. The capital femoral epiphysis becomes radiopaque relative to the osteoporotic adjacent bone by the 6th–8th week of symptoms. Eventual mottling of the head appears as new bone begins to form.	Typically occurs in children 3–10 years of age.
Slipped capital femoral epiphysis.	Groin and anteromedial aspect of the thigh and knee.	The child limps without recognized antecedent injury, but will occasionally report an abrupt onset of pain while running. The child walks with a unique abduction gait. The child appears otherwise well.	Internal rotation, extension, and abduction are limited by pain.	A frog-leg lateral or true lateral radiograph will show the slippage of the capital femoral epiphysis.	Typically occurs in children between 10 years of age and the end of growth. An unidentified endocrine disorder is suspect.
Degenerative joint disease of the hip.	Groin and anteromedial aspect of the thigh and knee.	Prolonged weightbearing increases the pain. Pain during resting hours can prevent sleep. Afflicted persons show a characteristic gait: The trunk leans out over the affected hip when stepping with that ex-	Internal rotation, extension, and abduction are limited by pain and, in time, by contracture.	Narrowing of the joint space associated with wearing of the cartilage. Eburnation of subchondral bone. Spurring at the cartilage margins.	Probable hereditary predisposition. Past history of injury, aseptic necrosis, slipped femoral epiphysis, septic arthritis, granulomatous arthritis or cryptogenic proliferative synovial disorder.

tremity. Findings of degenerative disease in other characteristically vulnerable joints: knees, distal interphalangeal joints of the fingers, trapeziometacarpal joints of the thumbs, facets of the spine, particularly the lumbosacral and cervical.				
Cryptogenic proliferative synovial disorders and granulomatous arthritis of the hip.	Groin and anteromedial aspect of the thigh and knee.	Same as degenerative arthritis, plus: conservative treatment for degenerative joint disease does not attenuate the disability; the cryptogenic proliferative synovial disorders typically appear in youth and in early middle age before the usual onset of symptomatic degenerative joint disease.	Internal rotation, extension, and abduction are limited by pain and, in time, by contracture. Those with granulomatous disease may develope draining sinuses and are typically chronically ill and immunodepressed, and may show other foci of granulomatous disease, particularly in the lungs.	All of the cryptogenic proliferative synovial disorders may show deep cystic erosions into the acetabulum and the femoral head, and in time the narrowing of the joint space, eburnation of subchondral bone, and spurring at the joint margins typical of degenerative joint disease.

Pigmented villonodular synovitis—may show increased soft tissue shadow about the joint.

Synovial osteochondromatosis—may show periarticular foci of calcification.

Granulomatous arthritis—may show an increased soft tissue shadow and, in time, the signs of degenerative joint disease and perhaps the distinctive changes of granulomatous infection of the acetabulum and/or the head of the femur. | Any of the reasons for chronic immunodepression will predispose to granulomatous arthritis. |
| Immune complex arthritis of the hip (rheu- | Groin and anteromedial aspect of the thigh and | The afflicted cannot bear weight during acute | Internal rotation, extension, and abduction are | No findings early. Eventual cystic subchondral | Probable hereditary predisposition to rheu- |

TABLE 14-1—Continued

The Disorder	Distribution of Pain	Usual Presentation	Distinctive Physical Findings	X-ray Findings	Prodromes and/or Predisposing Circumstances
matoid arthritis, psoriatic arthritis, arthritis of inflammatory intestinal disease, Reiter's syndrome, acute rheumatic fever, subacute lupus erythematosus and other collagen vascular disorders).	knee.	exacerbations. Pain during resting hours can prevent sleep.	limited by pain and, in time, by contracture. These diseases are usually polyarticular. They present with variable degrees of toxicity. Other manifestations of the associated illness are usually evident. (See Chapter 18.)	bone resorption and regional osteoporosis will accompany rheumatoid arthritis and may accompany psoriatic arthritis, arthritis of inflammatory intestinal disease, and Reiter's syndrome.	matoid arthritis, psoriasis, inflammatory intestinal disease, and the collagen vascular disorders.
Iliopsoas bursitis/tendinitis.	Groin and anteromedial thigh. When severe or persistent, pain will refer into the anteromedial aspect of the knee.	Pain inhibits active hip flexion and limits the range of extension.	Deep tenderness is palpable in the anteromedial thigh at the level of the distal border of the greater femoral trochanter. Hip extension limited by pain.	If recurrent, soft tissue calcifications may be evident near the lesser femoral trochanter.	Uncustomary exercise is occasionally admitted.
Obturator bursitis/tendinitis.	Groin and anteromedial thigh.	Pain at rest and abruptly whenever actively externally rotating or abducting the hip.	Abduction and external rotation against resistance while in the sitting position increases pain. Tenderness detected about the ischial spine by rectal examination.	If recurrent, soft tissue calcifications may be evident about the ischial spine.	Uncustomary exercise is occasionally admitted.
Trochanteric bursitis, myotendinous pain syndromes of the buttock and lateral thigh.	Lateral aspect of the hip and thigh. When severe or persistent, pain will refer into the lateral aspect of the knee.	Pain may inhibit walking.	Abduction and internal rotation against resistance may increase the pain. Tenderness will be palpable over the greater femoral trochanter, the tensor fasciae latae, the gluteus medius and minimus, or the iliotibial tract.	If recurrent, soft tissue calcifications may be evident about the greater femoral trochanter.	Uncustomary exercise is occasionally admitted.
Gluteal bursitis.	Buttock and posterior thigh. When severe or persistent, pain may refer into the lateral aspect of the knee.	Pain may inhibit walking.	Abduction against resistance and full passive flexion and adduction will increase the pain. Tenderness will be palpable over and posterior to the greater femoral trochanter.	If recurrent, soft tissue calcifications may be evident about the greater femoral trochanter.	Uncustomary exercise is occasionally admitted.

Condition	Location of pain	Effect on walking	Physical examination	Radiographic findings	Comments
Ischial bursitis/hamstring tendinitis.	Buttock and posterolateral aspect of the thigh. If severe or persistent, pain may refer into the lateral aspect of the knee.	Pain will limit full hip flexion and may inhibit walking.	Tenderness will be palpable over the outer border of the ischial tuberosity.	If recurrent, soft tissue calcifications may be evident over the ischial tuberosity.	Uncustomary exercise is occasionally admitted.
Osteochondritis dissecans.	Anywhere about the knee. May refer into the thigh and leg.	The child may limp or refuse to bear weight. Aching at rest can prevent sleep. Intermittent locking may occur when the necrotic fragment is extruded into the joint.	Knee examination may be entirely normal until degenerative joint disease develops. Occasionally, locking will be demonstrable.	Circumscribed radiopacity in the subchondral bone of one femoral condyle becomes evident after 6–8 weeks of symptoms.	Typically afflicts school children between 10 years of age and the completion of growth.
Aseptic necrosis of a pole of the patella (Larsen-Johansson's disease), and aseptic necrosis of the tibial tuberosity (Osgood-Schlatter's disease).	Anterior aspect of the knee. May refer into the thigh and leg.	Pain may inhibit walking and limit the range of flexion. Tenderness will interfere with kneeling.	Tenderness and swelling will be evident over the necrotic bone.	Initially normal. Fragmentation of the involved bone will eventually appear, often after symptoms abate.	Typically afflicts school children between 10 years of age and the completion of growth.
Prepatellar and superficial infrapatellar bursitis.	Anterior aspect of the knee. When severe or prolonged, pain may refer into the thigh and leg.	Pain limits flexion. When inflammation is intense, pain will inhibit walking.	Redness, tenderness, and swelling will be evident over the patella and/or the patellar ligament. Other aspects of the knee examination are normal. Diagnostic fluid can be aspirated from the affected bursa.	If recurrent, soft tissue calcifications may be evident over the patella and patellar ligament.	Habitual kneeling or previous contusion to the bursa.
Deep infrapatellar bursitis.	Anterior aspect of the knee. If severe or persistent, pain may refer into the thigh and leg.	Pain will inhibit walking and limit flexion.	Swelling about the patellar ligament and tenderness over and to either side of the lower half of the patellar ligament.	If recurrent, soft tissue calcification may be evident just proximal to the tibial tuberosity.	Uncustomary exercise may be admitted.
Anserine bursitis.	Medial aspect of the knee. If severe or persistent, pain may refer into the thigh and leg.	Pain will inhibit walking and may limit extension.	Swelling and tenderness will be evident over and inferior to the medial tibial condyle. Other aspects of the knee examination are normal.	If recurrent, soft tissue calcifications may be evident over and inferior to the medial tibial condyle.	Uncustomary exercise may be admitted.
Nonspecific myofascial pain syndromes of the knee (pain syndromes of the collateral liga-	Over the affected structure and, if severe or persistent, into the thigh and leg.	Pain may inhibit walking. If the quadriceps tendon or patellar ligament is affected, pain may limit flex-	The affected structure is tender. Other aspects of the knee examination are normal.	If recurrent, soft tissue calcifications may be evident over the involved structure.	Uncustomary exercise may be admitted.

TABLE 14-1—*Continued*

The Disorder	Distribution of Pain	Usual Presentation	Distinctive Physical Findings	X-ray Findings	Prodromes and/or Predisposing Circumstances
ments, the quadriceps tendon, the patellar ligament, or the hamstrings.)	may limit flexion. If the hamstring tendon is affected, pain may limit extension. Pain during rest may prevent sleep.				
Chondromalacia patellae.	Anteromedial aspect of the knee. May refer into the anterior thigh and leg.	Inhibits running, climbing, and descending. May ache after sitting for an hour or more with the knee near 90°.	Tender patellar margins. Pain during manipulative compression and elevation of the patella. Eventual effusion and/or Baker's cyst.	Usually normal. May show subchondral eburnation and spurring at the cartilage margins of the patella, and the patellar articular surface of the femur.	Habitual vigorous weightbearing activity. Perhaps a hereditary predisposition to degenerative joint disease, and an increased quadriceps-patellar ligament vector angle.
Degenerative joint disease of the knee.	Anywhere about the knee and, if severe or persistent, will refer into the thigh and leg.	Inhibits weightbearing. Limits range of motion. Aching at rest may prevent sleep. Findings of degenerative disease in other characteristically vulnerable joints: hips, distal interphalangeal joints of the fingers, trapeziometacarpal joints of the thumbs, facets of the spine, particularly lumbosacral and cervical.	Epicondylar bone of the femur and tibia protrude visibly and palpably. Occasional genu valgum or varum is evident. If secondary to trauma or the loss of proprioceptive and pain sensation associated with a neuropathy, the knee may be unstable. Effusions will appear during acute exacerbations of synovitis and after chronic inflammatory changes have developed in the synovium. Manipulation of the ligaments and palpation of the joint line will cause crepitus and occasionally provoke pain.	Narrowed joint space due to cartilage wear. Eburnation of subchondral bone. Spurring at the cartilage margins.	Probable hereditary predisposition. Previous injury, infection, cryptogenic proliferative synovial disorder or proprioceptive and pain sensory loss secondary to neuropathy.
Cryptogenic proliferative synovial disorders.	Anywhere about the knee and, if severe or persistent, will refer into the thigh and leg.	Same as degenerative joint disease, plus: a conservative treatment regimen fails to attenuate the disability; the cryptogenic proliferative synovial diseases typically appear in youth	Same as degenerative joint disease.	All of the cryptogenic proliferative synovial disorders may show deep cystic erosions into the femoral and tibial condyles and in time the narrowing of the joint space, ebur-	

and in early middle age before the usual onset of symptomatic degenerative joint disease.

nation of subchondral bone, and spurring at the joint margins typical of degenerative joint disease. Pigmented villonodular synovitis—may show increased soft tissue shadow about the joint. Synovial osteochondromatosis—may show periarticular foci of calcification.

CHAPTER 15
Summary of Orthopaedic Disorders Unique to Children

Two generalities and a collation of disorders may bring the uniquely pediatric aspects of this text into clearer focus. One generality deals with the non-traumatic orthopaedic disorders of childhood, and the other with the orthopaedic injuries of childhood. A list of the disorders presented in this text and their chapter reference follows each general discussion.

While the *non-traumatic disorders of adulthood* are typically degenerative, the non-traumatic disorders of childhood are typically developmental; and while therapy of the disorders of adulthood typically focuses upon restoration of function and retardation of degenerative tendencies, therapy of the disorders of childhood typically focuses upon correction of distorted anatomy and prevention of a propensity to accelerated degeneration.

The following are the developmental anatomic distortions presented in this text.

Anatomic Distortions Recognized Typically Within the First Three Months of Life:

Congenital hip: under "Non-Traumatic Afflictions of the Hip Joint" in Chapter 11.

Metatarsus varus: under this heading in Chapter 13.

Metatarsus primus varus: under this heading in Chapter 13.

Talipes equinovarus: under this heading in Chapter 13.

Anatomic Distortions Which May not Be Recognized until the Onset of Standing and Walking, about the End of the First Year:

Pronated Feet.

Hypermobile flat feet: under "Pronated Foot (Flat Foot)" in Chapter 13.

Rigid flat feet: under "Pronated Foot (Flat Foot)" in Chapter 13.

Pigeon-Toed Stance.

Anteversion of the femur: under this heading in Chapter 12.

Tibial torsion: under this heading in Chapter 13.

Metarsus Varus will occasionally not be recognized until the end of the first year.

The pain syndromes unique to childhood are largely the various forms of aseptic necrosis. These all may share a common etiology which as yet remains unknown though Osgood-Schlatter's and Sever's Diseases are currently thought to represent shear fractures through those epiphyseal growth plates. They have been called the osteochondroses. Table 15–1 lists the osteochondroses presented in this text.

Certain acquired inflammations and structural displacements are also unique

Table 15-1
Osteochondroses Presented in the Text

Presentation	Disorder
Dorsal back pain	Dorsal epiphysitis (Scheuermann's disease): under "Scheuermann's Disease" in Chapter 9.
Hip and knee pain	Aseptic necrosis of the capital femoral epiphysis (Legg-Perthes' disease): under "Perthes' Disease" in Chapter 11.
	Aseptic necrosis of the femoral condyles (osteochondritis dissecans): under "Necrosis within the Condylar Epiphyses of the Femur (Osteochondritis Dissecans)" in Chapter 12.
	Aseptic necrosis of the tibial tubercle: under "Necrosis within the Tibial Tubercle (Osgood-Schlatter's Disease)" in Chapter 12.
	Aseptic necrosis within the poles of the patella (Larsen-Johansson's disease): under this heading in Chapter 12.
Foot and ankle pain	Aseptic necrosis of the calcaneal epiphysis (Sever's disease): under "Calcaneus Apophysitis (Sever's Disease)" in Chapter 13.
	Aseptic necrosis of the talar navicular (Köhler's disease): under "Aseptic Necrosis of the Navicular (Köhler's Disease)" in Chapter 13.
	Aseptic necrosis of the head of the 2nd metatarsal (Freiberg's disease): under "Aseptic Necrosis of the 2nd Metatarsal Head (Freiberg's Disease)" in Chapter 13.

Table 15-2
Acquired Inflammations and Structural Displacements Presented in the Text

Presentation	Disorder
Wry neck	Atlanto-axial subluxation: under this heading in Chapter 1.
Hip and knee pain	Pyogenic arthritis of the hip: under this heading in Chapter 11.
	Non-specific synovitis of the hip: under "Non-Specific or Transient Synovitis" in Chapter 11.
	Slipped capital femoral epiphysis: under "Slipped Femoral Epiphysis" in Chapter 11.

to childhood. Four have been presented in this text. (See Table 15-2.)

Developing bones and joints respond to *injuries* differently in several respects than do fully developed and deteriorating bones and joints:

1. The greater remodeling potential of growing bones and its effect on treatment plans was summarized in the eighth principle under "General Principles of Treatment of Forearm Fractures" in Chapter 6. This principle allows acceptance of positions that would be unacceptable in adult injuries, often sparing children the rigors and dangers of surgery. Unfortunately, application of this principle cannot be reliably taught in a text. When in doubt, an orthopaedist must be consulted.

2. Developing joints are usually more likely to repair damage to their articular surfaces than are deteriorating joints.

Thus, the prognosis of fractures into joints is more favorable in children than in adults.

3. Growing joint capsules, ligaments, and muscles are more tolerant to prolonged immobilization than are deteriorating joint capsules, ligaments, and muscles. Thus, the need for prolonged immobilization is less likely to contraindicate closed methods of treatment in children than it is in adults. This fact typically applies to shaft fractures of the radius and ulna, of the femur, and of the tibia.

4. Epiphyseal fractures of long bones can interfere with the growth of the injured bone. These fractures occur through the zone of proliferation. (See Figure 15-1.) Robert B. Salter has categorized these epiphyseal fractures into five groups, each of which presents different diagnostic and prognostic peculiarities.

Salter I fractures are transverse fractures of the growth plate without injury to the bony metaphysis or epiphysis. When these fractures are undisplaced, they are not radiologically evident at the time of injury. Tenderness over the level of the growth plate of a long bone and a normal x-ray imply a Salter I fracture until developments prove otherwise. Repeat x-rays after 2 weeks will show bone resorption and calcium deposition characteristic of fracture healing, if the Salter I fracture has actually occurred. Salter I fractures must be reduced and immobilized until radiologic and clinical union are evident—2 months at the least. True Salter I fractures rarely interfere with growth.

Salter II fractures are transverse fractures of the growth plate which have split obliquely into the bony metaphysis. This

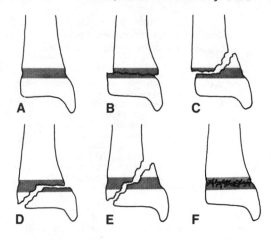

Fig. 15-1. The Salter classifications of epiphyseal fractures. A, normal. B, Salter I. C, Salter II. D, Salter III. E, Salter IV. F, Salter V: The crushed growth plate is usually not radiologically apparent. Within 1 year, part or all of the epiphysis is fused with the metaphysis.

fracture and the Salter I fracture are by far the most common of the epiphyseal fractures. The fracture separation of the distal radial epiphysis discussed in Chapter 6 under "Fractures of the Distal Third of the Forearm" is an example. The fracture into the metaphysis gives away the undisplaced fractures; hence, the Salter II fracture is rarely missed at the time of injury. Treatment and prognosis are identical to those of the Salter I fracture.

Salter III fractures are transverse fractures of the growth plate which have split obliquely into the bony epiphysis. No examples of this fracture have been given in this text. Why this fracture occurs and not the Salter I or II fracture is not known, but its occurrence may reflect subtle differences in direction of injuring force. Salter I, II, and III fractures all tend to occur in response to shearing forces. This fracture is more likely to lead to growth arrest than are the Salter I and Salter II fractures. Reduction must be anatomic. This injury should be referred to an orthopaedist.

Salter IV fractures extend axially into the bony metaphysis and into the bony epiphysis. The fracture may appear to extend axially from the bony epiphysis to the bony metaphysis directly through the growth plate, or it may appear to extend axially through the bony epiphysis, transversely across part of the growth plate, then axially into the bony metaphysis. However it appears, the danger of growth arrest is very great. Reduction must be anatomic. The injury must be referred to an orthopaedist.

Salter V fractures crush the growth plate. While this injury can accompany crush fractures of the bony epiphysis, the typical injury stands alone. Its initial clinical characteristics are indistinguishable from those of the undisplaced Salter I fracture:

1. Initial radiologic invisibility.
2. Initial tenderness at the region of the growh plate.
3. Eventual appearance of radiologic signs of bone healing (usually within 2–3 weeks).

The distinction occurs months later when it becomes evident that an injured bone is no longer growing and, indeed, that its bony epiphysis may have fused with its bony metaphysis. When this tragedy emerges, the clinician recognizes the injury to have been a Salter V fracture. Though the injury were recognized on the 1st day, nothing could be done to prevent the outcome. When the undisplaced-Salter I/Salter V clinical presentation appears, parents must be warned of the worst possibility while the injury is treated as a Salter I fracture.

The prognosis of epiphyseal fractures differs not only among the types, but also among the locations. Except following Salter V injuries, epiphyseal fractures in the upper extremity are rarely followed by growth failure. In the lower extremity, any epiphyseal fracture can be followed by growth failure, and the Salter III and IV fractures carry a very guarded prognosis. The Salter V fracture, of course, results inevitably in a tragic outcome.

Table 15-3
Epiphyseal Avulsions Presented in the Text

Muscle Strained	Epiphysis Avulsed
Iliopsoas muscle	The lesser trochanter of the femur
Straight tendon of the rectus femoris	The anteroinferior iliac spine
Sartorius	The anterosuperior iliac spine
Hamstring and adductor muscles	The ischial tuberosity

The epiphyseal fractures presented in this text are the following:

Fracture of the distal radial epiphysis: under "Fractures of the Distal Third of the Forearm" in Chapter 6.

Fracture of the distal femoral epiphysis: under "Epiphyseal Fractures" in Chapter 12.

Fracture of the proximal tibial epiphysis: under "Epiphyseal Fractures" in Chapter 12.

Fracture of the distal tibial epiphysis: under "Fractures of the Shafts of the Tibia and Fibula" and "Axial Compression" injuries of the ankle in Chapter 13.

5. Muscle strains about the hip may cause avulsion fractures of the epiphyses about the hip. The epiphyseal avulsions presented in this text are listed in Table 15-3.

The mechanism, recognition and treatment of these avulsion fractures are described under "Periarticular Myofascial Injuries" in Chapter 11.

CHAPTER 16

Regional and Local Anesthesia in the Outpatient Practice*

A bewildering number of local anesthetic agents have been synthetized since Koller first used cocaine in 1884. We have about six agents in common use today, which can be classified into two basic groups:

1. Ester compounds: cocaine, procaine, chloroprocaine (Nesacaine). These are hydrolized in the blood by the enzyme pseudocholinesterase. Cocaine in a 5% solution is only used topically. For local and regional blocks, the following are used: procaine in a 1–2% concentration acts rapidly and is eliminated rapidly; chloroprocaine (Nesacaine), in a 1–2% concentration, the latest of the ester compounds, is the most rapid acting and has the fastest elimination of all local anesthetic agents. In equipotent doses, it is the least toxic of all agents.

2. Amide compounds; lidocaine (Xylocaine) in 0.5–2.0% concentrations, mepivacaine (Carbocaine) in 1–2% concentrations, bupivacaine (Marcaine) in 0.25–0.5% concentrations, are all used for local or regional blocks. They are all broken down in the liver, and the degradation products excreted in the urine. Speed of onset is roughly equivalent in all of these, but the duration is shortest for lidocaine and longest for bupivacaine.

For practical purposes, the doctor should confine himself to one or two drugs with which he is familiar. Also, he should use the lowest concentration necessary which will do the job adequately. Example: lidocaine 0.5% for infiltration, and 1% for regional blocks.

Addition of Epinephrine

Epinephrine, by reason of its vasoconstrictor properties, cuts down on the rate of absorption, thus allowing the drug to act longer. For the same reason, the total dose can be increased. Epinephrine should never be used in the region of end arteries, such as fingers and toes. It should not be necessary to exceed 1 in 200,000 concentration, especially when using large amounts of the local agents. Adding 0.25 cc. of 1:1000 aqueous epinephrine solution to a 50 cc. bottle of local agent will give a 1:200,000 concentration.

Allergic Reactions

These are very rare, especially with the amide compounds. If there is a history of true allergy (rash, edema, anaphylactic re-

* Contributed by Patrick Bennett, M.D., D.A., F.A.C.A., Department of Anesthesiology, Group Health Coöperative of Puget Sound, Seattle, Washington.

action), one should definitely switch to another agent, preferably of a different group. Example: Nesacaine instead of lidocaine, and vice versa. As a test, 0.25 cc. of the offending agent may be injected intradermally, and the area inspected within 15 minutes for a rash. However, it is generally inconclusive testimony. A careful history will usually elicit the fact that the so-called reaction was not a true allergy, but a simple faint (vasovagal reaction), or was due to the epinephrine (tachycardia, headache, buzzing in the ears), or to an overdose of the anesthetic agent.

Toxic Reactions

These are due to overdose, but may also occur with relatively small amounts if they happen to be injected intravascularly. So, repeated aspiration during the injection is a very useful practice. Generally, they are manifested initially by increasing excitement (garrulousness, hostility, etc.) leading to convulsions, which may progress to cardiovascular collapse.

Treatment

1. *Prophylactic.* Careful monitoring of dose and repeated aspiration. If it is anticipated that the patient will require large amounts of drug, he should have an intravenous infusion set up with a plastic cannula. Also, light sedation will not only help to calm the patient, but will diminish the chances of convulsion occurring at a given dose. Valium in small amounts, 2.5 mg. intravenously (I.V.), is ideal for this purpose and may be repeated. Blood pressure and pulse should also be monitored; any increase in both will give early warning of the impending reaction. The operator may respond to this early warning by giving additional Valium I.V.

2. Convulsions are treated with oxygen 100% by mask, and Valium 5–10 mg. I.V. A barbiturate such as Nembutal 25–50 mg., or sodium pentothal 50 mg. I.V. may be added in refractory cases. However, great care should be taken that the patient is not precipitated into cardiovascular collapse.

3. Cardiovascular collapse is treated with:

a. One hundred percent oxygen by mask. However, if respiration ceases or becomes inadequate, manual ventilation will be necessary. Endotracheal intubation may be required if it is difficult or impossible to ventilate the patient properly with the use of the mask.

b. Increasing the flow rate of intravenous fluids.

c. Ephedrine 12.5 mg. I.V., which may be repeated to restore blood pressure.

d. Cardiac arrest is treated with a full CPR regimen.

Resuscitation equipment should always be on hand, and personnel should be familiar with its use.

Maximum Dose (Calculated for a 70 Kg. Person)

Lidocaine (Xylocaine).

1. Without epinephrine, 300 mg., which is 30 cc. of a 1% solution.

2. With epinephrine, 500 mg., 50 cc. of a 1% solution.

Chloroprocaine (Nesacaine).

1. Without epinephrine, 800 mg., 80 cc. of a 1% solution.

2. With epinephrine, 1000 mg., 100 cc. of a 1% solution.

Mepivacaine (Carbocaine).

Five hundred fifty milligrams, 55 cc. of a 1% solution.

Bupivacaine (Marcaine).

1. Without epinephrine, 175 mg., 70 cc. of a 0.25% solution.

2. With epinephrine, 225 mg., 100 cc. of a 0.25% solution.

For practical purposes, and to avoid repetitive qualifications, we will continue to specify dosages for a 70 Kg. person, and our agent will be 1% lidocaine. The doctor, however, should be aware that age, weight, and physical condition will have an important bearing on total dosage. A direct proportion can be used to calculate the dosage for other weights. The very young, the very old, and the very sick tolerate a lesser total dose—between 10 and 30% less.

Regional Blocks

The advantage of regional blocks is that relatively large areas of the body can be anesthetized by the injection of local anesthetic agents in specific areas close to an individual nerve or where bundles of nerves are congregated. The disadvantage of this method is that if the nerves are damaged by the needle, there will likewise be a relatively large area subject to paresthesia or numbness. Also, the nerves may lie deep and close to other vital structures, such as lungs, arteries, or the spinal cord, with possible damage to these areas. Consequently, if local infiltration will do the job without having to use excessive volumes, it would be folly for the occasional anesthetist to subject a patient to the potential hazards of these blocks. The object with regional blocks is to deposit the anesthetic solution as close as possible to the nerve without actually penetrating it. A momentary paresthesia is often necessary to confirm that the needle is in the correct area, but if it persists, the needle should be withdrawn gradually until this disappears.

For regional blocks requiring large volumes of solution, the simplest method is to draw up the maximum dose into a 30–50 cc. syringe with an extension tube and needle attached, and to inject the recommended amount after proper location of the needle and by alternating small increments with repeated aspiration. The needle is a 1½″, 22-gauge, except for the axillary blocks, where a ⅝″ or 1″, 24- or 25-gauge is used, preferably with a short bevel. For a sciatic nerve block, a 3½″, 22-gauge needle will be necessary. The remaining blocks will require smaller volumes and are more easily accomplished with a 10 cc., 3-ring syringe directly connected to a 1½″, 22-gauge needle.

Upper Arm Blocks

Winnie describes a fascial compartment surrounding the cervical and brachial plexus nerve roots and extending down into the axilla. Injection of local anesthetic into this area in sufficient volume will block all the nerves from the neck to the fingertips. However, depending on where the operation is to be performed, one can cut down on the volume by injection at one of the following appropriate sites:

1. *Interscalene*. (See Figure 16–1.) **Indications and Method.** This block may be used for operations on the shoulder and upper and lower arm. The cricoid cartilage is marked and a line drawn laterally across the neck. The patient is asked to turn his head to the opposite side and raise it slightly off the pillow, thereby causing the sternocleidomastoid muscle to stand out. A line is drawn along the lateral border of the clavicular head of the sternocleido- mastoid. The patient is then asked to lower his head back to the pillow, relaxing the sternocleidomastoid. The palpating fingers are inserted deep to the intersection of the two lines, and should lie on the surface of the anterior scalene muscle. They are now slipped a little further posteriorly and should lie in the groove between the ante- rior and middle scalene muscles. An "X" is placed over this spot. This should lie over the sixth cervical transverse process. The needle is inserted in a medial, dorsal, and caudad direction between the muscle planes until a paresthesia is elicited. If bone is encountered, the needle is with- drawn and reinjected at a slightly different angle. When a paresthesia is elicited, pref- erably to the elbow or hand, the local anesthetic is injected in increments alter- nating with repeated aspirations. Analge- sia should extend from the shoulder to the hand, the upper arm being best. Volume: 25 cc.

Specific Dangers. a. Epidural injection. b. Subarachnoid injection.

The signs will be very similar but more prominent with the latter because of the

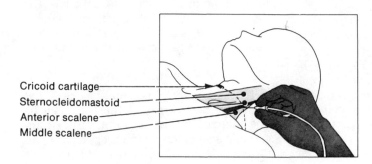

Cricoid cartilage
Sternocleidomastoid
Anterior scalene
Middle scalene

Fig. 16–1. The interscalene block.

wider spread of the agent due to mixing with the cerebrospinal fluid. The two basic and dreaded signs are:

(1) Apnea, due to blocking of the phrenic and the intercostal nerves.

(2) Hypotension, due to sympathetic nerve blockage.

Treatment.

(1) Apnea will require ventilation with bag and mask initially, but may require a respirator and an endotracheal tube later, as it may last several hours.

(2) Hypotension may respond to a rapid infusion of 1000 cc. of a balanced salt solution, such as Ringer's lactate, and the administration of a vasopressor, such as 12.5 mg. of Ephedrine, which may be repeated. In addition, if the hypotension persists, 10 mg. of Neo-Synephrine are added to 500 cc. of 5% dextrose and water, and an infusion is set up. The rate of infusion is titrated until a pressure of approximately 100 mm. Hg systolic is obtained. The infusion should be monitored very carefully, preferably with an infusion pump (Ivac). Extravasation of a large amount of this solution would severely compromise the circulation to the limb. The use of a plastic cannula and frequent checking of the infusion site are mandatory in this situation.

Both of these complications can be avoided by the caudad direction of the needle.

c. Intravascular injection, especially carotid and vertebral arteries, which will result in instantaneous convulsions. This complication can be avoided by repeated aspiration during the injection.

d. Blocking the phrenic, vagus, or recurrent laryngeal nerve. These are rare complications and are generally of no conse-quence. However, both sides should never be blocked simultaneously.

e. Injecting solution into the esophageal musculature will result in difficulty in swallowing.

2. *Supraclavicular.* (See Figure 16–2.) **Indications and Method.** This block may be used for operations on the arm, forearm, and hand. The same landmarks are used as for the interscalene block. The groove between the anterior and middle scalene muscles is located by palpation with the index and middle fingers. The fingers are then advanced caudad until the subclavian artery can be palpated, or until the lower finger reaches the clavicle. The upper finger is then lifted away and the needle is inserted close to the upper border of the lower finger, avoiding the external jugular vein, and is advanced directly caudad, between the muscles, and posterior to the subclavian artery. Once a paresthesia is elicited, the agent is injected in increments, alternating with repeated aspiration. Volume: 25 cc.

Specific Dangers.

a. Pneumothorax. If the needle is directed too far medially, the dome of the pleura will be pierced, and the needle will enter the lung, allowing air to escape into the pleura. This may pose quite a problem to individuals whose respiratory reserves are minimal.

Treatment.

(1) X-ray to confirm the diagnosis.

(2) If the pneumothorax is small and the patient shows no symptoms, no specific treatment is indicated, except that the patient is informed and told to report back if dyspnea develops.

(3) If symptoms are present, consultation may be required, and the insertion of

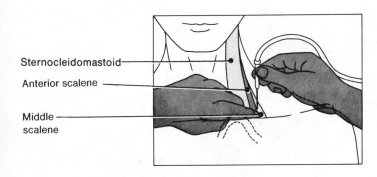

Sternocleidomastoid

Anterior scalene

Middle scalene

Fig. 16–2. The supraclavicular block.

a chest tube may be necessary with hookup to an underwater seal.

b. Injection into the subclavian artery or vein. Toxic effects are likely.

3. *Axillary.* (See Figure 16–3.) **Indications and Method.** This block is used primarily for operations on the hand, but may be extended for use in the forearm or upper arm if larger volumes are used. The arm is abducted to 90° and the elbow flexed to 90°. The arm is then externally rotated. The axillary artery is palpated at its highest point, with the fingers of the left hand. The needle is inserted close to the artery. A distinct click can be felt, especially if the needle is short beveled, when it penetrates the axillary sheath which surrounds the vessels and nerves. A paresthesia is not necessary if one is convinced that the sheath has been entered. Again, the agent is injected in increments, alternating with repeated aspiration. Volume: 30–40 cc. Pressure on the sheath distal to the needle stick will help direct the agent cephalad, resulting in a better block. One problem with this block is that while it is generally good for hand surgery, it may not block the musculocutaneous nerve, which arises higher in the plexus. The nerve supplies the flexors of the arm and the radial aspect of the forearm, down to the base of the thumb. Consequently, unless high volumes are used (50 cc.), it will not be adequate for Colles fractures or operations on the wrist. Sometimes this nerve can be blocked independently by injecting 5 cc. into the corocobrachialis muscle, which is a finger-sized muscle located in the axilla, anterolaterally to the artery.

Specific Dangers. Apart from the general complications of local anesthesia and intravascular injections, there are relatively few complications with this block. There have been rare cases of calcified hematomas following puncture of the axillary artery.

If a tourniquet is to be used, it will be necessary with all of the upper arm blocks, to block—in addition—the intercostobrachial nerve in the axilla. This is easily done by subcutaneous injection of 2–3 cc. superficial to the axillary artery.

Blocks of the Forearm and Hand (See Figure 16–4 through 16–8)

Elbow Block. The radial, median, and ulnar nerves can be blocked independently at the elbow and will provide analgesia to their respective areas in the hand. However, this will not be adequate for operations on the forearm, unless a subcutaneous block of the area above the elbow is also done to block the medial cutaneous nerve to the forearm. The arm is flexed 90°, and a line is drawn along the crease of the elbow. The arm is then extended, and injections are made on this line.

Radial Nerve. The needle is inserted approximately 1 cm. lateral to the biceps tendon, and 5 cc. are deposited in a fanwise manner down to the bone, unless paresthesiae are encountered. This generally blocks the musculocutaneous nerve as well.

Median Nerve. The needle is inserted medial to the brachial artery until paresthesiae are elicited; 5–10 cc. are injected.

Ulnar Nerve. The nerve is rolled under the palpating finger proximal to the sulcus in the back of the elbow. Two cubic centimeters are injected on either side of the nerve. It is not wise to inject directly into

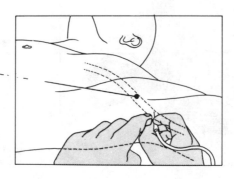

Sheath containing
axillary nerves,
the axillary vein,
and the
axillary artery

Fig. 16–3. The axillary block.

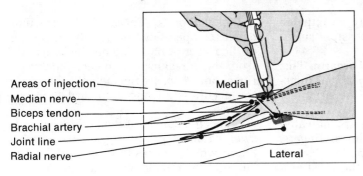

Areas of injection
Median nerve
Biceps tendon
Brachial artery
Joint line
Radial nerve

Medial

Lateral

Fig. 16–4. Block of the radial and median nerves at the elbow.

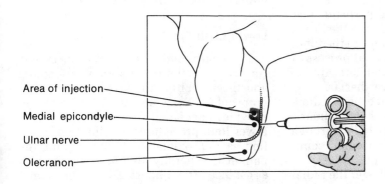

Area of injection

Medial epicondyle

Ulnar nerve

Olecranon

Fig. 16–5. Block of the ulnar nerve at the elbow.

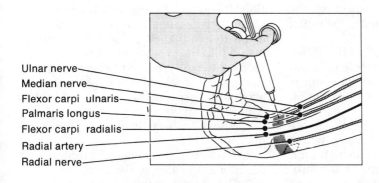

Ulnar nerve
Median nerve
Flexor carpi ulnaris
Palmaris longus
Flexor carpi radialis
Radial artery
Radial nerve

Fig. 16–6. Block of the median, radial, and ulnar nerves at the wrist.

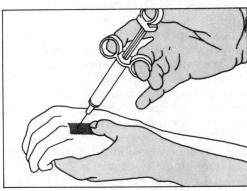

Fig. 16–7. Metacarpal block.

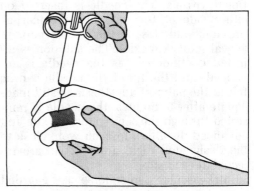

Fig. 16–8. Digital block of the finger.

the sulcus, as the nerve may be impaled against the bone, and also possibly suffer from compression.

Medial Cutaneous of the Forearm. This can be accomplished by superficial injection of the medial half of the arm just above the elbow.

Wrist Blocks. These blocks are indicated for specific areas in the palm or fingers. Each of the three blocks is made by injection into the volar aspect of the wrist at a level identified by a line drawn between the radial and ulnar styloid processes.

Ulnar. Needle is inserted perpendicular to the skin immediately radial to the flexor carpi ulnaris tendon and ulnar to the ulnar artery, at the level of the styloid process of the ulna. Four cubic centimeters are injected, with or without paresthesias.

Median. Needle is inserted perpendicularly between the tendons of the palmaris longus and flexor carpi radialis through the flexor retinaculum. Five cubic centimeters are injected at this site.

Radial. Needle is inserted over the radial artery, just proximal to the radial styloid, and directed dorsally, injecting 5 cc. superficially around the radial aspect of the wrist. The needle must not enter the radial artery.

The *specific danger* with all of the above is nerve damage following needle penetration of a nerve. Intravascular injection is guarded against by repeated aspiration during the injection.

Metacarpal Blocks. These blocks are useful for operations on the fingers, where digital injections are not suitable by reason of location of the operation, or compromise of blood flow due to compression of finger vessels. The needle is inserted on either side of the adjoining metacarpal, proximal and close to the metacarpophalangeal joint (knuckle). The solution is injected continuously as the needle is advanced until the tip of the needle can be felt in the palm. If anesthesia is still inadequate after 5 minutes, the needle is reinserted through the same puncture site and advanced distally into each web, close to the designated digit, and 1–2 cc. are injected at each site.

Intravascular injection is guarded against by repeated aspiration during the injection.

Digital Blocks. These blocks are indicated for operations on the distal portion of the finger or nail. The needle is inserted from the dorsal aspect on each side of the finger, and 2 cc. are injected at each site as the needle is advanced toward the volar surface.

A *specific danger* of digital blocks is the swelling of the proximal phalanx with solution which can result in impaired circulation to the remainder of the finger.

Epinephrine should not be used with either the metacarpal or the digital block.

Lower Limb Blocks

The fastest and most reliable anesthetic for the lower limb is undoubtedly spinal anesthesia. Fifty to seventy-five milligrams of 5% Xylocaine in 7.5% glucose will provide adequate anesthesia for most lower limb procedures. Its duration of action is approximately 2 hours, and the patient is generally able to go home with assistance after 4 hours. Disposable spinal trays and proper aseptic technique have virtually eliminated all possibility of infection. Likewise, the use of 25- or even 26-gauge needles has reduced spinal headaches to less than 1%. The doctor must be aware that the sympathetic nerves are also blocked two or three segments higher than the somatic block, so that hypotension can occur and pose a major problem. Absolute contraindications are:

1. Shock, especially due to hypovolemia.

2. History of neurological problems, especially in the area of the cord.

3. Patient not in full agreement.

4. Patient receiving anticoagulant medication.

Spinal anesthesia should never be attempted without (a) intravenous infusion in place, with a plastic cannula, (b) regular blood pressure and pulse monitoring, (c) resuscitation equipment on hand and expertise in its use, (d) proper observation area for patient postoperative recovery.

Technique of Spinal. (See Figure 16–9.) The patient is positioned for a lumbar puncture, and the needle is inserted between L_3 and L_4 vertebrae, which are at the level of the iliac crest. Following injection, the patient is immediately turned to a supine horizontal position, and the level of analgesia is checked with a needle. As the solution is hyperbaric (heavier than cerebrospinal fluid), putting the patient in the head-down position will cause the level of anesthesia to rise. For operations on the lower limb, it should never be necessary to get a higher level of analgesia than T_{10} (umbilicus). Raising the head of the table will prevent upward spread. However, hypotension may develop, and if it is below 90 mm. Hg, it is better not to raise the head as cerebral ischemia may result, but rather to treat the hypotension directly with intravenous fluids and vasopressors, as described above under "Treatment" for "Toxic Reactions."

The lower limb may also be blocked by the following two methods:

Femoral Nerve. (See Figure 16–10.) A line is drawn between the anterosuperior iliac spine and the pubic tubercle. Another line is drawn along the course of the femoral artery as it crosses the first line. The needle is inserted lateral to the femoral artery, immediately below the first line, and is directed posterior and cephalad in the direction of the umbilicus. On elicitation of paresthesiae, 25–30 cc. are injected. This volume blocks, in addition to the fem-

oral nerve, the obturator and the lateral femoral cutaneous nerves. For this reason, it is often called the three-in-one block.

Specific Dangers.

1. Puncturing the femoral artery with resultant hematoma. The risk of this complication occurring is decreased by continually palpating the artery with the other hand throughout the introduction of the needle, and the injection.

2. Intravenous injection. The risk of this complication occurring is decreased by repeated aspiration during the injection.

Sciatic Nerve (See figure 16–11.) The patient is placed on his side with the affected limb upward. A line is drawn from the posterosuperior iliac spine to the greater trochanter of the femur. A second line is drawn from the greater trochanter to the sacral hiatus. A perpendicular is dropped from the midpoint of the first line, and where it intersects the second line is the point of the needle insertion. A 3½″ needle is inserted perpendicular to the skin in all planes and advanced until a paresthesia is elicited or bone is encountered. Once the paresthesia is elicited 25 cc. are injected.

These two blocks (femoral and sciatic) will give anesthesia to the leg, but may still

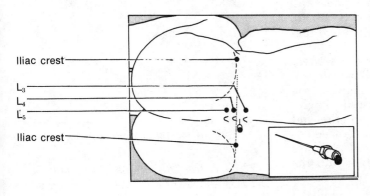

Iliac crest

L_3
L_4
L_5

Iliac crest

Fig. 16–9. Spinal block.

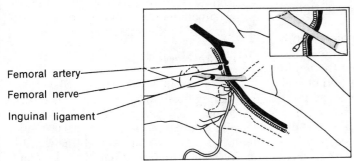

Femoral artery

Femoral nerve

Inguinal ligament

Fig. 16–10. Block of the femoral nerve at the hip.

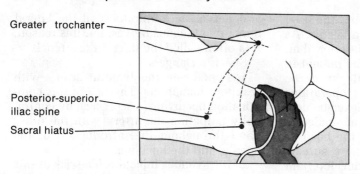

Greater trochanter

Posterior-superior iliac spine

Sacral hiatus

Fig. 16–11. Block of the sciatic nerve at the hip.

be inadequate to relieve tourniquet pain because unblocked nerve fibers may have reached the lower limb superficially. The sciatic nerve may also be blocked at the apex of the popliteal fossa, between the biceps and semitendinous tendons. The patient is placed prone, and the needle is inserted perpendicularly at the apex of the fossa until paresthesiae are elicited, and 25 cc. are then injected.

Foot Blocks

The anterior tibial (deep peroneal) and posterior tibial nerves can be blocked individually, and the saphenous, sural, and terminal cutaneous branches of the superficial peroneal nerve may be blocked by circumferential subcutaneous infiltration proximal to the ankle joint. Metatarsal and digital blocks (Figures 6–12 and 16–13) are performed as are the Metacarpal and digital blocks of the hand.

Anterior Tibial Block (Deep Peroneal Block). (See Figure 16–14.) A line is drawn across the front of the ankle, between the two malleoli. The needle is inserted lateral to the tendons of the tibialis anterior and extensor hallucis longus and advanced until a paresthesia is elicited, and 5 cc. are then injected. Risk of injection into the anterior tibio artery which may lie on either side of the nerve can be minimized by intermittent aspiration during the injection.

Posterior Tibial Block. (See Figure 16–15.) The needle is inserted midway between the medial malleolus and the tendo achilles. The nerve is posterior and lateral to the artery. The needle is advanced until a paresthesia is elicited, and 5 cc. are then injected. If no paresthesia is elicited, the needle is withdrawn, and a fan-wise injection made.

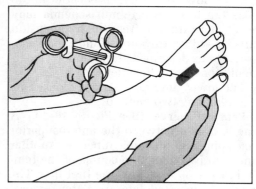

Fig. 16–12. The metatarsal block.

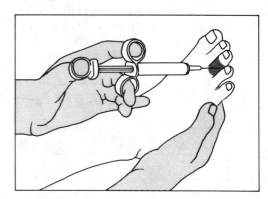

Fig. 16–13. Digital block of the toe.

Block of the Saphenous, Sural, and Terminal Branches of the Superficial Peroneal. This block is accomplished by circumferential subcutaneous infiltration of 10–15 cc. proximal to the ankle joint.

Intercostal Nerve Block

This is useful for fractured ribs, so a long-acting local anesthetic agent is desirable. Ten cubic centimeters of 0.5% bupivacaine (Marcaine) with 1 in 200,000 epinephrine are drawn up into a three-ring 10 cc. syringe which is then directly con-

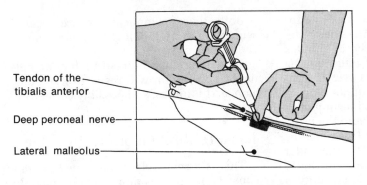

Tendon of the tibialis anterior

Deep peroneal nerve

Lateral malleolus

Fig. 16–14. Block of the deep peroneal nerve at the ankle.

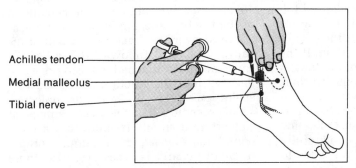

Achilles tendon

Medial malleolus

Tibial nerve

Fig. 16–15. Block of the tibial nerve at the ankle.

nected to a 22-gauge needle. The palpating finger is inserted into the intercostal space below the injured rib, proximal to the fracture line, and the skin is pulled up over the rib. The needle is inserted as close as possible to the finger and advanced until it strikes the rib. It is then walked off the lower border of the rib and advanced approximately ⅛". Following careful aspiration, 5 cc. are injected.

Specific Problems.

Intravenous Injection. The risk of this complication is minimized by repeated aspiration during injection of the anesthetic. Treatment is as advised on pages 2–3 of this chapter.

Pneumothorax. The risk of this complication is minimized by ensuring that the needle does not enter further than ⅛" beyond the lower border of the rib. The patient must be positioned stably—e.g., gripping the back of a straddled chair—and the needle must be pinched at the body wall between the thumb and index finger of the hand which is not manipulating the syringe.

Intravenous Regional (Bier Block)

This is suitable for most operations on the upper limb, but has a very limited application to the lower limb because of the huge volume of solution required. A double tourniquet is recommended, as a single tourniquet may be uncomfortable for the patient. Also, it is very important to reiterate than an I.V. infusion should be set up in the other arm and the patient's vital signs monitored. The double tourniquet is positioned in the upper arm and connected to the inflator, but not turned on. The pressure is set at approximately twice the systolic blood pressure, generally in the area of 300 mm. Hg. A small plastic cannula, 22-gauge, is inserted into a vein on the dorsum of the hand. Following aspiration of blood, it is flushed with 2 cc. of saline, preferably with a heparin-type lock. The cannula is taped in position. The arm is then raised vertically and exsanguinated by means of an Esmarch bandage. On reaching the tourniquet, the distal cuff is inflated and then the proximal one. Following satisfactory inflation of the latter, the distal cuff is then released. It is very important to check the tourniquet by palpation, to see if it is inflated, and not simply rely on the pressure gauge. Fifty cubic centimeters of 0.5% lidocaine *without epinephrine* are now injected, making sure that the lidocaine is not infiltrating. The cannula is then withdrawn and pressure maintained over the puncture site for approximately 3 minutes. Anesthesia develops within approximately 5 minutes and will last as long as the tourniquet is inflated. If the operation lasts over 15 minutes, and the patient is complaining of tourniquet pain, the distal tourniquet is then inflated, and after 1 minute the proximal tourniquet released. By this time, the agent will have anesthetized the arm under the distal cuff. It is very important not to release the tourniquet completely until a minimum of half an hour has elapsed following injection, as it takes that long for the bulk of the anesthetic to diffuse out of the vasculature into the tissue fluid. If the operation finishes before then, the tourniquet is kept inflated for the required time. If deflated sooner, the amount of anesthetic remaining in the vasculature can be enough to cause a toxic reaction. Following deflation, the patient should be carefully monitored for a further half an hour, to make sure no toxic reaction develops.

Specific Dangers.

1. Inadequate or non-inflation of the tourniquet prior to administrating the agent will result in a bolus dose injection of the local agent.

2. Premature release of the tourniquet will result in a similar effect.

Both these complications are treated with Valium up to 5 mg. I.V., intravenous fluids, and oxygen.

3. Inadvertent administration of an epinephrine solution will result in hypertension, arrhythmias, and possibly cardiac arrest.

Local Infiltration of Fracture Sites

This is a relatively easy procedure and consists of the injection of approximately 10 cc. of 1% lidocaine into the hematoma of the fracture site. An intradermal wheal is raised over the fracture site with a 25-gauge needle and, following this, a 1½″, 22-gauge needle is attached to the syringe and inserted into the fracture site. Following aspiration of blood, 10 cc. are injected. This procedure has the disadvantage of converting a simple fracture into a compound one. Consequently, surgical preparation of the area is necessary. Also, there are the dangers of intravascular absorption of the agent with its consequent effect. Also, for a Colles fracture, it will be necessary to inject not only the radial fracture site, but also the styloid process of the ulna, should that also be fractured.

CHAPTER 17

Mechanical Therapeutics Summarized

Orthopaedic treatments are essentially mechanical, whether done *to* a patient or *by* a patient. They apply forces to reconstruct and stabilize disrupted structures, or forces to mobilize and strengthen stiffened, weakened structures. Particular manipulations for reductions and mobilizations, and particular exercises for mobilization and strengthening have been described in the regional chapters, as their details are regionally determined. Certain principles of reduction and fracture follow-up, the techniques of casting, splinting, and the introduction of needles, the application of heat or cold, measurement of joint motion, and certain principles of exercise are gathered for more efficient summary in this chapter.

Principles of Reduction

Timing of a Reduction

All dislocations must be reduced as soon as possible, as pain will remain intense until they are, as neurovascular injury is the more likely the longer a joint is allowed to remain dislocated, and as cartilage exposed to air in compounded injuries will be damaged by desiccation if left exposed overlong. As detailed in the regional text, the acromioclavicular, the anterior sternoclavicular, the sacroiliac, and the interpubic joints are the only exceptions to this principle.

On the other hand, only compound fractures require prompt reduction always and then simply to minimize the risk of infection. Closed fractures may be reduced any time within a week of the injury, provided skin and neurovascular structures are not threatened by the abnormal position, and provided increased deformity is prevented by adequate splinting. When the economics of family and/or hospital support allow, a delay of 3–4 days can be advantageous. If, during those days, the extremity is kept elevated at or above heart level (not so high as to compromise distal arterial flow), the initial swelling secondary to bleeding and reactive transudation will greatly diminish, and the period of bleeding and rapid transudation will be passed. At that point, a skin-tight cast can be applied which is more likely to hold the desired position than is the padded and split cast which often must be applied when fractures are reduced on the day of injury.

Standards of Reduction.

Displacement is *absolutely unacceptable* only when it threatens skin or neurovascular structures, or disrupts the continuity of a joint surface, or delays healing. Displaced tibial fractures can threaten the tight overlying skin, displaced clavicular, humeral, wrist, elbow, knee, and ankle fractures can threaten adjacent neurovascular structures, and displaced condylar fractures disrupt continuity of joint surfaces. When lateral displacement exceeds the width of the bone, so that the ends of the bone no longer remain in contact, involuntary muscle contraction will cause shortening by axial displacement as well. Some axial displacement is desirable when a child's femur has been fractured, to compensate for the invariably accelerated growth of the fractured bone. Unless the femur is shortened by axial displacement, the extremity will ultimately grow undesirably longer than the uninjured extremity. In nearly every other instance, axial displacement is unacceptable, either because it subluxates joints between paired bones, or alters muscle balance, or because it can delay healing.

Displacement is *relatively unacceptable* when the expected remodelling is unlikely to restore a normal appearance to a subcutaneous bone. Remodelling will restore an appearance acceptable to most adults when displacement does not exceed half the width of the bone.

Mature bones cannot correct *angulation* by remodelling, though occasionally angulation is accepted when the only promising method of reduction and immobilization is less acceptable than the angulation itself—e.g., Colles fracture and fractured neck of humerus in the debilitated and arthritic (see Chapters 4 and 6). Angulation of the long bones will change the orientation of the articular surfaces of the nearest joint. In weightbearing extremities, such a change will usually create shearing forces across the joint, and will burden a portion of the surface with a greater proportion of body weight than it is structured to bear. Degenerative processes in that joint will thus be accelerated. In nonweightbearing extremities, the arc of motion will always be changed, and neuro-

vascular structures will occasionally be compromised by such angulation. *Growing bones* can correct some degree of angulation—an increasingly great degree, the closer the fracture line is to an epiphysis. (See Chapter 6.)

Any obvious *rotation*, whether in mature or growing bones, is unacceptable.

The Forces of Reduction

Most reductions are accomplished by an appropriate combination of traction with angular and rotational forces. The only exceptions are the reductions of metacarpophalangeal, metatarsophalangeal, and interphalangeal joints, which in our opinion are best effected by pure pushing forces. (See Chapter 6.) Traction forces usually must be strong and persistent, while angular and rotational forces usually must be gentle and brief. Traction must overpower any reactive muscle resistance and the lesser friction forces that bind impacted fragments. These forces are best overpowered by lengthy application of modest traction forces, rather than by an abrupt application of violence.

Forces Applied to Dislocations. With only four exceptions, closed reduction of large joint dislocations requires manual traction. The exceptions are the acromioclavicular dislocation, which is reduced by a binding dressing, and the dislocations of the spine and pelvis, and the central dislocation of the hip, all of which require open reduction or prolonged weighted traction in bed. (See Chapters 3, 10, and 11.) Good analgesia will greatly diminish the muscle resistance and often make the difference between success and failure when manipulating dislocations of the larger joints. The manipulation should await evidence of the patient's relaxation, and then should begin with fairly gentle traction—indeed, merely the weight of the dependent arm when manipulating an anterior dislocation of the shoulder. (See Chapter 3.) Gentle rotational and angular forces are then applied as described in the regional chapters, *stopping when mechanical resistance is encountered.* Tactlessly strong angular and rotational forces have caused fractures during efforts to reduce large joint dislocations. When these gentle maneuvers fail, stronger traction should be applied for many seconds, even for 1-2 minutes, before the appropriate rotational and angular forces are again gently applied. When these maneuvers fail, or when at any time the patient begins to resist, deeper analgesia must be effected before repeating the maneuver.

Forces Applied to Fractures. Unless the operator is uncommonly strong, impacted and over-riding fractures are more readily reduced by weighted traction, which can outlast the strongest patient, is usually not painful, and which leaves the operator free to apply well-controlled angular and rotational forces to the fracture fragments. (See "General Principles for Treatment of Forearm Fractures," Chapter 6.) The angular and rotational forces needed rarely require more strength than abides in the hands and wrists alone. Various gripping forces that bridge the fracture site are typically all that are required to complete the reduction of most forearm, wrist, hand, and ankle fractures. Modest arm forces may be required to complete the reduction of shaft fractures of tibia and fibula, one hand gripping above and the other below the fracture site. Angular and rotational forces must nearly always be initiated gently and gradually, and increased smoothly until the desired movement is produced. The only exception is the completion of the incomplete fracture, which is effected by an abrupt cracking force over the examiner's knee. (See Figure 17-1.) The examiner's hands grip the extremity, each 3-4″ to either side of the

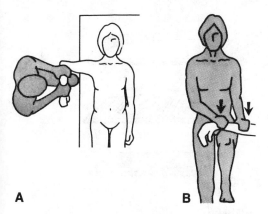

A   **B**

Fig. 17-1. *A* and *B*, completion of the incomplete fracture of a child's forearm.

fracture line, and both arms force the fractured extremity quickly downward across the knee. The force is not great, being about that necessary to break a dry stick of cedar shake ½″ in width and thickness. The trick lies less in the force itself, than in the quickness of its application and cessation. The movement begins abruptly from a position 2″ above the examiner's knee, and ends a split second after the fractured segment strikes the knee.

Principles of Immobilization

Splinting

Indications. A splint is usually chosen for temporary immobilization of an injury while awaiting definitive treatment, for immobilization of an injury that needs protection but not great stability, and for immobilization of joints affected by acute arthritis and periarticular pain syndrome when rest for the painful structures is indicated and when splinting can provide comfortable stability in the context of the person's expected activities.

Five splints are often used by primary clinicians:

1. The volar forearm splint—used for temporary immobilization of forearm and wrist fractures, for protection of wrist sprains, and for resting of an acutely arthritic wrist, an inflamed paracarpal tendon, or the involved tendon and/or bursa of the painful elbow syndromes.

2. The dorsal forearm splint—used for protection of fractures of the base or shaft of metacarpals 2 through 5, and for resting of inflamed flexor tendons when associated with a carpal tunnel syndrome.

3. The long arm splint—used for temporary immobilization of fractures about the elbow, and for protection of a sprained elbow.

4. The short posterior leg splint—used for temporary immobilization of ankle injuries until swelling subsides and proper evaluation for stability can be conducted, and for resting of an arthritic ankle joint or inflamed paramalleolar tendon.

5. The long posterior leg splint—used for temporary immobilization of disruptive injuries of the extensor apparatus and potentially or obviously unstable ligament inju-

ries of the knee, of fractures of the shaft and proximal condyles of the tibia, and, if a traction splint is unavailable, the condyles of the femur; for protection of a stable knee sprain; and for resting of the arthritic knee.

Technique. (See Figure 17–2.) Depending on the mass of the extremity, the splint must be 8 to 12 plaster strips in thickness. Such splints are made by piling plaster slabs on top of one another, then cutting the whole to the desired length (Figure 17–2A) or by laying out strips of the desired length back and forth from a plaster roll (Figure 17–2B). The width of the plaster is chosen so that half the girth of the extremity will lie within the splint. Arm splints are shaped at one end to fit around

the thenar eminence and to parallel the distal palmar crease. Other splints are left square at the ends. The finished plaster is then threaded into a slightly longer stockinette, and the ends of the stockinette are tucked inward over the ends of the plaster. Where the plaster must round a flexed joint, slits are made to allow a smooth overlap at the turn. The sheathed plaster is then immersed in warm water until thoroughly wet, then stripped of excess water and applied to the extremity with bias stockinette or elastic bandage. Alternatively, unsheathed plaster can be immersed in warm water until thoroughly wet, then stripped of excess water and laid on cast padding, and covered with cast padding. Slits as necessary are then made

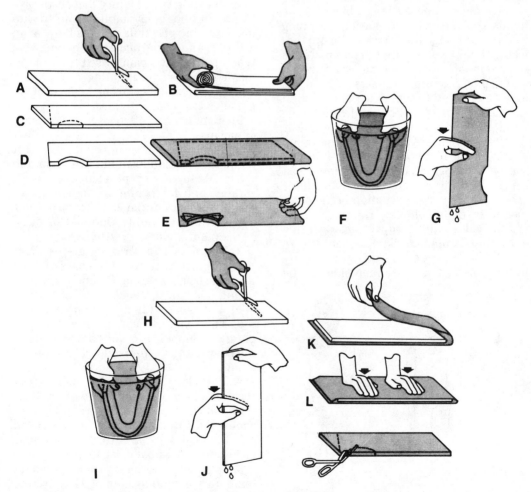

Fig. 17–2. Preparing a plaster splint. *A* through *G*, employing a stockinette liner. *H* through *M*, employing a cast padding liner.

through the padding and wet plaster together, and the splint is applied to the extremity with bias stockinette or elastic bandage. While the plaster hardens, the operator holds the included joint in the desired position, and molds the splint to the contours of the extremity. When the plaster is hardened, the circulation is evaluated, and if it is normal, the dressing is accepted; if it is impeded, the wrappings are removed and reapplied with a lesser firmness that will allow normal circulation.

Casting

Indications. Casts immobilize by rigidly enveloping the unstable structure and, in certain locations, by also maintaining the distracting force necessary to prevent over-riding of the fragments of oblique or spiral fractures. The wrist and elbow can be so positioned as to present the points of purchase necessary for a long arm cast to maintain the necessary distraction force on oblique and spiral fractures of the forearm. Likewise, the ankle and knee can be so positioned as to allow a long leg cast to maintain the necessary distraction force on oblique and spiral fractures of the leg, and the knee and hip can be so positioned as to allow a spica cast to maintain the necessary distraction force on an oblique or spiral fracture of the thigh. The elbow can be so positioned as to direct the weight of a long arm cast in the axis of the humerus, thus allowing for gravity distraction of an over-riding oblique or spiral fracture of the humerus. Casts alone can rarely maintain sufficient distraction force to correct or prevent over-riding of oblique and spiral fractures of metacarpal, metatarsal, and phalangeal bones.

Rigid envelopment alone provides quite adequate stability to transverse shaft fractures in apposition, to fractures of carpal and tarsal bones in anatomic position, and to unstable ligament injuries of elbows, wrists, fingers, knees, ankles, and the 1st metatarsophalangeal joints of the feet.

Six basic casts are often used by primary clinicians:

1. The short arm cast—used in appropriate forms for stabilization of finger splints, immobilization of knuckle fractures, carpal fractures, reduced carpal dislocations, distal third of forearm fractures, and reduced dislocations of the distal radio-ulnar joint.

2. The long arm cast—used in appropriate forms for immobilization of upper and middle third forearm fractures, for late immobilization of reduced elbow dislocations and condylar and supracondylar fractures of the humerus after the circulatory response to injury has stabilized and swelling subsided, and for the carpal and distal third of forearm fractures, when swelling, muscle mass, or obesity prevent the well-molded short arm cast from adequately limiting rotation.

3. The hanging arm cast—used to provide traction immobilization of humeral shaft and humeral neck fractures.

4. The short leg cast—used in appropriate forms for immobilization of unstable ankle injuries, fractures of the proximal phalanges of the great toes, avulsion fractures of the extensor hallucis, ruptures of the achilles tendon, subluxations of the peroneal tendons, and crack fractures of the calcaneus, and for comfort during healing of metatarsal fractures.

5. The long leg cast—used for immobilization of reduced fractures of the shaft of the leg, undisplaced fractures of the tibial condyles, non-disruptive injury to the extensor apparatus, and some unstable knee injuries.

6. The patellar weightbearing cast—used in preference to the long leg cast for immobilization of reduced transverse fractures of the leg when weightbearing is to begin. This cast prevents rotation while allowing knee motion.

Technique.

Application.

1. Casts are constructed from rolls of plaster applied circumferentially and slabs of plaster applied axially. It is usually easiest to apply a layer of circular plaster before applying any appropriate slabs. Application of slabs allows the cast to be reinforced over one region quickly. They are usually applied across wrist, knee, and ankle joints. Figure 17–3 illustrates orientations of slabs across these joints which we

have found effective. Figure 17–4 illustrates the application of roll plaster.

2. Plaster should be applied quite wet—wet enough to drip slowly.

3. Fast-setting plaster gets the job done sooner, but leaves less time for plaster molding, and in the hands of slow workers will produce an irregular, weak, and unsightly cast.

4. To avoid transverse ridging and its tendency to create ischemic pressure points on the skin, and to avoid the tourniquet effect, roll plaster should be laid on, not stretched on.

5. To keep the core of the larger rolls from sliding out and creating an unmanageably twisted rope of plaster, both ends of the roll are pinched when squeezing excess water from the roll before application, then the roll is kept on the limb and rolled around it.

6. As limbs taper and curve, the direction of plaster application can be controlled only by creating pleats whenever the contour of the limb directs the plaster away from the intended course. The roll is lifted from the extremity and unrolled several inches to create a slack which can then be pleated to create the desired direction of application.

7. To prevent air and water from accumulating between plaster layers and creating a weak structure of concentric spirals, each layer must be rubbed into the previous layer. This rubbing is done with the entire palm for large surfaces, the thenar eminence for smaller surfaces, and the fingertips for the smallest surfaces. If plaster is too dry to start with, or sets too fast for the practitioner's skill, this effort to fuse the layers will be foiled.

8. All plaster is applied over a stockinette, never directly to the skin.

9. The "skin-tight" casts hold the reduction more securely than do thickly padded casts. However, they can be applied only

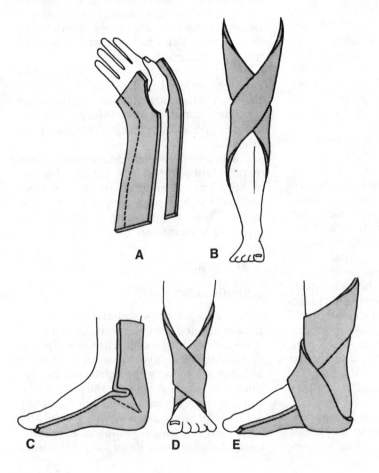

Fig. 17–3. *A* through *E*, use of plaster slabs to reinforce casts at joints.

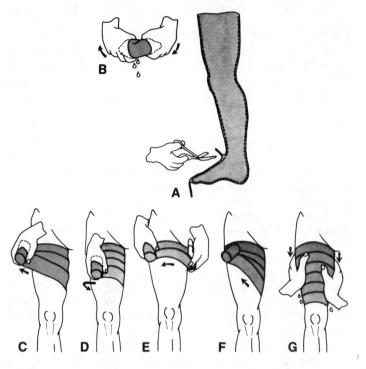

Fig. 17–4. Application of roll plaster. *A*, applying and fitting the stockinette. *B*, pinching the ends of the wet plaster roll. *C* and *D*, plaster must not be pulled on as in *C*, but rolled on as in *D*. *E* and *F*, directing the lie of the plaster. *F*, the contour of the extremity guides the plaster in a wrong direction. *E*, by pleating, the plaster can be guided as desired. *G*, stroking the plaster to fuse the layers and to smooth the surface.

after the period of progressive swelling has passed, or in some cases before it begins, and they must be applied with expert adherence to the precautions listed in the next section.

10. The position of the extremity during application and the areas of the cast which require special molding are unique to each injury and/or cast and are described in the regional chapters.

Cast Precautions. Three risks accompany the use of casts: generalized ischemia of a limb as swelling accrues, necrosis of skin at pressure points, and prolonged joint stiffness after long periods of immobilization. These risks are countered by the following precautions:

1. The circulation to the casted part must be carefully monitored for at least the first 2 days after application of the cast. When casts are applied on the day of injury, the danger of circulatory impairment does not diminish until the 3rd or 4th day.

The following is a speculative but clinically consistent conceptualization of the physiology of this circulatory risk.

Circulation, through any tissue, stops when tissue pressure (P_t) just exceeds capillary blood pressure (P_c).

$$P_t = P_c + dP_c \qquad (1)$$

Tissue pressure in confined tissue spaces rises as blood and/or transudate enter those spaces. All tissues are elastic to a point, and the strength of their resistance to stretch at any point is the upper limit of tissue pressure.

When coagulation and vessel constriction fail to seal a bleeding vessel, *bleeding stops* only when tissue pressure equals blood pressure of the bleeding vessel. Venous blood pressure in an extremity at rest at heart level is less than or equal to capillary blood pressure. Blood pressure in a bleeding artery in an extremity at heart level is directly proportional to the brachial blood pressure and to the caliber of the bleeding artery, and barring shock, is always sustantially greater than capillary blood pressure.

Transudation "stops" (i.e., ions and water pass in and out at equal rates) when tissue pressure (P_t) equals transudate pressure (P_{tr}). Stated differently, transudate flow (F_{tr}) is directly proportional to filled capillary volume (V_c) within the recipient tissue and to transudate pressure (P_{tr}) less tissue pressure (P_t).

$$F_{tr} \sim V_c(P_{tr} - P_t) \qquad (2)$$

Transudate pressure equals capillary blood pressure (P_c) less capillary oncotic pressure (P_{oc}) plus tissue oncotic pressure (P_{ot}).

$$P_{tr} = P_c - P_{oc} + P_{ot} \qquad (3)$$

Thus:

$$F_{tr} \sim V_c(P_c - P_{oc} + P_{ot} - P_t) \qquad (4)$$

Transudation of water and ions increases after injury in response to a reactive vasodilation (an increase in V_c) and to an increase in tissue (extravascular) colloid which can cause tissue oncotic pressure to rise to equal and even exceed the capillary oncotic pressure.

When the elastic compliance of the injured tissue is exhausted prior to cessation of transudate flow, the tissue pressure will rise rapidly to meet transudate pressure at which point transudate flow will cease. When extravascular colloid just exceeds intravascular colloid, as it may when the tissue fluid includes whole blood, flow of transudate will continue until tissue pressure just exceeds the capillary blood pressure, at which point the circulation will also cease.

When arterial bleeding is not stopped by vessel constriction and coagulation, it will continue until tissue pressure equals the pressure of the bleeding vessel, which, barring shock, will substantially exceed the capillary blood pressure. By this means, circulation to the tissues effecting the tamponade will be stopped whether an extremity be casted or not.

While the elastic compliance of fascial sheaths is minimal, and that of skin considerable, the elastic compliance of the cast is zero. The tissues of an uncasted extremity will thus expand to accommodate quite a volume of transudate before their compliance is exhausted. However a casted extremity will expand only to the internal volume of the cast. The bulk of colloid leakage into extravascular tissue occurs early after injury. The continued transudation of water and ions dilutes the extravascular colloid and thus, in time, will restore the supremacy of the capillary oncotic pressure, and allow tissue pressure to meet transudate pressure before rising to capillary blood pressure. The volume constraints of the cast prevent this dilution of extravascular colloid and its restoration of the supremacy of the capillary oncotic pressure. Thus, the tissue pressure in casted extremities can rise rapidly to capillary blood pressure, and circulation cease.

When only minimal capillary or venous bleeding has occurred, and capillary permeability to colloid has not increased substantially, capillary oncotic pressure (P_{oc}) will continue to exceed tissue oncotic pressure (P_{ot}), and an early application of a skin-tight cast can prevent swelling by allowing a quick rise in tissue pressure (P_t) to a transudate pressure (P_{tr}) which is less than capillary blood pressure (P_c). Such a favorable opportunity can be expected when a patient arrives more than 1 hour after the injury and presents a minimally swollen extremity.

When casts are applied on the day of injury, unless the favorable opportunity described in the previous paragraph is sus-

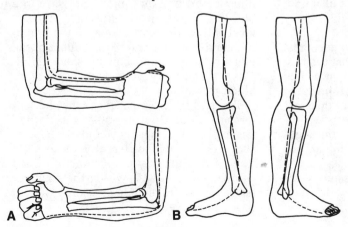

Fig. 17–5. Splitting casts. The *dotted line* indicates where we split our casts. *A*, long arm cast. *B*, long leg cast.

A   B

pected, the problem of progressive swelling must be anticipated by two acts: Two layers of cast padding must be applied over the entire area to be casted, and the cast must be split over its entire length after it hardens. Figure 17–5 illustrates the best line for splitting the usual casts. When the favorable opportunity is suspected, a skintight cast may be applied. In all cases, circulation to the casted extremity must be vigilantly monitored.

The elderly and the chronically ill are particularly vulnerable to these circulatory risks as they are likely to continue bleeding and to lose the supremacy of the local capillary oncotic pressure. (Their vessels are sclerotic and more friable, and their plasma albumin may be low.) Hence, we urge that such persons be admitted to hospital for 1 or 2 days after casting for observation and rest, with the extremity suspended at heart level. Persons who live a great distance from medical care should be admitted to hospital, or should find temporary lodging nearby until the period of bleeding and transudation is safely past. Persons whose compliance cannot be trusted must be admitted to hospital.

Other individuals who are not admitted must be instructed to return immediately should any of the following signs of circulatory impairment appear:

a. Coolness and sluggish capillary return in the fingers or toes of the casted extremity.

b. Cyanosis or pallor of the fingers or toes of the casted extremity.

c. Tingling of the fingers or toes of the casted extremity.

d. Pain in the casted extremity, worsened by movement of the fingers or toes.

2. A constant point of pressure will cause local cutaneous ischemia, and slight axial movement occurring under a cast will in time cause erosions over bony prominences and beneath irregularities of the undersurface of the cast. To avoid these problems, the stockinette must fit snugly without wrinkles, the plaster must be applied smoothly over the stockinette, and must be separated from the skin of bony protrusions by padding. In addition to the circulatory precautions taught to patients, the following skin precautions are also taught. Patients are to return immediately, should they experience burning pain inside a cast, or any other sensation which they interpret to feel like an abrasion, or a boil. When faced with any such complaint, the primary clinician is obliged to window the cast over the area of concern. If a cutaneous injury is evident, the injured area is cleansed and dressed with a non-adhesive dressing over which is applied several layers of padding, and finally the piece of plaster which was cut out of the cast. This piece of plaster is then held snugly in place with circumferential plaster. If the window is left open, with the intention of having better access to the wound, tissue will swell up through the window, causing erosions at the margins of the window and ultimately impairing circulation to the skin of that area.

3. Joints immobilized but a few hours may be transiently painful when moved again—particularly degenerated joints. After weeks of immobilization, they stiffen, and efforts to move them beyond a greatly limited arc are obstructed by mechanical resistance as well as pain. What process this stiffness represents is not thoroughly understood. The following is a useful conceptualization that at least fits the clinical facts: As long as blood continues to flow, fluids that transude from normal capillaries into soft tissues return again to the circulation through lymphatic channels and through more distal capillary segments where transudate pressure reverses as a consequence of the continued drop in capillary blood pressure and the rise in capillary oncotic pressure which results as proximal transudation of water and ions in excess of albumin creates a relatively protein-rich intracapillary fluid distally. (This physiologic process is distinct from the pathologic process discussed above under precaution 1, which we postutate is determined by the rise in tissue oncotic pressure which follows some injuries.) During movement of a part, its soft tissues are stretched in the direction of movement and thus compressed at right angles to that direction, and fluid is thereby displaced out of its lymphatic and capillary channels into more proximal channels. When the movement stops, the compression ceases, and the vascular

channels again fill with tissue fluid, and so blood and lymph continue to flow, and so, the pump effect of movement may keep soft tissues decongested. During immobilization, this pump effect is prevented, tissue capillaries congest, and the capsules, ligaments, and tendons they serve likewise congest, are thickened by this congestion, and consequently shortened. (Forces that stretch a piece of leather in one dimension will at the same time shorten it in perpendicular directions.) Such a mechanism may account for the stiffness that results when any joint is immobilized for an extended period.

Should tissue fluid in immobilized soft tissues become relatively protein rich and remain so, as it will in injured soft tissue, fibroblast activity will be accelerated, and the congested tissue will become increasingly fibrotic. Such a phenomenon could account for the fact that injured joints that have been immobilized are much more resistant to remobilization than are uninjured joints that have been immobilized. Perhaps a similar process occurs in degenerated as well as injured tissues. If so, it could also account for the fact that immobilized degenerated joints are much more resistant to remobilization than are growing joints.

Thus, the benefits and hazards of prolonged immobilization must be weighed before initial treatment is chosen, and thus a regimen of remobilization as well as strengthening must follow the period of immobilization. The regional chapters include several examples of the dilemma of immobilization and the compromises those dilemmas force: E.g., in those dilemmas involving degenerative joint disease, precision of reduction is sacrificed to maintain a range of motion (see "Treatment of fractures of the upper end of the humerus" in Chapter 3, and Colles' Fractures in Chapter 6); growing joints can be immobilized for longer intervals than can degenerated joints without great risk of lasting stiffness (see principle number 12 under "General Principles for Treatment of Forearm Fractures" in Chapter 6).

To remove a cast and discharge a person before following the person through a well-guided restorative program is incomplete treatment. Each regional chapter includes descriptions of exercises used to remobilize and recondition iatrogenically stiffened extremities.

Radiographic Monitoring

Fractures are examined by x-ray under seven different circumstances:

1. On first contact, to make the diagnosis and plan the treatment.

2. After manipulation, to assess the accuracy of reduction.

3. At intervals during early healing to detect slippage.

4. At later intervals to assess progress in healing.

5. When clinically stable, to assess bone bridging and thereby the strength of the fracture line and the degree of further protection necessary.

6. When remodelling is thought to be complete, to assess the integrity and form of the final structure.

7. In the event of further violence to the healing extremity, when the cast loosens or breaks, or when pain returns about the fracture site, to assess for reinjury.

Except, of course, in technically undeveloped regions, where x-ray is not available, all fractures requiring reduction should be examined by x-ray under circumstances 1, 2, and 7. Not all fractures need be examined by x-ray under circumstances 3 through 6. The experienced bone setter, one who may set several bones each month, will need x-rays for reliable assessment less often than the clinician who may set only four or five bones in a year. The next several paragraphs outline the principles applying to circumstances 3 through 6 upon which the experienced bone setter may rely when deciding whether or not to x-ray, and enumerate general rules upon which the occasional bone setter may base a decision regarding x-ray examination.

Third Circumstance. Fractures are variably stable after reduction, and experienced bone setters can assess the stability quite reliably by postreductive manipulation. When a reduced fracture is determined to be stable, if properly immobilized, it will rarely if ever slip, and the experienced bone setter may not re-x-ray these fractures for slippage.

The timing of x-ray for slippage is determined by the speed of healing. Fractures that heal quickly must be x-rayed 1 week after initial immobilization, as they become very difficult to remanipulate thereafter, and as they are unlikely to slip thereafter. On the other hand, fractures that heal slowly should be x-rayed 2 weeks after reduction, as slippage is most likely to occur within that interval. When slow-healing fractures show slight but acceptable slippage at 2 weeks, further x-rays should be made at 3 and at 4 weeks. Most slow-healing fractures can be remanipulated within 4 weeks of the initial immobilization.

Among the common fractures reduced in an outpatient setting, the following are likely to be unstable, and the occasional bone setter should x-ray these fractures for slippage routinely:

Fractures that Heal Quickly.

1. Fractures of the shafts of the phalanges of the fingers.

2. Fractures of the carpal bones.

3. Fractures of the distal third of radius and ulna when committed to an anatomic reduction.

4. Fractures of both bones of the forearm in mid- or proximal third. (Although these fractures heal quickly enough to require x-ray for slippage at the end of the 1st week, healing is usually not sufficiently strong for the fracture to be considered clinically stable until 12 weeks, except in very young children.)

5. Fractures of the neck of the radius.

6. Pericondylar fractures of the humerus.

7. Fractures of the tarsal bones.

8. Malleolar fractures.

9. Intra-articular fractures: diagonal fractures of the base of a phalanx of a finger or the great toe, the Bennett fracture of the 1st metacarpal, axial fractures of the head of the radius, condylar fractures of the humerus and tibia.

10. Nearly all fractures in children.

Fractures that Heal Slowly.

1. Isolated fractures of the shaft of the ulna. (These can angulate in time, narrowing the interosseous space, and subluxing the radio-ulnar joint, and thus impairing the mechanism of forearm rotation.)

2. Fractures of the shaft of the humerus.

3. Isolated fractures of the shaft of the tibia.

4. Fractures of both bones of the leg in adults.

Fourth Circumstance. Progress of healing is monitored by x-ray examination only for those fractures that heal slowly. For this purpose, we recommend x-ray at 6 weeks and every 6 weeks thereafter until clinically stable and bone bridging appears substantial.

Fifth Circumstance. Following the x-ray for slippage, fractures that heal quickly are next x-rayed when clinical stability is demonstrated or presumed. Clinical stability of shaft fractures can and should be demonstrated by manipulation: Gentle manipulation should produce neither pain nor motion. Fractures that heal quickly are generally clinically stable by 6–8 weeks after the initial immobilization. Fractures of the shaft of both bones of the forearm are the exception: except in very young children, clinical stability is not looked for until 12 weeks.

Sixth Circumstance. Unless union has been delayed, nearly all fractures treated in the outpatient setting will be remodelled by 1 year after the initial immobilization. We recommend that nearly all fractures be re-x-rayed at that time. Assessment of subsequent injuries is often simplified if one can compare the film of the injury with a post-remodelling film.

The Introduction of Needles

General Principles

During the evaluation and treatment of orthopaedic disorders, primary clinicians may introduce needles for one of three purposes: (1) anesthesia; (2) injection of analgesics and/or corticosteroids into well-localized foci of pain process; (3) arthrocentesis for aspiration and for intra-articular injection of corticosteroids. An understanding of some general as well as local principles will facilitate the applications of this mechanical mode. Local principles are concerned with the details of particular applications and are described and diagrammed in the final paragraphs of this section. We commend the following general principles as well:

Anesthesia. (See Chapter 16.)

Injection of Focal Pain Processes. These processes are the varieties of inflammatory and non-inflammatory myofascial pain syndromes. (See the regional chapters and Chapter 18.) While the mechanisms of remission of an inflammatory myofascial pain process, after an injection of corticosteroid, seem at least superficially clear to us, the mechanism of remission of a non-inflammatory myofascial pain process after injection of saline, xylocaine, or corticosteroid, or simply after dry needling remains utterly obscure—obscure because the pathophysiology of the non-inflammatory myofascial pain process is obscure. Chapter 18 makes some reference to this process. Whatever the mechanism, the efficacy of needling non-inflammatory myofascial pain syndromes, with or without injection of fluids, seems clinically established.

A variety of corticosteroids are available for local soft tissue and intra-articular use. We use aqueous suspensions of methylprednisolone (Depo-Medrol) and triamcinolone (Kenalog, or Aristocort Forte). Both are packaged in multiple-dose vials—Depo-Medrol in 40 mg./cc. and 80 mg./cc. concentrations, Kenalog in 10 mg./cc. and 40 mg./cc. concentrations, and Aristocort Forte in 40 mg./cc. concentration. Surprisingly, we have detected no clear difference in response among the various concentrations, implying that the weakest, and hence cheapest, solution may be generally sufficient. The volume used depends upon the volume of the structure to be injected. The regional chapters specify the volume used for each disorder.

We commend the following general technique (see figure 17–6):

1. Discover the center of the painful focus by careful thumb or fingertip palpation, and mark it with crossed fingernail indentation.

2. Cleanse the area with 70% ethyl alcohol.

3. Choose the narrowest-gauge needle of the desired length. (Length must be adequate for the needle to reach through subcutaneous fat to the painful myofascial focus.)

4. Draw up the solution to be injected, if any—corticosteroid when an inflammatory process is evident, and either saline, 1% Xylocaine, corticosteroid, or nothing when an inflammatory process is not evident. Use a 20- or 18-gauge needle to draw the material from the vial, then exchange for that needle the needle chosen for the injection.

5. Holding the syringe like a pencil, pass the needle abruptly through the skin at the intersection of the crossed nail indentations.

6. Slowly pass the needle inward perpendicular to the surface until deep pain is stimulated, or as far as bone—if bone immediately underlies the painful structure. If the painful focus is not identified with the first needle passage, the needle is partially withdrawn and redirected at another angle, and so the exploration is continued until the needle is seated in a zone that provokes pain.

7. Once the painful zone is identified by the needle, inject the chosen fluid. If dry needling has been chosen in lieu of a fluid, pass the needle in and out 10 to 20 times within the painful zone.

8. The frequency of injections depends upon the area to be injected, and the response to therapy. The regional chapters specify the frequency for each disorder.

Arthrocentesis for Aspiration and/or Intra-Articular Injection of Corticosteroid. Aspiration is performed as part of the evaluation of a joint effusion (see Chapters 12

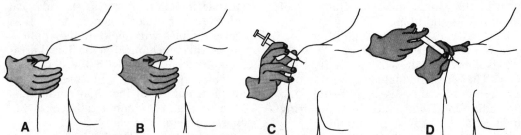

Fig. 17–6. Injection of focal pain processes. Anteroposterior view of the shoulder. *A*, discovery of painful focus. *B*, marking the point with the thumbnail. *C*, passing the needle. *D*, injecting the solution.

and 18), and to relieve the painful pressure of a tense effusion, thus easing the patient and facilitating further examination. Corticosteroids are injected into *aseptically* inflamed joints when one or two joints only are disablingly afflicted. Not all joints are equally vulnerable to the afflictions that may require aspiration or corticosteroid injection. In our experience, the primary clinician is most likely to introduce needles into the following joints, listed in decreasing order of vulnerability: injuries with effusion—knee, elbow, hip, ankle, shoulder; degenerative joint disease with exacerbation of synovitis—trapeziometacarpal joint of the thumbs, knees, hips, L_5-S_1 and L_4-L_5 facet joints, 1st metatarsophalangeal joints of the feet, ankles, and subtalar joints; rheumatoid arthritis—knees, metacarpophalangeal (MP) and interphalangeal (IP) finger joints, wrists, ankles, and hips.

We commend the following general technique (see Figure 17-7):

1. Identify joint lamdmarks by fingertip palpation, and mark the point for needle entry with crossed fingernail indentations. These points are designated for each joint in the final portion of this section.

2. Cleanse the area with ether or acetone, followed by 70% alcohol, or by detergent antiseptic, followed by 70% alcohol.

3. Create a 1% Xylocaine wheal over the point for needle entry, using a No. 27 needle. A fast method for knee injection without aspiration does not require an anesthetic wheal—see the description of knee injections in the local section which follows.

4. For joint aspiration, use a No. 19 or No. 18 needle; for knee and hip joints, use a 50 cc. syringe; and for ankle, shoulder, elbow, and wrist joints, a 20 cc. syringe; for all smaller joints, a 5 or 10 cc. syringe.

5. For corticosteroid injection, use the narrowest-gauge needle of the desired length; MP and IP joints can usually be injected with a 3/4″ No. 25 needle; wrist, elbow, shoulder, L_4-L_5, and L_5-S_1 facets, knee and ankle joints can usually be injected with a 1″ or 1½″ No. 22 needle; hip joints of relatively thin persons can usually be entered from the anterior approach with a 1½″ No. 22 needle, but 3″ are often required for heavier individuals.

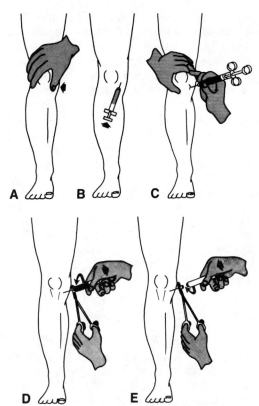

Fig. 17-7. Aspirating the knee. *A*, identifying the joint space. *B*, anesthetizing the skin. *C*, passing the needle. *D*, removing the filled syringe. *E*, replacing the emptied syringe.

6. Draw corticosteroid into a 2½ or 5 cc. syringe, from 0.25 to 2 cc., depending on the size of the joint to be injected: MP and IP joint—0.25 cc.; wrist—0.5-1 cc.; elbow —0.5-1 cc.; shoulder—1 cc.; ankle—0.5-1 cc.; knee—1 cc.; hip—1-2 cc. Draw the corticosteroid into the syringe from the vial using No. 20 to No. 18 guage needle, then exchange for it the needle intended for the injection.

7. Never touch or breathe on the skin after preparation, and never touch or breathe on any portion of the needle. When applying the needle to the syringe, use the needle guard which surrounds disposable needles, or a hemostat if handling needles not so packaged. When aspirating a joint, the syringe may have to be detached from the needle hub and emptied several times, leaving the needle in the joint. Use a hemostat to hold the needle hub while twisting off the syringe. The

point of the hemostat must not be handled or allowed to touch non-sterile materials. When laid back on the injection tray, the point must not touch any portion of the towel that has been touched by the examiner's hands. When using this method correctly, gloves, masks, and drapes need not be used. Indeed, this method is more sterile if used properly than is the more involved protocol when used clumsily, and it is more easily and quickly employed.

8. Introduce the needle with a steady determined thrust, not an abrupt push. Hold the syringe like a pencil, and use only the force of the fingers and occasionally the wrist. Elbows and shoulders should be braced and motionless. Use the other hand to steady the syringe hand, or to compress the joint when indicated.

Local Principles

The local principles of anesthesia are detailed in Chapter 16, and the local principles of injection of focal pain processes are detailed in the regional chapters. Arthrocentesis of the following joints is illustrated in Figures 17–8 to 17–18. Note the identified landmarks and the orientation of the needle.

Generalizations Concerning Musculoskeletal Rehabilitation

The rehabilitative regimens outlined in the regional chapters are founded on some generalizations of physiology and art which this section will summarize.

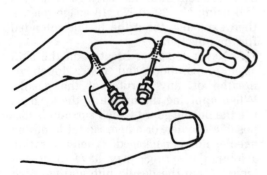

Fig. 17–8. Placing a needle into the metacarpophalangeal and interphalangeal joints.

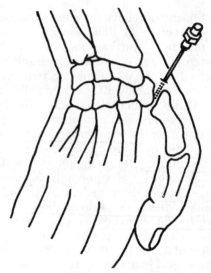

Fig. 17–9. Placing a needle into the trapeziometacarpal joint.

Physiology

The conceptualization of the pathophysiology of stiffness has been described above under "Cast Precautions" (point 3). This problem is a major concern of musculoskeletal rehabilitation. A second major concern is weakness, and a third is pain. These three problems perpetuate one another in a vicious circle which we call the *circle of passive congestion.* Once started, this circle can be further driven by and will itself drive another vicious circle, which we call the circle of reticular activation.*

The Circle of Passive Congestion. (See Figure 17–19.) Under "Cast Precautions" (above) congestion was postulated to result from immobilization and to lead to stiffness by thickening and shortening of capsules, ligaments and tendons. Pain terminals in these structures respond to stretch, and their thresholds are lowered by certain metabolites that accompany the inflammatory process. The joint stiffened by

* The following material concerning the physiology and art of musculoskeletal rehabilitation has been largely taken from the editor's chapter regarding Musculoskeletal Rehabilitation in the text, C. J. Leitch and R. V. Tinker, *Primary Care,* F. A. Davis & Co., Philadelphia, 1978. Dr. Leitch and the publishers have graciously permitted use of this material here.

congestion alone will be painful at the mechanical limit of motion, and the joint stiffened by the congestion that accompanies inflammation will be painful well before the mechanical limit is reached. In either case, the pain on movement will tempt the patient voluntarily to immobilize the joint, and may induce involuntary reactive muscle contractions that will further immobilize the joint. The resultant immobilization will lead to disuse atrophy of controlling muscles, a further cause for

immobility, and will augment or at least continue the congestion, and so this circle will turn.

The Circle of Reticular Activation. (See Figure 17-19.) It is fairly well established that each segment of the segmental reticular apparatus of the brain stem and spinal cord integrates sensory messages from primary sensory neurons to its own and var-

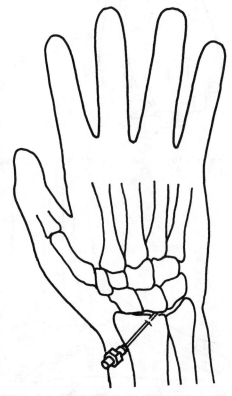

Fig. 17-10. Placing a needle into the radiocarpal joint through the dorsal aspect of the wrist.

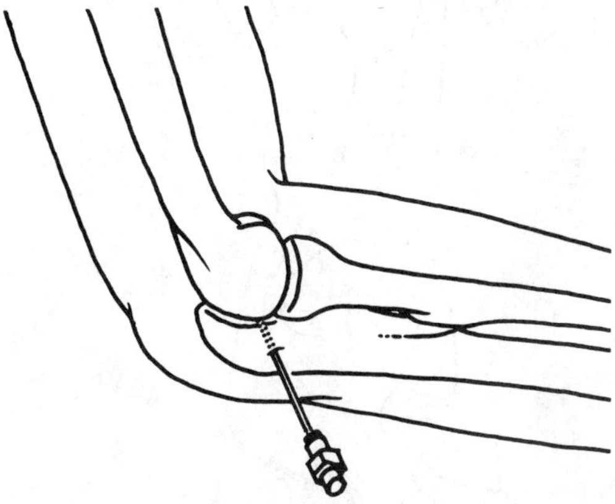

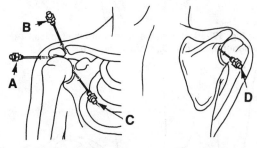

Fig. 17-11. Placing a needle into the ulnohumeral joint through the radial aspect of the elbow.

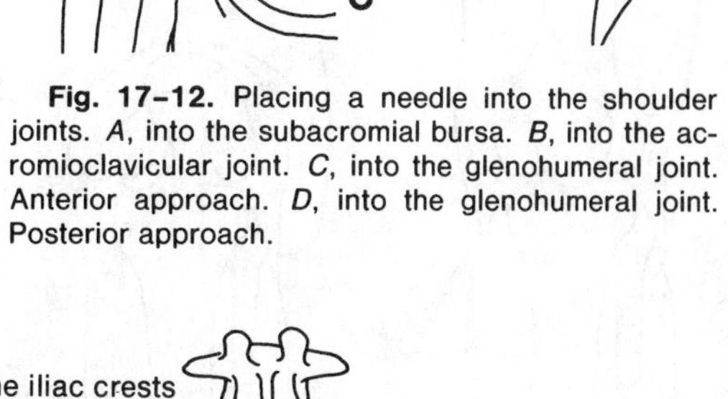

Fig. 17-12. Placing a needle into the shoulder joints. *A*, into the subacromial bursa. *B*, into the acromioclavicular joint. *C*, into the glenohumeral joint. Anterior approach. *D*, into the glenohumeral joint. Posterior approach.

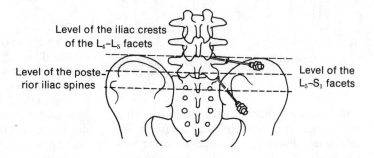

Level of the iliac crests of the L₄-L₅ facets

Level of the posterior iliac spines

Level of the L₅-S₁ facets

Fig. 17-13. Passing a needle into the L₄-L₅ and L₅-S₁ facet joints.

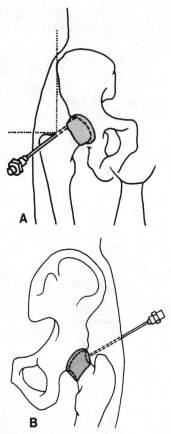

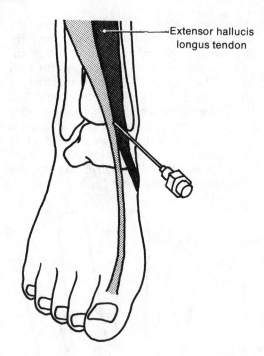

Fig. 17–16. Passing a needle into the tibiotalar joint.

Fig. 17–14. Passing a needle into the hip joint. *A*, anterior approach. *B*, lateral approach.

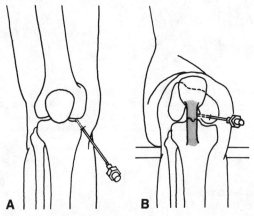

Fig. 17–15. Passing a needle into the knee joint. *A*, medial approach, with the knee extended. *B*, anterior approach, with the knee flexed to 90°.

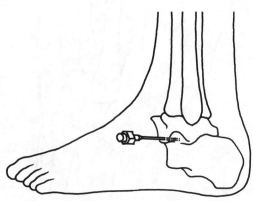

Fig. 17–17. Passing a needle into the subtalar joint by way of the sinus tarsi. Note the position relative to the lateral malleolus. The depression of the sinus tarsi is palpable there, especially when the ankle is inverted.

iably distant segments with messages from suprasegmental centers to generate facilitatory or inhibitory messages to lower motor neurons and to secondary sensory neu-rons in its own and variably distant segments. The degree to which pain messages can activate the reticular apparatus determines the intensity of reactive muscle contraction which follows from it. The greater the intensity of the pain, the longer its duration, and the more excitable the reticular apparatus, the greater the consequent activation of the reticular apparatus. The excitability of the reticular apparatus is determined by sensory messages, including the pain messages themselves, and by suprasegmental messages determined by neurophysiologic events that represent such complexities as the anamnestic, cognitive and affective patterns of an individual. Suprasegmental excitation of the reticular apparatus may well be greater among the cold, the fatigued, the anxious, the depressed, the hysterical, and the passively angry. Indeed, it has been our clinical impression that reactive muscle tone

often evident during pain processes is likely to be greatest among such individuals. As muscle contraction is sustained, pain processes begin in the contracted muscles, and the consequent pain messages contribute to the continued activation of the reticular apparatus, and so this circle turns.

Through pain, each circle, the circle of passive congestion and the circle of reticular activation, can energize the other.

Principles of the Art

The regimens of musculoskeletal rehabilitation are pitted against these vicious circles. These regimens must balance the need to oppose disuse atrophy and the stiffness of myofascial congestion against the need to facilitate a decrease in reactive muscle tone. The former requires active movement to the point of pain and muscle fatigue, while the latter requires a tranquil quiescence of the disordered part and of the total organism. How to balance these needs effectively is an art which cannot be taught. Thus it is that in the regional chapters we have so often recommended the services of a tactful physical therapist during the rehabilitative process. Some basic

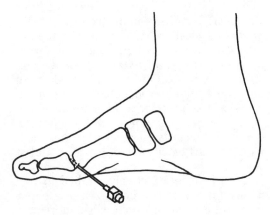

Fig. 17–18. Passing a needle into the first metatarsophalangeal joint.

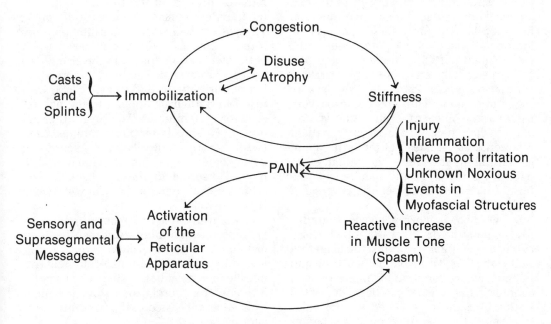

Fig. 17.19 Circles of passive congestion and reticular activation.

principles of the art, however, can be taught, and will be useful to primary clinicians when monitoring the simpler rehabilitative regimens themselves, or through their office helpers, and when working with and judging the work of physical therapists.

1. Muscle strengthens in proportion to load moved. It is usually safe and effective to choose a resistance that will fatigue the muscle within 20 repetitions.

2. Joints begin to remobilize when regularly moved, barely through the point of pain.

3. Active exercise is preferred to passive exercise because it is independent, strengthens while it mobilizes, and is less likely to do harm than are passive movements in the hands of an inexpert manipulator.

4. Tactful passive exercise or assisted active exercise is necessitated by weakness, timidity, harmful discoordination, or a pain process that is worsened by active movement (e.g., traumatic hemarthrosis or acute arthritis).

5. As discussed above under "Cast Precautions," congestion is moderated by movements that rhythmically compress the congested structures. Stretch applies a compressive force perpendicular to the axis of stretch. Joint movement to the mechanical limit of motion and manipulation in joint play will apply such compression. Manipulations in joint play require the least patient participation, and when performed skillfully are less likely to irritate congested tissues than are exercises in range of motion. Thus, they can be very useful at the outset of a rehabilitative program, when pain, stiffness, and patient reluctance are greatest. Often, after a single skillful manipulation, the patient is capable of performing and inspired to perform a therapeutically beneficial range of motion.

6. Wet heat is more analgesic than dry heat, unless the dry heat is applied over a cutaneous counter irritant, such as methyl salicylate. Analgesic balm, Ben-Gay and Deep Heat, are common examples of such counter irritants. Heat can burn, hence the heat source must be tested on the volar forearm of the therapist, must not be applied to insensitive or ischemic skin, and if prevented from cooling by a continuous source of energy, must not be occluded. For example, a common and blistering error is to lie upon a heating pad. Wet heat is best applied as a local bath, but may be applied as a hot wet towel and kept hot with a heating pad that has been insulated in plastic. Note that local heating, immersion of the disordered part alone, is more effective than total heating, immersion of the whole body, as it can be kept hotter longer without harm to the patient.

7. Cold is less likely to congest an area than is heat, and can be analgesic. The analgesic benefit is more likely to be appreciated after rather than during the application. Cold is unequivocally preferred to heat during the first 2–7 days after an injury, and is often more analgesic than heat on a shoulder afflicted by the tendinous cuff syndrome, perhaps because that tight space does not accept congestion kindly. For nearly all other problems, heat or cold must be chosen only after a trial of each.

Cold can be effectively applied in two ways: (a) Water can be frozen in a paper cup and the ice, held in a washcloth, massaged over the painful area. To avoid thermocutaneous injury, the ice must be kept moving throughout the treatment. Five to ten minutes of massage is usually effective. The patient will suffer a burning pain before the analgesic effect is achieved. (b) A bath towel can be folded to the size of the area to be treated, dampened thoroughly but not drippingly, and frozen. The frozen towel may then be applied to the painful area for 5–10 minutes. To prevent thermal injury, a damp towel must intercede between the frozen towel and the disordered part. For example, the individual with a painful disorder of the low back can lie with his back upon a damp towel over a frozen towel.

8. Painfully reactive muscle tone must be kept at a minimum. Any manipulation or motion, active or passive, which is followed by an increase in painfully reactive muscle tone must be avoided or its harmful influence on muscle tone somehow neutralized as suggested in the next three paragraphs.

9. Topical and systemic analgesics facilitate a decrease in painfully reactive muscle tone. Topical analgesics include heat, cold, and gentle massage. Systemic analgesics include drugs such as salicylates and narcotics, and various inductors of intense concentration on other matters, such as hypnotic instructions, erotic stimulation, perhaps acupuncture, and skilled meditative practices.

10. Fatigue must be recognized, relieved, and subsequently avoided when it appears to augment pain. The word "fatigue" in this context is meant to refer not to muscle fatigue, but to a total personal fatigue.

11. Anxiety and depression must be recognized and relieved. Efforts to facilitate the patient's recognition of the anxiety or depression and to enlist the patient's active assistance in its dissipation may or may not be useful. An empathic acknowledgement of the therapist's suspicion of anxiety or depression often leads to the distinction. Patients who respond promptly on the next visit with emotive or factually detailed agreement may well benefit from further exploration and empathic acknowledgement of the origins of his anxiety. The patient who denies it or admits it without emotion or further detail will probably not benefit from further exploration of that kind at that time. The patient's denial or bland acceptance forces the therapist to consider that his intuition may be wrong. If not wrong, then at least in that context, the therapist will have to work alone and more authoritatively, or, as some would say, more magically.

Whether attention to these affective deterrents to rehabilitation becomes a joint project with the patient or not, drugs may be useful. When anxiety is provoked by pain or the horror of an accident, the axiolytics, Valium or lithium, may augment the benefit of analgesics and may greatly facilitate the physical therapy. Dexedrine, cautiously monitored, may be of benefit when depression appears to be reactive to the pain, the injury, or some other contemporary insult. When depression appears to be endogenous, the tricyclic antidepressants, imipramine or amitriptylline, may lead within 1–3 weeks to a brightening of the mood and a more active compliance with the rehabilitative program.

Antitherapeutic Motives

Litigious resentment, hysteria, economic and interpersonal passivity, and the sociopathic intent to dissemble can be powerful deterents to rehabilitation. When these deterrents are active, the goals of the therapist are often drastically at odds with those of the patient, empathy is hard or impossible to muster, and the therapeutic alliance rarely develops. Nowhere in human therapeutics do diagnostic sophistication, objectivity, and good humored courage weigh more heavily in the therapeutic balance. An everpresent danger is the temptation for the therapist to become an advocate, if not for the patient then for the ethics of chivalry, personal objectivity and responsibility, or social honesty. Neither the patient nor the therapist benefits by such advocacy. Clear, utterly direct, and impecably correct descriptions of the pathology, intended therapy, and expected results from enthusiastic compliance will occasionally prove therapeutic for the resentful or hysterical patient and rarely for the passive patient. The sociopath may initially respond to such a frustration of his intentions with threats and belittling accusations, but when a distinct need for a therapist's services coexists with the malingering intent, continuing firmness by the therapist will occasionally be rewarded by a tolerable, though always unstable, therapeutic alliance.

The Measurement of Joint Motion

While a qualitative sense of joint motion is often adequate for diagnostic and planning purposes, a quantitative measure of joint motion provides a more securely objective measure of the effect of therapy and a better documented report of disability to courts and private or governmental claims adjustors.

Joint motion is measured with a *goniometer* (Greek: *gonia*, angle + *metron*, measure). One limb, the static limb, of the goniometer, is aligned with a reference axis along the body part just proximal to

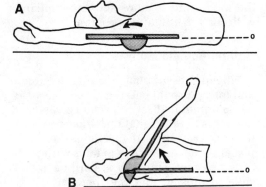

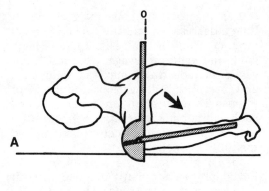

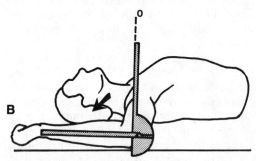

Fig. 17–20. *A,* shoulder elevation through flexion. Measurement is made in the sagittal plane of the trunk. *B,* shoulder extension. Measurement is made in the sagittal plane of the trunk.

Fig. 17–22. *A,* internal rotation of the shoulder at 90° abduction. Measurement is made in the sagittal plane of the trunk. *B,* external rotation of the shoulder at 90° abduction. Measurement is made in the sagittal plane of the trunk.

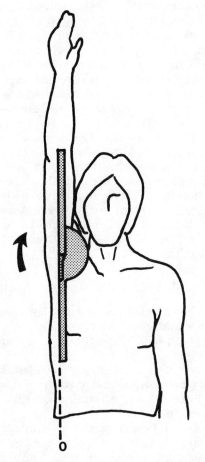

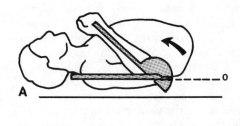

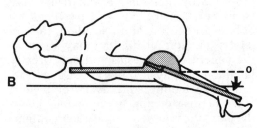

Fig. 17–21. Shoulder elevation through abduction. Measurement is made in the frontal plane of the trunk.

Fig. 17–23. *A,* elbow flexion. Measurement is made in the sagittal plane of the arm. *B,* elbow extension. Measurement is made in the sagittal plane of the arm.

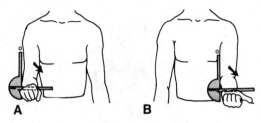

Fig. 17–24. *A*, forearm pronation with the elbow at 90° flexion, and the forearm in the sagittal plane of the trunk. Measurement is made in the frontal plane of the trunk. *B*, forearm supination with the elbow at 90° flexion, and the forearm in the sagittal plane of the trunk. Measurement is made in the frontal plane of the trunk.

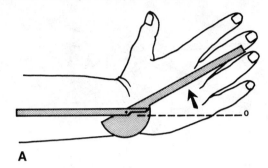

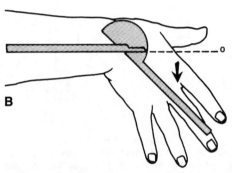

Fig. 17–26. *A*, radial deviation of the wrist. Measurement is made in the frontal plane of the forearm. *B*, ulnar deviation of the wrist. Measurement is made in the frontal plane of the forearm.

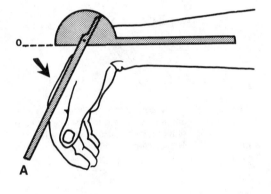

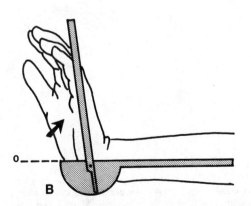

Fig. 17–25. *A*, wrist flexion. Measurement is made in the sagittal plane of the forearm. *B*, wrist extension. Measurement is made in the sagittal plane of the forearm.

the joint, and the other limb, the dynamic limb of the goniometer is aligned with the moving axis along the body part just distal to the joint.

The joint motion is measured from a position as close in line to the reference axis as the moving axis can attain, to a position as far from the reference axis as the moving axis can attain, within the intended plane of motion. The reference axis is always designated 0°.

Figures 17–20 through 17–34 name the motion, the plane of its measurement, designate the reference axis, and show the proper alignment of the goniometer for each measurement.

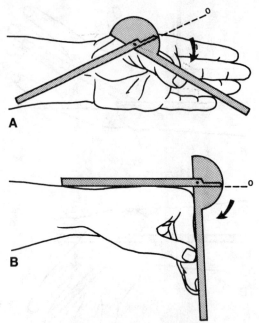

A

B

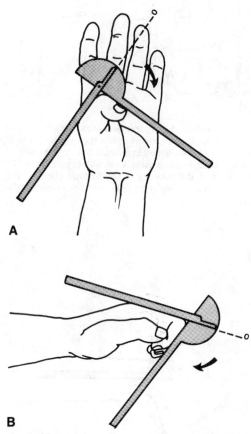

A

B

Fig. 17–27. *A*, flexion of the 1st metacarpopha-langeal joint. Measurement is made in the frontal plane of the forearm and hand. *B*, flexion of the 2nd, 3rd, 4th, and 5th metacarpophalangeal joints. Measurement is made in the sagittal plane of the forearm and hand.

Fig. 17–28. *A*, flexion of the 1st interphalangeal joint. Measurement is made in the frontal plane of the hand. *B*, flexion of the 2nd, 3rd, 4th, and 5th interphalangeal joints. Measurement is made in the sagittal plane of the hand.

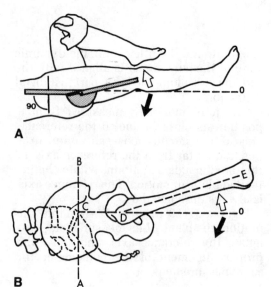

A

B

Fig. 17–29. *A*, skeletal landmarks used to orient the goniometer when measuring hip extension and flexion. The 0° axis is perpendicular to a line connecting the point of the anterior-superior iliac spine with the point of the posterior iliac spine. *B*, hip extension. Measurement is made in the sagittal plane of the trunk. The example illustrates limitation of extension to a point short of the zero axis (note open arrow).

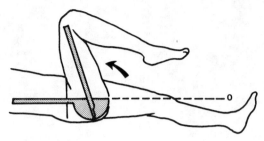

Fig. 17-30. Hip flexion. Measurement is made in the sagittal plane of the trunk.

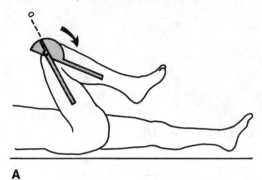

A

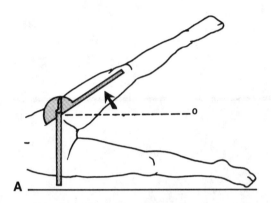

A

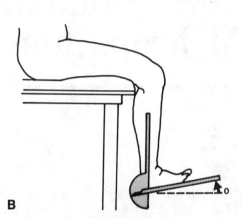

B

Fig. 17-33. *A*, knee flexion. Measurement is made in the sagittal plane of the thigh. *B*, ankle dorsiflexion. Measurement is made in the sagittal plane of the leg.

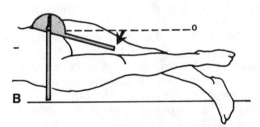

B

Fig. 17-31. *A*, hip abduction. Measurement is made in the frontal plane of the trunk. *B*, hip adduction. Measurement is made in the frontal plane of the trunk.

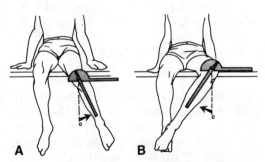

A   B

Fig. 17-32. *A*, internal rotation of the hip. Measurement is made in the transverse plane of the thigh. *B*, external rotation of the hip. Measurement is made in the transverse plane of the thigh.

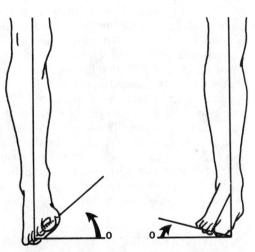

Fig. 17-34, Supination and pronation of the foot. Supination is measured in the transverse plane of the foot. Pronation is measured in the transverse and frontal planes of the foot.

CHAPTER 18

Non-Traumatic Arthropathies

The non-traumatic arthropathies are the articular and periarticular pain syndrome that emerge without any necessary association with an injury. While the regional chapters describe with fair detail the pathology and clinical distinction among the acute traumatic arthropathies, their references to the non-traumatic arthropathies, while anatomically specific, are pathologically quite general. The regional chapters intend to teach the distinction between the general categories *articular pain syndrome*, and *periarticular pain syndrome*. Once a regional disorder is determined to represent a non-traumatic arthropathy, its specific form must be determined. To teach this determination is the first purpose of this chapter. The second purpose is to provide a summary of the analgesic/anti-inflammatory drugs commonly used in the treatment of periarticular and articular pain syndromes, so as to avoid tedious repetition throughout the text.

The Non-Traumatic Arthropathies

Of the various forms of non-traumatic arthropathy, only the periarticular pain syndrome, degenerative joint disease, gouty arthritis, and rheumatoid arthritis present to primary clinicians with any regularity. The other forms occur so infrequently that primary practitioners have rare opportunities to practice their differentiating skills. The primary practitioner needs a terse essential view of the total problem that can be readily called from memory when circumstances require a differential determination. The following discussion attempts to present this view in three parts:

1. The pathogenesis and clinical features of the six fundamental non-traumatic arthropathies;

2. a summary of the clinical and laboratory characteristics that distinguish the arthropathies;

3. an outline of the treatment of each.

Pathogenesis and Clinical Features

Periarticular Pain Syndromes. **Periarticular Inflammatory Disorders.** Occasionally, as a consequence of recognized trauma or overuse, but usually without recognized correlative events, an inflammatory process will emerge in bursae, tendons, or their synovia in the neighborhood of joints. These disorders are diagnosed only when they produce overlying visible signs of inflammation.

Periarticular Cryptogenic Pain Syndromes. As mentioned in Chapter 3, the bulk of periarticular pain syndromes do not manifest visible evidence of inflammation. The pain-producing process is unknown. Theories of ischemia and congestion have been proposed, but have not been validated. In this text, we have referred to these pain syndromes as myofascial or myotendinous pain syndromes, or specifically when the shoulder is involved, as the tendinous cuff syndrome.

Degenerative Arthritis. Compressive and frictional forces wear hyaline cartilage over time. The worn cartilage is abraded thin, fibrillated, and ulcerated. The rate of wear is directly proportional to the magnitude of the wearing forces and the degree of "mismatch" between articulating surfaces, and inversely proportional to the inherent resistance of the cartilage to the wearing forces. The inherent resistance emerges partly from developmental influences (heredity, childhood health and nutrition), and partly from traumatic circumstance (damaged cartilage is more vulnerable to wearing forces than is intact cartilage). Wearing forces on weight bearing cartilage (hips, knees, ankles, and subtalar joints) are obviously proportional to weight and to weightbearing time, while wearing forces on non-weightbearing cartilage (upper extremity joints, facet joints, and metatarsophalangeal joints of the feet) are proportional to compressive and shearing forces during habitual activities. Manipulative activities generally apply greater compression and shear to the distal interphalangeal (DIP) and proximal interphalangeal (PIP) joints of the fingers than to the metacarpophalangeal (MP) joints of the fingers. Some activities are more wearing than others (organists experience greater wearing forces on the distal IP joints of the fingers when playing their instrument than do trombonists when playing theirs). Because most of us do more pushing with our thumbs than with our fingers, the first MP and trapeziometacarpal joints are more subject to wear than are the other MP and carpometacarpal joints of the hand. The normal gait pattern and the deforming effect of shoes conspire to apply greater shearing stress to the MP joint of the first toe than to the MP joints of the other toes. Due to their mobility and to the angulating forces applied to them in daily activity, the facet joints of the lumbosacral and cervical spines are more subject to wear than are the other facet joints of the spine.

Not only does the nature of habitual activity determine exposure to wear, but so also does the manner by which an activity is conducted. When muscle tone is crudely coordinated so that a joint is stressed with untimely support from its controlling muscles, the stress of the activity imparts to the joint excessive movement in play, thus subjecting it to greater shearing forces. Neurogenic arthropathy (the Charcot joint) is the extreme example of this principle: Deprived of proprioceptive and pain sensation, the joint is exposed to stresses which are unopposed by protective muscle responses. The subtalar joint degeneration that accomapanies chronic foot strain, and the increased lumbosacral facet degeneration that accompanies marked lumbosacral lordosis are more prevalent examples.

Bone development can cause joint malalignment. Unrecognized and sometimes hereditary events can lead to such developments: For example, the rotational lumbosacral facet malformation, and marked genu valgum. Recognized injuries can also lead to such developments: Epiphyseal injuries may interrupt the growth of one condyle but not the other; malunited fractures can disturb the alignment of articulation (the radiohumeral joint may be malaligned by an angulated fracture of the proximal radial neck, and the radio-ulnar articulation may be malaligned by the impacted Colles fracture).

The joints most subject to degenerative disease are the following: (a) weightbearing joints—hip, knee, ankle, and subtalar joints; (b) joints subject to the compressive and shearing forces of habitual activity—DIP and PIP joints of fingers, MP and trapeziometacarpal joints of the thumb, metatarso-phalangeal joint of the great toe, and the facet joints of the lumbosacral and cervical spines. Unless made more vulnerable to wear by injury, wrist, elbow, and shoulder joints rarely develop degenerative joint disease.

The periarticular tissues respond to cartilage wear as follows:

1. Adjacent bone hypertrophies and becomes more dense (spurring and eburnation).

2. The synovium may become mildly inflamed from time to time in reaction to cartilagenous debris, and a mild to moderate joint effusion and an increase in pain will result.

3. The fibrous capsule thickens and shortens.

The characteristic clinical features are the following:

1. The onset is insidious, and much cartilage wear can occur without symptoms emerging.

2. The disease is not systemic, and, as explained in the prior paragraphs, afflicts those joints most subject to stress and, because of injury, habits of posture or movement, or developmental distortions, those joints most vulnerable to the wearing effects of stress.

3. Older individuals are more likely to be afflicted than are younger individuals.

4. Afflicted joints tend to stiffen as fibrous capsules tend to thicken and shorten.

5. Pain accompanies forces that compress afflicted joints or that move afflicted joints to their limit of play.

6. Episodes of mild acute synovitis punctuate the chronic stiffness and stress pain.

7. Inactivity increases pain, particularly when a joint is inflamed—hence, the severe night pain that may follow intense activity.

8. X-ray findings are the following: (a) the joint space narrows as cartilage thins. (b) bony margins become overgrown. (c) subchondral bone becomes more dense than normal (eburnated).

Characteristics 1, 4, and 5 suggest why some individuals afflicted with considerable cartilage wear, as evidenced by x-ray, suffer little distress and others with lesser wear may be disabled. If the fibrous capsule maintains normal pliance, and muscle tone remains coordinately responsive, capsular stress is kept to a minimum. When weight is moderate and the shocks of weightbearing are absorbed by coordinate muscles responses, compressive forces and the pain accompanying them are minimal.

Immune Complex Disease. Arthritis is a prominent feature of seven fundamental immune complex diseases. Rheumatoid arthritis is by far the most prevalent of the seven. The other six are: ankylosing spondylitis, rheumatic fever, systemic lupus erythematosus, arthritis of inflammatory intestinal disease, psoriatic arthritis, and Reiter's syndrome. All are presumed to result when some process or processes of the immune response become disordered.

While all are systemic diseases, and some can be very difficult to distinguish one from another, the distinction can usually be made by attention to the following clinical patterns:

Rheumatoid Arthritis.

1. Articular pain and inflammation is dominant.

2. Proximal IP and MP joints of the hands are more commonly afflicted than other joints.

3. The erythrocyte sedimentation rate is elevated, and macroglobulins called the rheumatoid factor can usually be isolated.

4. Antinuclear antibodies are present, but usually in low titer.

5. Renal disease is not part of the process.

Ankylosing Spondylitis.

1. The disease usually emerges as sacroliac and lumbosacral facet arthritis.

2. In time, the dorsal and cervical facets become involved.

3. The erythrocyte sedimentation rate is elevated, but the rheumatoid factor is usually not detected.

4. The histocompatibility antigen, HLA-B27, is found in a majority of these afflictions.

5. Men are more likely to be afflicted than women.

Rheumatic Fever.

1. Arthritis is migratory.

2. Erythemas are fairly common.

3. Carditis is more common than in the other diseases.

4. Salicylates produce a uniquely rapid

remission.

Systemic Lupus Erythematosus.

1. Arthritis is rarely deforming.

2. Typical skin manifestations are prevalent (variably inflamed, scaly, erythematous discs).

3. Urinalysis typically shows findings of inflammatory renal disease, and liver function tests may be abnormal.

4. Women are more likely to be afflicted than men.

Arthritis of Inflammatory Intestinal Disease.

1. Affects those afflicted by ulcerative colitis, regional enteritis, or Whipple's disease.

2. Arthritis typically affects large joints asymmetrically and does not lead to permanent change.

3. The arthritis may resemble the early form of ankylosing spondylitis.

4. Rheumatoid factor is usually not found.

5. When the disease resembles the early form of ankylosing spondylitis, the histocompatibility antigen, HLA-B27, can usually be found.

6. The arthritis parallels the action of the bowel disease.

Psoriatic Arthritis.

1. Typically accompanies *generalized* psoriasis.

2. DIP joints are more commonly afflicted than are PIP joints, and the nails of the afflicted fingers show nail plate pittings and nail bed thickenings.

3. Arthritis is frequently asymmetric.

4. Occasionally the arthritis will extend to the sacroiliac and lumbosacral facet joints.

5. Rheumatoid factor is usually not found.

6. When sacroiliac and lumbosacral facets are involved, the histocompatibility antigen, HLA-B27, can usually be found.

Reiter's Syndrome.

1. The arthritis is one of four disorders that constitute this syndrome, the other three being: non-specific urethritis, conjunctivitis, or uveitis, pustular and ulcerative dermatoses, and mouth lesions.

2. The arthritis affects large joints asymmetrically and in time may affect the sacroiliac and lumbosacral joints in a manner resembling early ankylosing spondylitis.

3. The arthritis may lead in time to permanent joint changes.

4. The histocompatibility antigen, HLA-B27, can be found in the majority.

The text will discuss the characteristics and treatment of rheumatoid arthritis and ankylosing spondylitis in somewhat greater detail. Because the other disorders are rare always and involve other systems, they will not be discussed further in this chapter.

Pathogenesis of Rheumatoid Arthritis. The synovium develops a granular inflammation which, in time, extends a granular membrane called a pannus. This pannus erodes cartilage, bone, capsule, and ligament. An inflammatory effusion distends the joints which are actively afflicted.

Characteristic Clinical Features of Rheumatoid Arthritis.

1. The disease afflicts three times as many women as men.

2. Typically, the disease emerges in young adulthood, but can emerge at any age.

3. Onset is usually insidious, but may be acute.

4. While arthritis is often prevalent at the onset, occasionally the disease begins with a systemic syndrome of fever, fatigue, weight loss, paresthesiae, and arthralgias.

5. Typically, many joints are involved, but occasionally the disease will begin as a monarticular arthritis.

6. In order of decreasing prevalence, joints most commonly afflicted are the following: MP joints of the fingers, PIP joints of the fingers, wrist joints, elbow joints, knee joints.

7. Inflammation and thus pain and stiffness wax and wane. Exessive activity will provoke an inflammatory relapse.

8. Stiffness is greatest after a period of inactivity (like a night's sleep), and least after a period of mild to moderate activity.

9. X-ray findings are these: (a) Early changes are usually limited to periarticular osteoporosis. (b) In time, the bony margins of joints, where synovial membranes meet cartilage, will show erosion. (c) In late stages, the joint space will be narrowed.

10. The erythrocyte sedimentation rate

is elevated, and rheumatoid factor can usually be detected in serum and/or joint fluid. Joint fluid shows inflammatory changes (See Table 18–1.)

11. As progression of the synovial proliferation leads to erosion of cartilage and periarticular structures, joint deformity and disability will occur.

Pathogenesis of Ankylosing Spondylitis. A proliferative chronic synovitis like that of rheumatoid arthritis afflicts the sacroiliac and the lumbosacral facet joints and, in time, ascends to afflict the length of the spine. As the facet synovitis progresses, the annulus fibrosus of each intervertebral disc begins to ossify and, in time, to fuse the vertebrae one to another. When the process extends to the dorsal spine, it also afflicts the costovertebral joints, which greatly restricts thoracic ventilatory excursions. The ultimate deformity is a fused spine in the shape of a shallow C, from occiput to sacrum. Carditis may occur late and uveitis may occur early.

Characteristic Clinical Features of Ankylosing Spondylitis.

1. Men are afflicted 10 times more often than women.

2. Onset is typically gradual, and experienced as pain and stiffness in the low back.

3. In time, the dorsal and cervical spines become stiff and painful as well.

4. The erythrocyte sedimentation rate is usually elevated, the rheumatoid factor is usually not found, and the histocompatibility antigen, HLA-B27, is found in the great majority.

5. X-ray findings are these: (a) Early changes are erosion and eburnation about the sacroiliac joints. (b) In time, lumbar and eventually dorsal and cervical facet joints show similar changes. (c) In late stages, the annulus fibrosis will show evidence of ossification, and the anterior and posterior ligaments will show calcium deposits.

6. Eventually, the spine will be fused.

Metabolic Arthritis. The intra-articular crystalization of two metabolic salts, *monosodium urate monohydrate,* and *calcium pyrophosphate dihydrate,* is associated with acute arthritis. In time, these salts can accumulate in cartilage and periarticular tissue, and will accelerate the development of degenerative joint disease. The intra-

Table 18–1
Differential Characteristics of Joint Fluid

Characteristic	Degeneration	Aseptic Inflammation	Septic Inflammation
Gross appearance.	Yellow, transparent, with high viscosity.	Yellow, translucent, with low viscosity.	Yellow to green, opaque, with low viscosity or with the viscosity of pus.
Leukocytes/mm³	200–2000. Less than 25% are polymorphonuclear leukocytes.	2000–100,000. 50% or more are polymorphonuclear leukocytes.	10,000->100,000. 50–75% are polymorphonuclear leukocytes.
Mucin clot.	Firm.	Friable.	Friable.
Glucose.	Near to the blood glucose.	Lower than the blood glucose.	Much lower than the blood glucose.
Rheumatoid factor.	Absent.	Present in rheumatoid arthritis.	Absent.
Crystals.	Absent.	Urate crystals in gout. Calcium pyrophosphate crystals in pseudogout.	Absent.
Culture.	No organisms.	No organisms.	Specific organism usually, but not always recovered.

articular urate crystals are definitively associated with *acute gouty arthritis,* and the intra-articular calcium pyrophosphate crystals are definitively associated with *pseudogout.* The degenerative joint disease associated with urates is called *chronic tophaceous arthritis,* and the degenerative joint disease associated with calcium pyrophosphate crystals is called *chondrocalcinosis.* It is generally presumed that intraarticular crystals are phagocytosed by polymorphonuclear leukocytes, which are thus provoked to release substances which induce a synovial and periarticular inflammatory process. Each disease can emerge primarily or secondarily. The primary forms appear to be hereditary. Secondary gout emerges when hyperuricemia complicates neoplastic disease. That complication is most likely to occur when rapid cellular turnover or rapid destruction of neoplastic cells with cytotoxic drugs accelerates the production of urates. Secondary gout also emerges when renal disease or thiazide diuretics decrease the excretion of urates. Chondrocalcinosis emerges as a late complication of primary pseudogout or as a complication of a variety of endocrine and metabolic disorders, the most common of which is diabetes mellitus. Characteristic clinical features of acute gouty arthritis and chronic tophaceous gout are the following:

1. Men are afflicted nine times more often than women.

2. The first onset in men usually occurs in early middle life, while in women it usually occurs after the menopause.

3. The onset of acute arthritis is very rapid.

4. The current textbook description of acute gouty arthritis refers to an inflammation of the MP joint of the great toe, and of the tarsometatarsal, intertarsal, ankle, and knee joints, associated with demonstrable urate crystals in the affected joints.

5. In addition to this pathognomonic form of acute gouty arthritis, we believe other forms of acute and subacute articular and periarticular disease are disproportionately prevalent in association with hyperuricemia and remit when serum uric acid levels are decreased. These are recur-

rent and chronic prepatellar and olecranon bursitis, various myotendinous and tenosynovial pain syndromes, and vertebral facet joint arthritis.

6. In time, x-rays of recurrently affected joints show disproportionate degenerative change.

7. Serum uric acid will be elevated above 8 mg.%.

8. Microscopic examination of joint fluid under polarized light will demonstrate the intra- and extracellular negatively birefringent needle-like urate crystals.

9. Colchicine typically induces a dramatic remission.

Characteristic clinical features of pseudogout and chondrocalcinosis are the following:

1. The disease is equally prevalent between the sexes.

2. The first onset usually occurs after the 6th decade.

3. Onset of acute arthritis is very rapid.

4. Large joints are typically involved— the knees more often than any other.

5. In time, x-rays will show calcification of articular cartilage and all the signs of degenerative joint disease.

6. Serum uric acid is normal.

7. Microscopic examination of joint fluid under polarized light will demonstrate the intra- and extracellular weakly positively birefringent calcium pyrophosphate crystals.

8. Colchicine is typically ineffective.

Septic Arthritis. Infections of joints will be discussed in detail in Chapter 19, along with the infections of bone. However, the differentiation of septic arthritis from the other forms of non-traumatic arthropathy should be reviewed in this broader context.

Acute septic arthritis must be suspected whenever the following clinical characteristics appear:

1. Usually only one, and rarely more than two joints are affected.

2. The onset is very rapid.

3. The affected joint is very painful, hot, red, and fluctuant.

4. Signs of acute systemic illness are prominent: All patients usually manifest a hectic fever with chills and sweats; a child

so afflicted will be prostrate, will vomit, and may be delirious; adults, on the other hand, may seem merely fatigued and will be capable of bringing themselves to an outpatient clinic.

5. Joint fluid will be cloudy or frankly purulent. Thousands of leukocytes will be evident per cubic millimeter, and the majority will be polymorphonuclear leukocytes.

6. Bacteria may or may not be evident by Gram stain and culture of joint fluid. (See Chapter 19).

Tuberculous or mycotic granulomatous arthritis must be suspected whenever a subacute or chronic arthritic picture appears. Though primary clinicians encounter these joint infections very rarely, the diseases should be considered whenever a monoarticular arthritis of subacute or chronic form emerges in an immunodeficient or otherwise debilitated person. Recovery of the organism from joint fluid confirms the diagnosis. When these diseases are suspect, a search for other sites of infection must be made, and orthopaedic consultation must be obtained.

Cryptogenic Proliferative Synovial Disorders. A variety of rare cryptogenic proliferative synovial disorders can superficially resemble degenerative joint disease. Two forms are histologically distinct, *pigmented villonodular synovitis,* and *synovial osteochondromatosis.* Other much less distinct examples are grouped in a general category called *chronic synovitis.* These disorders tend to emerge in the larger joints, particularly the hip and knee joints. Though rare, they must be considered in three circumstances:

1. A joint not usually afflicted by degenerative disease looks as if it is. Example: The elbow.

2. Any joint appearing to be afflicted by degenerative disease continues to be disablingly painful, in spite of compliance with the usually beneficial conservative measures.

3. X-rays show: (a) increased soft tissue shadow (pigmented villonodular synovitis). (b) erosion of adjacent bone (any of the disorders). (c) multiple periarthritic foci of calcification (synovial osteochondromatosis).

When these diseases are suspect, the patient must be referred to an orthopaedist. The prognosis is always guarded, and surgical treatment is often attempted.

Differential Diagnosis Summarized

Temporal-Spatial Characteristics. The non-traumatic arthropathies generally present in one of five temporal-spatial patterns. The differential diagnosis of each pattern is distinct from but overlaps the others.

Rapid Onset, One or a Few Joints.

Typical presentation: septic arthritis, gout and pseudogout, periarticular myofascial pain syndromes.

Occasional presentation: immune complex arthritis.

Rare presentation: degenerative joint disease.

Rapid Onset, Many Joints.

Occasional presentation: immune complex disease, periarticular myofascial pain syndromes.

While septic arthritis may present with a brief systemic prodrome characterized by multiple arthralgias, arthritis rarely establishes in more than one or two joints.

Gradual Onset, One or a Few Joints.

Typical presentation: degenerative joint disease, cryptogenic proliferative synovial disorders, granulomatous septic arthritis.

Rare presentation: immune complex arthritis.

Gradual Onset, Many Joints.

Typical presentation: rheumatoid arthritis.

Rare presentation: degenerative joint disease, periarticular myofascial pain syndromes.

Progressive Disorder, Punctuated by Acute Exacerbations and Decreasingly Complete Remissions, One or More Joints.

Typical presentation: gout, pseudogout, immune complex disease, periarticular myofascial syndromes.

Rare presentation: degenerative joint disease.

Physical Characteristics.

Acute Articular Inflammation. Generalized periarticular redness, heat, and swelling, with evidence of effusion; generalized periarticular tenderness; joint is immobilized by pain.

Typical presentation: acute septic arthritis, acute gouty arthritis, pseudogout.

Occasional presentation: immune complex disease.

Rare presentation: degenerative arthritis.

Acute Periarticular Inflammation. Redness, heat, and swelling, well localized to a particular myofascial structure, without evidence of effusion unless into a bursa. Range of motion is greatly restricted by pain.

Typical presentation: periarticular myofascial pain syndromes, gouty bursitis/tendinitis/tenosynovitis, septic cellulitis/tenosynovitis/bursitis.

Subacute Articular Inflammation. Generalized periarticular tenderness and swelling, with evidence of joint effusion. The joint may be warm. Range of motion is limited by pain.

Typical presentation: immune complex arthritis, granulomatous septic arthritis.

Occasional presentation: degenerative joint disease, chondrocalcinosis, chronic tophaceous gout.

Subacute Periarticular Inflammation. Marked tenderness, well localized to a particular myofascial structure, without evidence of effusion unless into a bursa. Range of motion is limited by pain.

Typical presentation: periarticular myofascial pain syndromes.

Occasional presentation: gouty bursitis/tenosynovitis/tendinitis.

Subacute Articular Inflammation. Generalized periarticular tenderness and swelling, with evidence of joint effusion. The joint may be warm. Range of motion is limited by pain.

Typical presentation: immune complex arthritis, granulomatous septic arthritis.

Occasional presentation: degenerative joint disease, chondrocalcinosis, chronic tophaceous gout.

Subacute Periarticular Inflammation. Marked tenderness, well localized to a particular myofascial structure, without evidence of effusion unless into a bursa. Range of motion is limited by pain.

Typical presentation: periarticular myofascial pain syndromes.

Occasional presentation: gouty bursitis/tenosynovitis/tendinitis.

Chronic Articular Inflammation and/or

Degeneration. Deformed joint, crepitation with movement, variable tenderness in the joint line, variable pain with joint play, range of motion constricted by contractures as well as pain.

Typical presentation: degenerative joint disease, chronic rheumatoid arthritis, chondrocalcinosis, chronic tophaceous gout, granulomatous septic arthritis, cryptogenic synovial disorders.

Chronic Periarticular Inflammation. Variable tenderness over particular periarticular structures, bursal effusion if chronic bursitis, range of motion restricted by contracture as well as pain if myotendinous or tenosynovial pain syndromes.

Note. As emphasized in the regional text, when a joint is disabled, the location of pain and the particular constraint on motion imposed will be of one distinct pattern if the joint itself be affected and of another distinct pattern if periarticular myofascial structures be affected.

Laboratory Characteristics.

Blood Changes.

Polymorphonuclear leukocytosis: Acute septic arthritis, acute gouty arthritis, acute exacerbations of rheumatoid arthritis.

Anemia: immune complex disease, granulomatous septic arthritis.

Accelerated erythrocyte sedimentation rate: any acute arthritis, granulomatous septic arthritis, immune complex disease.

Normal erythrocyte sedimentation rate: degenerative joint disease, chondrocalcinosis and chronic tophaceous gout in the absence of acute exacerbation, periarticular myofascial pain syndrome unless septic.

Antinuclear antibody titers: rheumatoid arthritis—low titer; systemic lupus erythematosus—high titer.

Rheumatoid factor: rheumatoid arthritis, present in 60–70%.

Joint Fluid Changes. The normal synovium exudes a small amount of clear, colorless, mucoid material, which lubricates and thus diminishes the friction wear on articular cartilage. Degeneration, aseptic inflammation, and septic inflammation each affects the synovium uniquely, and each effect results in the production of a joint fluid with unique characteristics. In addition, three changes specific to three arthritic forms can be detected: the presence of rheumatoid factor in some joints affected by rheumatoid arthritis; the presence of urate crystals or calcium pyrophosphate crystals in the metabolic arthritides; and the presence of specific bacteria by culture in the septic arthritides. Table 18-1 compares the joint fluid characteristics which we find most distinctive.

Treatment

Fundamental Protective and Rehabilitative Treatment. The treatment of all arthropathies and periarthropathies is founded upon the appropriate application of the following regimen:

1. In the face of acute inflammation, the joint must be rested. Weightbearing must cease, and the joint should be kept in a position of function: toes—their spontaneous position when motionless; ankle—with the foot at right angles to the leg; knee—15° flexion; hip—straight or slight flexion; fingers—as though gripping a soft ball; wrist—slight dorsiflexion; elbow—forearm at 90° to the arm, and in neutral rotation; shoulder—with the arm at the side; spine—position of comfort. These positions may be maintained voluntarily or by splints. The ankle, fingers, wrist, and elbow nearly always require splints. The shoulder can be supported in a sling. A pillow under the knee is often sufficient for knee immobilization, though a posterior splint or cylinder cast will be required when ambulation with crutches is unavoidable.

To prevent a tenacious stiffness, strict immobilization should not exceed 1 week.

2. Ice application can be quite comforting during acute inflammation. The following method of icing is easy and not messy: A bath towel is folded to appropriate size to cover the joint and is dampened thoroughly and placed in a freezer. When frozen, it is removed, and wrapped in a damp towel and bent over the affected joint. It remains cold on the joint for 20–30 minutes. If more than one towel is frozen, ice treatments can be applied continuously. Heat should be avoided in the acute stage, except when the process is septic. Acute septic processes have been treated with both modalities. In our opinion, re-

sults do not appear to favor one mode over the other.

3. As the inflammation subsides, joint exercise should begin. We recommend the exercise be supervised by a physical therapist as the path is subtle between exercises which are too vigorous and thus likely to provoke an exacerbation, and exercises which are too timid and are unlikely to restore range of motion and strength.

The exercises begin with active assisted range of motion and progress to active resisted range of motion. Exercises appropriate to each joint have been described in the regional chapters. It is not unusual for pain to increase during exercise, but whenever that increase in pain persists after completing an exercise, or whenever visible signs of inflammation reappear, the exercise must be moderated or stopped until the inflammatory response has again remitted.

4. Partial weightbearing may begin when pain has subsided sufficiently to allow the upright position. Weightbearing must be less than that which provokes pain and will progress as range of motion and strength return. At the outset, only the weight of the extremity itself should be transferred to the ground. Crutches of various types are available. Physical therapists can help patients select the most secure and comfortable kind for their needs. When weightbearing is near full, a cane in the opposite hand may be used in lieu of crutches. Most people do not use a cane correctly unless taught. Physical therapists will teach correct use of the cane.

Summary of Drugs Used in Treatment of Rheumatic Disorders

These drugs are grouped in seven classes:

1. Salicylates.
2. Non-salicylate, non-steroidal' anti-inflammatory agents.
3. Gout-specific drugs.
4. Gold salts.
5. Corticosteroids.
6. Antimalarials.
7. Cytotoxic agents.

Antimalarials are used in the treatment of immune-complex arthritis fairly often in the American community. We have become accustomed to a regimen which excludes these antimalarials because we are discouraged by their damaging accumulation in the retina. Cytotoxic agents are used infrequently by physicians who are accustomed to their dangers, and then only in those immune-complex disorders that are progressing discouragingly in spite of compliant observance of other regimens. We do not use them, and we do not recommend that primary care clinicians use them. All the other drugs we find useful under various circumstances will be discussed in the next several paragraphs.

Salicylates (Aspirin)

Mechanism of Action. The full analgesic effect of salicylates occurs at lower dose than does the anti-inflammatory effect. Salicylates produce this analgesic effect by inhibiting the activation of pain terminals by various substances which accumulate in affected tissues during inflammation and other processes.

High doses of salicylates, in some as yet unknown manner, are thought to inhibit several of the molecular interactions that drive the *exudative events* of the inflammatory process. Thus they stabilize capillary permeability, attenuate those events which lead to vasodilation, and impede granulocyte adherence. However, they do not impede synovial *proliferative events* and the consequent joint destruction.

Contraindications, Side Effects, and Cautions. Allergy is the only absolute *contraindication* to salicylate usage. Erythemas, urticarias, and/or respiratory congestive syndromes are the usual manifestations of salicylate allergy. Patients chronically troubled by asthma or allergic nasal polyposis are most vulnerable to the respiratory congestive allergic response. The usual *side effects* are central nausea and vomiting, and upper gastrointestinal distress and bleeding. The low analgesic blood levels can cause urate retention. Variable doses of salicylate can provoke hemolysis in persons whose red blood cells are deficient in glucose 6-phosphate dehydrogenase. The high anti-inflammatory doses will augment urine excretion of potassium and urate. Blood levels just greater

than anti-inflammatory levels provoke tinnitus and reversible hearing loss. Blood levels somewhat greater than anti-inflammatory threshold are likely to provoke a reversible liver injury.

Salicylates block the effect of a number of drugs and potentiate the effect of others. The primary clinician is most likely to encounter four drug interactions, and must consider these prior to any prescription of salicylate:

1. Alcohol and aspirin potentiate each other's tendency to provoke upper gastrointestinal bleeding.

2. Indomethacin, phenylbutazone, and aspirin potentiate each other's tendency to provoke upper gastrointestinal bleeding and ulceration.

3. Aspirin displaces Coumadin from its plasma protein carrier, thus increasing its anticoagulant activity.

4. Aspirin blocks the effects of the uricosuric drugs probenecid and sulfinpyrazone.

When considering the use of aspirin, the following *precautions* should be observed: The drug should not be given in any dosage to persons who have suffered an allergic response in the past, who are known to be habituated to alcohol, who are known to be glucose 6-phosphate dehydrogenase deficient, or who claim to be intolerant of its side effects. The low analgesic doses should not be given to those who have suffered gout. Aspirin and the nonsalicylate, non-steroidal anti-inflammatory agents should not be used together. When given to patients using Coumadin, the aspirin dosage must be constant and the prothrombin time must be monitored very closely until a Coumadin dosage compatible with the aspirin dosage is determined. During treatment with aspirin, the patient must be alert to the emergence of rash, obstructive respiratory symptoms, increasing upper gastrointestinal distress, and evidence of gastrointestinal bleeding. The emergence of any such symptoms necessitates prompt investigation. Allergic reactions necessitate discontinuance of the drug, and other reactions necessitate a decrease in dosage or a temporary discontinuance. When undesirable side effects continue to recur, the drug must be discontinued.

Indications and Dosage. We recommend that the drug be given with antacids at mealtimes and at bedtime. Aspirin is a first drug of choice for the following disorders (Dosage is calculated for the 60–80 kg person):

Cryptogenic periarticular myotendinous pain syndrome.	Analgesic doses are used (less than 3 grams/day)—1–2 300 mg. tablets 3 or 4 times daily.
Degenerative joint disease.	
Periarticular inflammatory pain syndromes (bursitis, tendinitis, tenosynovitis)	Anti-inflammatory doses are used (more than 3.5 grams/day) —3–4 300 mg. tablets every 4–6 hours, for a total of 4 doses each day.
Rheumatoid arthritis	
Arthritis of inflammatory intestinal disease and psoriatic arthritis when resembling rheumatoid arthritis	

Non-Salicylate, Non-Steroidal Anti-Inflammatory Drugs (Indomethacin, Phenylbutazone, Propionic Acid Derivatives, and Tolmetin)

Some of these drugs can be useful when aspirin cannot be used, and some are specifically indicated for certain rheumatic disorders against which aspirin is less effective.

Their mechanisms of action are even less clear than is that of aspirin, and we will not summarize the meager insights in this text.

Contraindications, Side Effects, and Precautions. Indomethacin is absolutely contraindicated for use in children under 14 years of age, in pregnant and nursing mothers, and in those who have suffered a prior allergic reaction or one of the rare cryptogenic disabling or life-threatening reactions (e.g., optic neuritis, retinopathy, hearing impairment, hepatitis, pancreatitis, hemolysis, aplastic anemia, agranulocytosis, thrombocytopenia, depression, hallucinations, seizures). In persons known to have suffered gastric or duodenal ulcers in the past, the drug should be used only as a last resort and to avoid greater dangers from other drugs. When these constraints are observed, the drug is fairly safe as the dangerous side effects are quite rare. Unfortunately, the drug has

to be discontinued very often as unacceptable nuisance side effects are common: upper gastrointestinal distress and occult bleeding, headache, dizziness, drowsiness, confusion, sodium and water retention.

Phenylbutazone is absolutely contraindicated for use in persons who have suffered a prior allergic reaction or life-threatening toxic reaction. As it tends to be ulcerogenic, and as it very frequently results in increased sodium and water retention, persons who have suffered gastric or duodenal ulcers in the past, or whose myocardial reserve is compromised, should be given the drug very cautiously, and then only when other alternatives are less acceptable. While the side effects of phenylbutazone occur less often than do the side effects of indomethacin, its toxic effect on the marrow is not rare, and its rare toxic effects on liver, kidney, and myocardium are at least as life threatening as the effect on the marrow. The emergence of life-threatening side effects is especially rare during the 1st week of usage. Thereafter, the incidence rises. Phenylbutazone potentiates the effect of some drugs and enhances the detoxification of others. The following interactions must be kept in mind when using phenylbutazone:

1. Phenylbutazone inhibits plasma protein binding of Coumadin and sulfonylureahypoglycemic drugs, thus potentiating their action.

2. While stimulating the enzymes that effect its own metabolism, it also stimulates the enzymes that metabolize a number of other drugs, of which those used most often by primary clinicians are phenobarbital, diphenylhydantoin, tolbutamide, and digitoxin.

The drug must be withdrawn the moment allergic or any of the life-threatening side effects emerge. Thereafter, it should not be resumed. Nuisance side effects often abate after a reduction in dosage, or a temporary discontinuance.

The *propionic acid derivatives* (ibuprofen (Motrin), naproxen (Naprosyn), and fenoprofen (Nalfon)) and *tolmetin* (Tolectin), are absolutely contraindicated only in those who have suffered a prior allergic reaction. Side effects occur less commonly than do the side effects of aspirin, but can in higher doses be as serious: upper gastrointestinal distress, ulceration, and bleeding; headaches; salt and water retention; heightened irritability, and rarely some of the more serious central nervous system effects experienced with indomethacin.

Indications and Dosage.

Indomethacin. To minimize the risk of gastrointestinal irritability, we recommend that indomethacin be given with antacids at mealtimes and at bedtime.

Indomethacin is a first drug of choice for:

Gouty arthritis Pseudogout	200 mg. (50 mg. every 4–6 hours for 4 doses) the first day. 150 mg. (50 mg. every 8 hours for 3 doses) each of the next 3 days.
Ankylosing spondylitis Arthritis of inflammatory intestinal disease and psoriatic arthritis when resembling ankylosing spondylitis Reiter's syndrome	25 mg. 2–3 times/day augmented by 25–50 mg./day each week as tolerated and until satisfactory response is achieved or a daily dose of 200 mg. has been given for 1 week without benefit.

Indomethacin is a second drug of choice for:

Periarticular inflammatory disorders (bursitis, tendinitis, tenosynovitis) Degenerative joint disease, particularly disease of the hip Rheumatoid arthritis, unless the patient is younger than 14 years of age Arthritis of inflammatory intestinal disease and psoriatic arthritis when resembling rheumatoid arthritis	25 mg. 2–3 times/day augmented by 25–50 mg./day each week as tolerated and until satisfactory response is achieved or a daily dose of 200 mg. has been given for 1 week without benefit.

Phenylbutazone (Butazolidin), Oxyphenbutazone (Tandearil). To minimize the risk of gastrointestinal irritability, we recommend that phenylbutazone or oxyphenbutazone be given with antacids at mealtimes and at bedtime. When used for longer than 1 week, a complete blood count must be obtained twice weekly for the first 4 weeks, once weekly for the next 4 weeks, and once every 2–3 weeks thereafter.

We no longer consider phenylbutazone to be a first drug of choice.

Phenylbutazone may be considered as a second drug of choice for:

Ankylosing spondylitis Arthritis of inflammatory intestinal disease and psoriatic arthritis when resembling ankylosing spondylitis Reiter's syndrome	100 mg. daily for one week, then increase by 100 mg./day each of the next 2 weeks if necessary to achieve the desired effect. The chronic dose should not exceed 300 mg./day. The daily dose may rise to 400 mg. for a few days at a time when that increment subdues an acute relapse.
Gouty arthritis Pseudogout	600 mg. the 1st day (100–200 mg. every 4–6 hours until 600 mg. have been given), 400 mg. the 2nd day (100 mg. every 4–6 hours until 400 mg. have been given), 200 mg. the 3rd day (100 mg. every 12 hours), 100 mg. daily the next 4 days.

Phenylbutazone is the third drug of choice for:

Periarticular inflammatory disease (bursitis, tendinitis, tenosynovitis)	600 mg. the 1st day (100–200 mg. every 4–6 hours until 600 mg. have been given), 400 mg. the 2nd day (100 mg. every 4–6 hours until 400 mg. have been given), 200 mg. the 3rd day (100 mg. every 12 hours), 100 mg. during the next 4 days.

Propionic Acid Derivatives. These drugs are to be used only when aspirin is contraindicated or intolerable. Whether to use these drugs or to proceed to indomethacin or phenylbutazone will be a matter of judgment. The analgesic effect is as great as that of aspirin, and greater than that of indomethacin, and phenylbutazone. The anti-inflammatory effects are less than those of indomethacin and phenylbutazone and at high doses equivalent to that of aspirin. Side effects at the anti-inflammatory dose may prove as troublesome as will those of aspirin. The drugs are about four times more expensive than aspirin, and three times more expensive than indomethacin and phenylbutazone.

Recommended dosages are as follows:

Periarticular myotendinous pain syndromes Degenerative joint disease	Ibuprofen 1200 mg./day (400 mg. tablets 3 times daily). Naproxen 250 mg. tablets twice daily. Phenoprofen 800 mg. daily (one 200 mg. tablet 4 times daily).
Periarticular Inflammatory Disorders (Bursitis, Tendinitis, Tenosynovitis) Rheumatoid Arthritis Arthritis of Inflammatory Intestinal Disease and Psoriatic Arthritis when Resembling Rheumatoid Arthritis	Ibuprofen 2400 mg./day (two 400 mg. tablets 3 times daily). Naproxen 500 mg. the first dose and 250 mg. every 12 hours thereafter. Phenoprofen 1600 mg. daily (two 200 mg. tablets 4 times daily).

Tolmetin. This drug may be used in lieu of aspirin or indomethacin when they are contraindicated or intolerable. Side effects are similar to, but less likely to occur, and usually less intense than, those of aspirin and indomethacin. Tolmetin is four to five times more expensive than aspirin and three to four times more expensive than indomethacin.

The following dosage is recommended: 1200 mg. daily (two 200 mg. tablets three times daily).

Gold Salts

Two drugs are currently used, aurothioglucose (Solganal) and gold sodium thiomalate (Myochrysine). Both drugs are rapidly absorbed from muscle and show a serum half-life of about 5 days. Both drugs are selectively bound to synovium as well as to liver, kidney, adrenals, and portions of the reticuloendothelial system. Most of the gold is excreted in the urine; some is excreted in stool.

Mechanism of Action. How gold inhibits the inflammatory process is not known, though in clinical studies it has been observed to inhibit a number of enzymes. Unlike all other agents used to treat rheumatoid arthritis, evidence suggests that it may actually retard the destructive progression of the disease in some individuals.

Contraindications, Toxic Reactions,

and Precautions. Gold is *contraindicated* for use in pregnant women, in persons whose renal function is impaired, and in persons who have previously failed to benefit from a proper trial, or have suffered one of the toxic reactions.

About 30% of persons treated with gold will develop *toxic reactions*. These reactions appear in one of four systems:

Skin—pruritus, purpura, erythema multiforme, exfoliative dermatitis.

Gastrointestinal—stomatitis and, rarely, enterocolitis and hepatitis. Gastrointestinal reactions will often be heralded by a sore mouth and throat and/or a metallic taste.

Renal—proteinuria and, rarely, the nephrotic syndrome or acute tubular necrosis.

Hematologic—thrombocytopenia, agranulocytosis, and aplastic anemia are rare but lethal.

The following *precautionary* search for toxic manifestations must be made prior to each injection:

1. The patient must be asked about pruritus, metallic taste, and sore mouth or throat.

2. The patient should be examined for rash or stomatitis, should the history suggest a need or seem unreliable.

3. The urine must be examined for protein and red cells.

4. A complete blood count, including a platelet count, must be performed. Polymorphonuclear leukocytes are usually the first to suffer a toxic depression. When the percentage of polymorphonuclear cells and band cells multiplied by the total white count is less than 2,000, *granulocytopenia* must be presumed and the gold stopped either permanently or until a different cause for the granulocytopenia, like an acute viral illness, appears very likely. Platelets may rarely become depressed before polymorphonuclear leukocytes. When the platelet count is less than 200,000, *thrombocytopenia* must be presumed, and the gold must be stopped, either permanently or until a different cause for the thrombocytopenia becomes evident. Rheumatoids can develop Felty's syndrome (splenomegaly, pancytopenia, hyperactive marrow, in the context of

rheumatoid arthritis) which does not contraindicate the use of gold. A drop in red blood cells without other hematologic abnormality is rarely, if ever, attributable to gold toxicity. Nutritional deficiency or iron loss is much more likely to be the cause. Eosinophils may rise shortly before the skin or gastrointestinal manifestations of toxic reaction appear. When the percentage of eosinophils multiplied by the total white count is greater than 500 cells/cu. mm., *eosinophilia* must be presumed, and the gold must be stopped, either permanently, or until other cause for eosinophilia appears very likely (e.g., seasonal respiratory allergy).

Once it is judged that a toxic reaction has occurred, gold must be discontinued permanently, hence it behooves the physician to base the interpretation upon thoughtful observation. It is a shame to deprive a person who has benefited from gold because winter itch, canker sores, or intestinal flu has been misinterpreted to represent gold toxicity. All the symptoms and signs of gold toxicity can be caused by other processes. A physician must assume responsibility for considering all the possible processes before blaming the change on gold toxicity. Such judgments are indeed among the most worrisome that physicians must make.

Gold is administered as follows: Both drugs are prescribed in terms of milligrams of gold. Both drugs are given intramuscularly. Begin with 10 mg. the 1st week, then augment the dose to 25 mg. the 2nd week and the 3rd week. The 4th week, give 50 mg., and continue to give 50 mg. weekly thereafter, until a total of 1000 mg. gold have been given. If the patient has not improved by the time 1000 mg. gold have been given, the drug should be discontinued. However, if the patient has improved, the weekly 50 mg. dosage should be continued until 2000 mg. have been given. Thereafter, the dosage should be decreased to 25 mg. and given at increasing intervals: Every week for four doses, then every 2 weeks for four doses, then every 3 weeks for four doses, etc. The interval is thus increased until the longest interval is found that can maintain a remission. Should the disease relapse, we shorten the interval. For this purpose, we consider a relapse to be represented by visible evidence of acute arthritis. When a remission has held for 12 months with the dosage given bimonthly, we discontinue the drug. If a relapse occurs after the drug has been discontinued, it may be resumed. If more than 1 year has passed since the last dosage, the initial regimen can be used. If less than 1 year has passed, we recommend 50 mg. be given monthly and the interval gradually decreased until weekly doses are given, at which point the initial regimen may be followed. Calculation of the total dosage given should include all the drug given from the day of its resumption. Once again, the drug is permanently discontinued whenever a toxic reaction should appear.

Drugs Used Only in the Treatment of Gout

Colchicine. Although the use of colchicine in treatment of pseudogout has occasionally been followed by a remission, its efficacy against gouty arthritis is otherwise so specific that it is viewed even as a reliable diagnostic tool: if it induces a remission, the arthritis is gout.

Colchicine is contraindicated for use in those with a measurable degree of hepatic or renal insufficiency, lest dangerous toxic levels of the drug accrue.

The high doses usually prescribed for acute gouty arthritis are very likely to produce nausea, vomiting, and diarrhea. When used prophylactically for long periods, the drug has rarely produced alopecia, myopathy, agranulocytosis, and aplastic anemia.

Precautionary screening for liver and renal disease and for prior experience with the drug should precede the decision to use colchicine. When used prophylactically for long periods, the patient should be warned to report any patches of baldness, any inexplicable muscle distress, or sore mouth and throat, and complete blood counts should be made whenever the patient complains of sore mouth or throat.

The generally accepted prophylactic colchicine regimen requires that 0.5 or 0.6 mg. be given three times daily for the first 3 weeks, starting with the first dose of a uricosuric or xanthine oxidase inhibitor, then 0.6 mg. twice daily during the first 2 weeks with one of those agents, then 0.6 mg. daily thereafter with one of those agents. To minimize the risk of marrow suppression, we recommend long-term use of prophylactic colchicine only for those who suffer several relapses of acute gout in a year, or those who manifest evidence of chronic tophacious gout.

Its gastrointestinal side effects make colchicine a less desirable drug for the treatment of gouty arthritis than indomethacin or phenylbutazone. The generally accepted colchicine regimen for acute gouty arthritis requires that 0.5 or 0.6 mg. be taken by mouth every hour until pain is relieved or gastrointestinal symptoms emerge. A total of 4–8 mg. is usually therapeutic. Each patient usually becomes sick with the drug at the same dose each time. Thus, once a patient has learned his or her toxic dose, the drug can be stopped when a total dose of 1 mg. less than the toxic has been taken. The earlier in onset the drug is started, the sooner is the remission induced. The drug may not seem effective if taken too late after the onset. Ideally, full remission of the arthritis should be expected within 72 hours. Patients who cannot take oral medication can be given colchicine intravenously; 1–3 mg. may be given in 10 cc. normal saline. The dose may be repeated every 4 hours until pain is relieved, gastrointestinal symptoms emerge, or a total of 6 mg. has been given. If colchicine extravasates around the vein, an intense subcutaneous inflammation will result. Colchicine by either the oral or intravenous route should not be repeated until 3 days have elapsed since the last therapeutic dosage, lest severe gastrointestinal toxicity occur.

Uricosuric Drugs. One of two uricosuric drugs is commonly used in the United States and Britain—probenecid (Benemid) and sulfinpyrazone (Anturane). Both drugs lower the serum uric acid level by interfering with renal tubular reabsorption of urate.

Both are *contraindicated* for use in patients with prior history of peptic ulcer disease, or ureteral uric acid lithiasis. If either drug has appeared to produce an allergic reaction in the past, its further use is contraindicated, but use of the other of the two drugs is not. Sulfinpyrazone is contraindicated for use in persons who suffered marrow suppression while using the drug previously.

Gastrointestinal irritation is more likely to result from use of sulfinpyrazone than probenecid. Allergic skin rashes are more likely to result from use of probenecid than sulfinpyrazone. Only sulfinpyrazone has produced marrow suppression.

A *precautionary* inquiry must be made concerning previous use of the drugs, peptic ulcer disease, or uric acid lithiasis. During treatment, the urine output must be kept at or above 2 liters per day, and the urine should be kept alkaline, using 10–12 grams of sodium bicarbonate if necessary, unless sodium is contraindicated for other reasons.

As sulfinpyrazone is relatively more dangerous than probenecid, probenecid remains the uricosuric of choice in all except those who have manifested an allergic skin rash while using it. Uricosurics are preferred to xanthine oxidase inhibitors, as long as they work, as their dangers are less.

After 1 week of colchicine and during an arthritis-free interval, either uricosuric is started. Following are the dosage regimens:

Probenecid. One 500 mg. tablet is taken daily for one week, then the dose is increased each week by one 500 mg. tablet daily until the serum uric acid is less than 8 mg.%. Usually 1000–1500 mg. daily is required to achieve that therapeutic effect. The dosage which eventually proves effective is continued indefinitely.

Sulfinpyrazone. One 100 mg. tablet is taken the first day, and the dose is increased every other day by one 100 mg. tablet, until the daily dose totals 400 mg. Then the serum uric acid is measured. If less than 8 mg.%, the dose is maintained indefinitely. If the uric acid is more than 8 mg.%, the dosage is increased each week by 100 mg. daily after determining the serum uric acid. The dosage which eventually proves effective is then continued indefinitely.

Xanthine Oxidase Inhibitor. Allopurinol

(Zyloprim) is the xanthine oxidase inhibitor used to combat hyperuricemia. By inhibiting xanthine oxidase, allopurinol decreases uric acid synthesis.

Allopurinol is *contraindicated* for use in those who have suffered an allergic reaction to the drug in the past. If any other alternative exists, it should not be used in persons whose liver or renal function is impaired, or who suffer ureteral xanthine lithiasis.

Allergic skin rashes and/or fever afflict about 3% of persons given the drug. A form of hepatitis has occurred infrequently. Both effects require discontinuance of the drug. Leukopenia, leukocytosis, and eosinophilia have occurred. If their occurrence cannot be attributed to any other process, and if they persist, the allopurinol must be discontinued.

Precautionary inquiry must be made concerning prior use of the drug, and knowledge of impaired liver or renal function. During its usage, rash must be watched for and complete blood counts made every 3 months. Early in its use while serum uric acid is still more than 8 mg.%, urine output should be kept at 2 liters daily, and urine should be alkalinized to prevent uric acid lithiasis.

Allopurinol is specifically *indicated* when gout emerges in the context of increased uric acid production, such as occurs when neoplasms are treated with cytotoxic drugs. When used with a uricosuric, the two potentiate each other and disperse tophaceous accumulations more rapidly than either alone. The drug is also indicated when uricosurics fail, or are contraindicated.

The following dosage regimen is generally recommended: After 1 week of colchicine, one 300 mg. tablet is taken daily for 2 weeks. At the end of that time, the serum uric acid is measured. If still above 8 mg.%,

the daily dose is increased by 100 mg. each subsequent week until the serum uric acid is less than 8 mg.%. The dosage which eventually proves effective is then continued indefinitely.

Corticosteroids

Corticosteroids are the most effective anti-inflammatory agent available. However, the side effects and complications are many and serious, and the euphoria induced can be most seductive. Patients who have used the drug are very hard to wean. In rheumatoid arthritis, we restrict the oral use of corticosteroid to periods of severe generalized rheumatoid activity, refractory to all other measures. It is our general practice to give Prednisolone 5 mg., not more than four times daily for a period of 7–10 days, and then to resume the safer agents if further anti-inflammatory effect is necessary. The same short course of oral corticosteroid can be effective in treatment of the other acute arthritides and periarticular inflammatory disorders. We reserve corticosteroids for use against these disorders when other agents are contraindicated.

Six corticosteroids are commonly available. Their names and dosage equivalents are listed in Table 18–2.

Table 18–2
Corticosteroids

U.S.P. Name	Trade Name	Approximate Equivalent Dose
		mg.
Hydrocortisone	Solu-Cortef	20.0
Prednisone	Meticorten	5.0
Prednisolone	Meticortilone	5.0
Triamcinolone	Aristocort and Kenacort	4.0
Dexamethasone	Decadron	0.75
Methylprednisolone	Medrol and Depo-Medrol	4.0

CHAPTER 19

Infections of Bones and Joints

Acute Septic Infections (Acute Septic Arthritis and Acute Osteomyelitis)

The great majority of bone and joint infections in North America are primary, developing as a consequence of direct contamination during compound injury and orthopaedic surgery. Primary practitioners add to these complicating infections when they introduce contamination into joints by performing arthrocentesis with clumsy technique.

Secondary infections, which develop by contiguous or blood-borne spread from antecedent infections, are most prevalent among premature infants. They occur rarely in healthy children and adults, and thus are rarely encountered in primary care offices. Bone infections are more likely to occur while bones are still growing. Joint infections, as well as bone infections, develop more commonly in those who suffer sickle cell disease, in diabetics during periods of poor control, in those who suffer recurrent or persistent skin, dental, respiratory, or genitourinary infections, and in those convalescing from total joint replacements, oral surgery, and genitourinary surgery.

Bone infections usually emerge in the metaphysis of long bones. The most common sites are the upper end and neck of the femur, the lower end of the femur, the upper end of the tibia, and the upper end of the humerus.

Joint infections probably start in periarticular soft tissues. The earliest effusion accompanying infection is often sterile. Presumably, the fluid becomes septic only after the infection has perforated the synovial capsule.

The organisms that most commonly infect bones and joints are *Staphyloccus aureus*, beta hemolytic *Streptococcus, Pneumococcus,* and in infants and young children, *Hemophilus influenzae* and the *Salmonella* organisms. Rarely *Salmonella osteomyelitis* occurs during or at varying intervals after typhoid fever. (Weeks to years may lie between the known episode of typhoid fever and the recognized onset of osteomyelitis.) Newborns and those affected with sickle cell disease are likely to become infected by Gram negative enteric bacilli, particularly the *Escherichia coli,* and *Pseudomonas*. In our central urban adult practice, we encounter gonorrheal arthritis at least as often as all the other acute septic forms together. While the diagnosis is immediately suspect when other symptoms of gonorrhea are reported, it appears often enough without a recognizable gonorrhea prodrome. We assume persons so affected are carriers. Its local manifestations and prognosis are indistinguishable from the other acute septic arthritides.

Characteristic Clinical Features

The characteristic clinical features of acute septic arthritis have been summarized in Chapter 17. Like joint infections, the clinical characteristics of acute osteomyelitis are unique to each age:

Onset. Infants usually become abruptly and desperately ill with hectic fever, rapid pulse, vomiting, and occasionally convulsions. Less commonly, an infant will become gradually ill, showing the illness only by loss of appetite, lethargy, fretfulness, and variable fever.

Older children will usually become rapidly ill, manifesting hectic fever, rapid pulse, and variable degrees of prostration. They will not appear as desperately ill as infants, however.

Adults usually do not appear acutely ill and may complain of migrating arthralgias and myalgias prior to localization of pain in one extremity.

Local Signs. Eventually, all persons will develop signs of inflammation at the site of bone infection within the metaphysis of one of the long bones. The signs at the site of infection usually develop in the following order:

1. Infants and young children manifest a flaccid extremity, indeed, so flaccid as to mimic a lower motor neuron paralytic illness such as poliomyelitis. Older children and adults complain of pain and resist passive and active motion.

2. The area over the infected metaphysis becomes tender.

3. The area over the infected metaphysis becomes reddened, indurated, and swollen.

4. If the infection erodes into overlying soft tissue, the area will become fluctuant and may eventually develop a draining sinus.

5. The neighboring joint may develop an aseptic hydroarthrosis as it participates in the inflammation surrounding the bone infection.

6. If the infection erodes into a neighboring joint, the joint will develop all the signs of septic arthritis.

Systemic and Distant Evidence of Infection. Persons in any group may manifest a polymorphonuclear leukocytosis, an elevated erythrocyte sedimentation rate, and a neighboring or distant site of antecedent infection.

Radiologic Signs. X-rays are remarkably normal during the first 1–2 weeks of infection, although bone scans quickly show an increased uptake in the zone of infection. Eventually, the following changes will appear:

1. An initial break in bony trabeculae of the metaphysis will appear and will progress to become large radiolucent lytic zones.

2. Periosteal new bone formation will appear at the epiphyseal end of the metaphysis.

3. The cartilage of the growth plate and/or joint surface may show multiple areas of scalloped erosion.

Prophylaxis. Antibiotic prophylaxis is indicated prior to surgeries which are generally accompanied by bacteremia: total joint replacement, oral surgeries, urologic surgeries. Ampicillin and methicillin are given together 12 hours prior to surgery and continued through the end of the third day postoperative. Thirty milligrams of each antibiotic/kg./24 hours are given in four divided doses about 6 hours apart. Those allergic to penicillin are given Cephazolin 30 mg./kg./24 hours in four divided doses about 6 hours apart.

Evaluation and Treatment

The earlier acute septic arthritis or acute osteomyelitis is diagnosed and treatment begun, the better the outcome. Prompt treatment of osteomyelitis before it has eroded into overlying soft tissues or through the growth plate or into a joint usually results in definitive resolution of the infection and healing of the bone without joint damage, pathologic fracture, interference with growth, or development of chronic osteomyelitis. Delay will permit the development of any or all of those disabling complications.

The responsibilities of the primary practitioner are prompt diagnosis, thorough initial evaluation, initiation of antibiotic therapy, and referral to or consultation with an orthopaedist. We recommend the following protocol:

1. Presume the diagnosis of acute septic arthritis when the characteristics summarized in Chapter 17 are evident. Remember that early in the course of infection the joint fluid may be sterile, thus the presence of numerous polymorphonuclear leukocytes necessitates the diagnosis—even when Gram stain and initial cultures fail to identify an organism— until proven otherwise by subsequent events.

2. Presume the diagnosis of acute osteomyelitis when an infant presents as described in the earlier paragraphs, or when a child or adult complains of particularly severe pain in one extremity and manifests focal bone tenderness over a metaphysis of that extremity, with or without the visible signs of inflammation, in association with the septic syndrome in children, and in association with migratory arthralgias and myalgias and variable fever in adults. Do not wait for visible or x-ray evidence of infection. By the time such signs appear, the critical therapeutic advantage will have been lost. If bone scan is available it may provide supportive evidence at this point.

3. Aspirate, examine, and culture any joint effusion. Include culture for *Gonococcus*.

4. Obtain several blood cultures, a reliable urine culture, an endocervical culture from women, and a urethral culture from men.

5. Aspirate, examine, and culture the exudate within a soft tissue fluctuance. Including culture for *Gonococcus*.

6. Admit the patient to a hospital and begin the following antibiotic regimens:

Newborns. Penicillinase-resistant penicillin (Methicillin, Nafcillin, Oxacillin) 300 mg./kg./day in divided doses every 2–4 hours, intravenously (i.v.), up to 18 grams/day; and Kanamycin 15 mg./kg./day in divided doses every 12 hours, intramuscularly, or Gentamycin 5–7.5 mg./kg./day in divided doses every 8–12 hours, intramuscularly.

Children and Adults. Penicillinase-resistant penicillin (methicillin, nafcillin, oxacillin), 300 mg./kg./day in divided doses every 2–4 hours, i.v., up to 18 grams/day.

If afflicted by sickle cell disease, the patient must also receive ampicillin 300 mg./kg./day every 2–4 hours, i.v., up to 18 grams/day.

If the patient is allergic to penicillin, we give cefazolin 100 mg./kg./day every 4–6 hours, i.v., up to 6 grams/day, though cross reactions do rarely occur.

When gonorrheal arthritis is strongly suspected, the patient must receive Crystalline Penicillin G, 10–20 million units daily, i.v., in four divided doses.

Antibiotics are changed as culture eventually dictates. The appropriate antibiotic regimen is continued for 2 weeks after the patient is asymptomatic and the sedimentation rate is normal.

7. Request an orthopaedist's participation on the 1st day of admission. Often when treatment is initiated early, no treatment other than that recommended above is required. Occasionally, a joint needs repeated aspiration when the joint becomes painfully distended. Intra-articular catheter irrigation several times daily is infrequently required.

8. Once the inflammation has subsided, restorative exercises as summarized in Chapter 17 and the appropriate regional chapters are begun.

Chronic Septic Arthritis

When acute septic arthritis has been inadequately treated, it will assume a chronic form which is difficult to distinguish from the granulomatous and noninfectious forms of chronic arthritis. The joint surfaces are usually badly damaged. The joint may be unstable, and an effusion is always obvious. The diagnostic protocol summarized in Chapter 18 must be adapted to whichever joint is involved. When diagnosis remains obscure or chronic septic arthritis is confirmed, the patient must be referred to an orthopaedist for treatment. Surgical treatment is often required, and prognosis is always poor.

Chronic Septic Osteomyelitis

The primary practitioner usually encounters this disease when a patient presents with a relapse following a long period of quiescence (10-plus years). Usually, the relapse presents as a new or an increased drainage from a cutaneous sinus in the midst of a deforming scar over a deformed bone. Pain is often denied. When, as less frequently occurs, the infection presents as pain without drainage, the problem becomes a diagnostic question: Myotendinous pain like that of shin splints of the leg and the tendinous cuff syndrome in the shoulder, fatigue fracture in the lower tibia, bone tumors, a granulomatous infection, developmental disturbances of the head of the femur such as Legg-Perthes disease and slipped femoral epiphysis, and developmental disturbances of the condyles of the femur such as osteochondritis desiccans can all look at first glance very similar to chronic osteomyelitis. Careful palpation and manipulation can usually exclude shin splints (see Chapter 13) and tendinous cuff syndrome (see Chapter 3), while x-ray will eventually detect the fatigue fracture, and always detect tumor and granulomatous infection. The x-ray changes characteristic of chronic osteomyelitis are very similar to those of granulomatous infection:

1. Bone deformity residual from a previous infection and/or fracture.

2. Areas of dense necrotic bone may be surrounded by relatively radiolucent areas of living bone.

3. Subperiosteal new bone formation will appear as laminar layers of bone outside the cortex.

Longstanding, active, chronic septic osteomyelitis usually results in anemia, loss of appetite and weight, loss of stamina, and eventually secondary amyloidosis. When osteomyelitis relapses only briefly after long intervals of quiescence, these deteriorations in health do not develop.

Evaluation and Treatment

The primary practitioner must make the diagnosis and distinguish between the long-standing active form and the brief episodic form. The long-standing active form should be referred to an orthopaedist as surgical treatment will almost certainly be necessary. The primary practitioner can treat the brief episodic form. Treatment of that benign nuisance should proceed as follows:

1. When the disease presents as pain-free, modest drainage, it may be treated by superficial wound care only.

2. When the disease presents as a painful relapse and/or has a copious discharge, it should be treated by immobilization, superficial wound care, and antibiotics.

3. Superficial wound care includes frequent dressing changes accompanied by irrigation of the wound with aqueous neomycin solution 1 mg./cc. We instruct our patients to carry out this treatment whenever exudate appears on the dressing.

4. If a reliable culture can be obtained by aspirating from a deep site through a well-prepared area of intact skin, we await sensitivities and prescribe the appropriate antibiotic. If a reliable culture cannot be obtained, we prescribe a penicillinase-resistant penicillin.

Granulomatous Bone and Joint Infection

Mycobacterium tuberculosis, coccidioidomycosis, histoplasmosis, *cryptococcosis,* and North American blastomycosis are likely to spread from antecedent lung and skin infections to bone or joint. Except for those treating the impoverished chronically ill, or those in endemic areas, primary practitioners in North America may encounter these infections once or twice in a lifetime. Granulomatous arthritis presents as does chronic septic arthritis. An initial impression of degenerative joint disease will not prove compatible with the evidence of inflammation, nor with the relatively rapid progress in joint and/or bone destruction. Whenever an indolent arthritis fails to clear or a bone aches relentlessly without evidence of other cause, granulomatous infection must be included in the differential diagnosis, along with chronic septic arthritis, degenerative joint disease, rheumatoid arthritis, and persistent cryptogenic synovial disorders.

The primary practitioner should carry out the following protocol:

1. Culture any aspirated fluid from infected joints for tuberculosis and fungus.

2. Examine for cutaneous lesions.

3. Obtain chest x-ray, purified protein derivative of tuberculin, coccidioidin, and histoplasmin skin tests, culture any sputum for tuberculosis and fungus, obtain a urinalysis and culture the urine for tuberculosis and fungus if the urinalysis is compatible with infection.

4. Instruct the patient to rest and avoid stressing the infected extremity.

5. Refer the patient to an orthopaedist and, if other system involvement is evident, to a physician used to treating these uncommon granulomatous infections within the week. Send x-rays and all joint fluid studies completed to these physicians.

Granulomatous osteomyelitis, like septic osteomyelitis, tends to involve the metaphyses of the long bones and the bodies of the vertebrae. They present initially with bone pain and eventually may show evidence of overlying chronic inflammation. As the infection erodes, it can emerge into overlying soft tissue and produce a "cold abscess" and draining sinuses, and it can erode into a neighboring joint to produce a granulomatous arthritis as well. In time, an infected vertebral body will collapse, producing a gibbus. Pathologic fractures can occur through infected long bones. Infection of long bones in children will disturb growth of that bone, accelerating it if the growth plate remains intact, and stopping it if the growth plate is destroyed. The differential diagnosis of nontraumatic focal pain and tenderness over bone must consider the following disorders: adjacent myofascial pains (tendinous cuff syndrome, Chapter 3, and shin splints, Chapter 13); fatigue fracture of the lower end of the tibia; developmental disturbance of the head of the femur (Legg-Perthes disease and slipped femoral epiphysis, Chapter 11); developmental disturbances of the condyles of the femur (osteochondritis dissecans, Chapter 12); tumors; chronic septic arthritis presenting with pain and an atypical history.

The primary practitioner must attempt to make the differential diagnosis, culture any exudate that can be aspirated for tuberculosis and fungus, and should then refer to an orthopaedist all disorders except the myofascial pain syndromes, and the fatigue fracture.

CHAPTER 20

Diseases of Bone

Except for osteoporosis, bone diseases are rarely encountered by urban North American primary clinicians. Clinicians working in some impoverished areas of North America are more familiar than the rest of us with the nutritional deficiency diseases scurvy and rickets, and clinicians whose panels include an abundance of children are more familiar with renal rickets. Australian and British clinicians may be more familiar with Paget's disease of bone than are North American clinicians. Most primary clinicians will encounter a few primary bone tumors and a number of metastatic bone tumors in a lifetime of practice, and will often be obliged to consider bone tumors as a possible cause of extremity and back pain.

In our view, mastery of three areas of knowledge of bone disease is essential if one is to deliver orthopaedic primary care efficiently and safely:

1. The characteristic clinical features of bone pain;

2. a simplified classification of bone diseases that will provide a conceptual order that will facilitate recall;

3. a fair understanding of the pathogenesis, clinical features, and treatment of osteoporosis and Paget's disease.

This chapter will present these generalizations in a form which we believe has been quite useful.

Characteristic Clinical Features of Bone Pain

The following clinical characteristics imply bone disease until careful evaluation proves otherwise:

1. Dull pain is often relentless.

2. The augmentation of pain by movements can be shockingly intense.

3. Compressive and shearing forces directed to the site of pathology will usually augment the pain. Compressive forces can be applied to the spine by downward thrusting on the shoulders of the sitting patient. The maneuver must be initiated gently, and may be performed more firmly if gentle manipulation is painless.

4. Concussion of the involved bone will usually augment the pain. Concussive forces can be applied to vertebral bodies by fist or rubber hammer percussion over the spinous processes. Concussive forces can be applied to long bones by axial fist percussion at the distal joint—e.g., jarring the heel of a fully extended lower extremity can evoke pain from bone pathology at

any point along the tibia or femur; jarring over the patella with the knee flexed to 90° can provoke pain from bone pathology at any point along the femur.

Confirmation of bone pathology can sometimes be made by x-ray in anteroposterior and lateral projections, but a "normal" standard x-ray does not rule out bone pathology. Tomograms and radio-isotope scans should be employed when standard x-rays fail to clarify the matter.

A Simplified Classification of Bone Diseases

We believe it is impossible and quite unnecessary for primary clinicians to learn and remember even the names and the essentials of all the bone diseases listed in the standard nomenclature. It is quite enough if the clinician be able to categorize the disease as one of three forms: developmental disorder, maintenance disorder, destructive disorder. The following are examples of these general disorders with which we believe the primary clinician should be fairly familiar:

Developmental Disorders

Rickets, nutritional and renal.
Scurvy.
Achondroplasia.
Osteogenesis imperfecta.

Maintenance Disorders

Osteoporosis.
Paget's disease.
Osteitis fibrosa cystica associated with primary hyperparathyroidism.
Osteomalacia associated with secondary hyperparathyroidism and developing usually as a result of intestinal malabsorption of calcium, or excessive renal loss of calcium.

Destructive Disorders

Infections.
Neoplasms.
Because most primary care clinicians will be obliged to respond to the effects of osteoporosis several times yearly, and because Paget's disease occurs to an asymptomatic degree in nearly 3% of the North American population, and as such can be confused for other problems, we feel obliged to summarize the essentials of these disorders from the primary clinician's point of view in this text. A summary of infections from the primary clinician's point of view is presented in Chapter 19. Our attempt to summarize the developmental disorders, the other maintenance disorders, and tumors would add nothing to the summary which may be found in many texts. Our reading list has particularly singled out H. L. Jaffe's text.

Senile Osteoporosis

Pathogenesis and Differential Diagnosis

Senile osteoporosis is the commonest form of osteopenia, and the commonest cause of back pain in the elderly.

While *osteomalacia* represents a deficiency of calcium in a normal bone matrix, *osteoporosis* represents a deficiency of matrix as well as calcium. Throughout life, bone matrix with the calcium apatite crystals bound to it, is continuously being resorbed and reformed in response to the organism's changing needs for free calcium and phosphate, and in response to changing stresses upon bone. With increasing age, reformation of bone decelerates while resorption continues at the same pace. Some evidence suggests that bone resorption accelerates with age, but the possibility remains unconfirmed.

The cause for this imbalance between re-formation and resorption is unknown. Within all the speculation five postulates continue to attract interest:

1. Osteoblasts, which form bone, and osteocytes, which nourish bone, may age in advance of osteoclasts, which resorb bone.

2. Senescent endocrine changes may favor catabolism over anabolism.

3. Partly as a consequence of an increasing lactase insufficiency, with age, and partly as a consequence of a decrease in calcium foods in the spontaneous diet of the elderly, calcium absorption may decrease.

4. Decreasing activity with age deprives osteoblasts and osteocytes of the stimulation which results from bone stress.

5. The senescent marrow may generate

a substance which inhibits osteoblastic and osteocytic activity.

While *senile osteoporosis* is by far the commonest cause of osteopenia in the elderly, other diseases can produce the same clinical and roentgenographic skeletal picture.

Osteoporosis is somewhat more prevalent among those with *leukemia* than it is among the general elderly population, and while *myeloma* and *metastatic carcinoma* are classically associated with an irregular cystic resorption of trabecular bone, they may be associated with a more uniform resorption, roentgenographically indistinguishable from senile osteoporosis. Some event proceeding from the presence of malignant cells in the marrow may inhibit osteoblastic and osteocytic activity.

Hyperparathyroidism whether primary or secondary is associated with increased resorption of bone. Calcium intake and other factors still unknown determine whether this increased resorption leads to *osteopenia,* or whether bone reformation will accelerate to compensate for the increased resorption. The osteopenia may take the classic cystic form, *osteofibrosis cystica,* or may take the more diffuse form, osteomalacia, roentgenographically indistinguishable from *osteoporosis.*

Thus, when suspecting *senile osteoporosis,* the primary clinician must intentionally consider these other causes. Often a careful history and physical examination, including complete blood count, urinalysis, and chest x-ray, will suffice to remove suspicion of these other causes. The tumors most likely to metastasize to bone are the carcinomas of the thyroid, lung, kidney, prostate, and breast. When symptoms and signs of these tumors are absent, when symptoms of hypercalcemia and renal dysfunction are absent, when a complete blood count and urinalysis and chest x-ray are normal, and when diet is normal and bowel function not suggestive of malabsorption, we are content with a diagnosis of *senile osteoporosis.* When we are in doubt, determination of serum calcium, phosphorus, and alkaline phosphatase, an estimated sedimentation rate and a serum electrophoresis will help to make the differentiation. Table 20–1 summarizes the results expected for each form of osteo-

Table 20–1
Laboratory Differentiation Among the Causes of Osteopenia

Forms of Osteopenia	Serum Calcium	Serum Phosphate	Alkaline Phosphatase	Estimated Sedimentation Rate	Serum Protein Electrophoresis	Bone Marrow
Senile osteoporosis	N*	N	N	N	N	N
Multiple myeloma and leukemia	Increased	Variable	Increased or normal	Increased	Globulin spiking	Plasma cells or leukemia cells
Carcinomatosis	Increased	Variable	Increased or normal	Increased or normal	Alpha 2 globulin may be increased	Malignant cells may be evident
Osteomalacia (negative calcium balance associated with vitamin D deficiency or vitamin D unresponsiveness, gastrointestinal malabsorption, renal tubular malfunction, or chronic renal failure)	Decreased or normal	Decreased except in chronic renal failure when it may be increased	Increased or normal	N	N	N
Hyperparathyroidism	Increased	Decreased	Increased or normal	N	N	N

* N, Normal.

penia. When doubt still remains, examination of an undecalcified bone biopsy may make the distinction.

Characteristic Clinical Features of Senile Osteoporosis

1. The patient is usually older than 60 years of age.

2. More women are affected than are men, and they are affected younger than are men. The deceleration in bone formation may begin 1–2 years prior to the menopause.

3. Back pain is severe and relentless, and worse during resting hours.

4. As the dorsal vertebrae become wedged anteriorly, a dorsal kyphosis gradually develops.

5. X-rays, particularly the lateral view of the dorsal and lumbar spines, show diffuse osteopenia of cancellous bone. The cortical plates of the vertebral bodies, both superiorly and inferiorly, may appear quite dense in contrast to the relative radiolucency of the atrophic cancellous bone. Disc spaces may be widened, and discs may bulge through the cortical plates. The dorsal vertebrae will appear anteriorly wedged, and compression fractures of dorsal and lumbar vertebrae are often evident.

6. Osteoporotic patients are uniquely vulnerable to fractures of the distal end of the radius and ulna, the neck of the humerus and fractures of the neck and trochanteric region of the femur, as well as the compression fractures of the vertebral bodies.

Treatment

As yet, there is no clear evidence that any treatment can restore normal bone density, though symptoms can be relieved, and a neutral calcium balance restored. We recommend a regimen that is slightly modified from the standard recommendaton. Though it may seem pharmacologically homeopathic, we have found that it works and have avoided worries about toxicity.

1. Diet should be reviewed and modifications advised as indicated to insure adequate protein, calcium, and vitamin intake (particularly vitamins C and D). When diet alone cannot provide adequate calcium, as will generally be true when patients cannot or will not drink milk, patients may be instructed to take calcium lactate tablets grains 10 3–4 times daily, between meals, or all at once at bedtime. Though we have not prescribed vitamin D supplements, the contemporary standard protocol recommends that all patients be advised to take vitamin D 50,000 units twice weekly. We will prescribe multivitamins for those whose diet remains generally deficient. We recommend one multivitamin daily.

2. The patient should be advised to take fluoride with meals. The contemporary standard protocol recommends that 20 mg. sodium fluoride be taken twice daily with meals. We have found too many of our patients suffer gastric distress on this dosage, even when they take the medication with meals, and have thus prescribed sodium fluoride 2.2 mg. (1 mg. of fluoride) 3 times daily with meals. Recent patients have appeared to experience the same benefit from this seemingly homeopathic dose as did earlier patients from the larger dose. We suspect that the benefit from fluoride has to do with its ability to catalize those events that restore balance between bone reformation and bone resorption, rather than with its participation in the structure of the apatite crystal.

3. When patients are quite disabled, we will give aqueous methyl testosterone 25 mg. intramuscularly, once in 10 days for three such doses. The rationale for use of this hormone is its anabolic influence.

4. The original rather strong recommendation that estrogens be used after the menopause to prevent or treat osteoporosis has recently been somewhat weakened by evidence that the incidence of endometrial cancer is increased among women who have used estrogen after the menopause. Though we have preferred not to use estrogens for either purpose, the current standard protocol recommends mestranol 50 micrograms/day cyclically or Premarin 0.625 mg./day cyclically, to begin wtihin the 1st year following the menopause, and to continue indefinitely. Personal history

of hypertension or recurrent thrombophlebitis, or of breast or endometrial carcinomas, or family history of breast or endometrial carcinomas contraindicate estrogens for this purpose.

Role of the Primary Practitioner

1. The primary practitioner must insure that the diagnosis is well founded on careful history, examination, and appropriate laboratory studies.

2. When the diagnosis of senile osteoporosis is secure, the primary practitioner should carry out the treatment protocol as advised above.

3. When the diagnosis remains uncertain, the primary practitioner should refer the patient to an orthopaedist or an endocrinologist accustomed to studying the bone diseases.

Paget's Disease of Bone

Paget's disease is a disorder of bone maintenance, of unknown cause. Bone resorption and re-formation are both accelerated. Whether one precedes the other, remains unknown, but one postulate views the disease as a benign neoplasia of osteoblasts. The new bone matrix is abnormal in composition, and the architecture of the new bone is not organized in appropriate response to bone stresses.

The disease usually starts in one bone and occasionally progresses to involve the skull, vertebrae, and several long bones. Long bones are typically involved at their metaphyses. Three percent of persons over 50 years of age manifest the disease in a single bone and may or may not complain of symptoms. The primary practitioner is quite likely to encounter these individuals. Very few persons develop the widespread disease. A primary practitioner may encounter two or three such in a lifetime of practice.

Paget's disease of bone can present as one of six problems, each of which requires a particular differential analysis:

1. Bone pain with x-ray evidence of a well-localized abnormality of bone architecture and/or pathologic fracture suggests osteogenic sarcoma or metastatic carcinoma as well as Paget's disease.

2. Disease near a joint may so distort the joint surface as to provoke the changes and symptoms of degenerative joint disease.

3. Encroachments on spinal and cranial neural foramina will produce a variety of spinal and cranial neuropathies, suggestive of degenerative spondylitis, disc syndrome, and brain tumor, as well as Paget's disease.

4. An otosclerotic-type conductive deafness can be caused by Paget's disease.

5. When a person with more extensive Paget's disease is forced by illness or injury to remain immobile for an extended period, bone resorption will exceed bone reformation, resulting in a marked rise in serum calcium, with all its attendant symptoms and dangers.

6. A great increase in vascularity within and about Paget's bone lesions creates a demand for a high cardiac output, which may precipitate cardiac failure when the cardiac reserve is at all compromised.

The *diagnosis* can be made by x-ray when the process is advanced. Early in the illness, only areas of radiolucency compatible with tumor, infection, and osteitis fibrosa cystica as well as early Paget's disease will be evident. Blood calcium and phosphorus are normal, unless a person with extensive disease has been immobile for an extended period, in which case the calcium will become markedly elevated. Alkaline phosphatase will be elevated when the disease is active and normal when the disease is quiescent.

When doubt remains after careful history, examination, and the laboratory and x-ray studies just summarized, the diagnosis can be made only by bone biopsy.

Treatment

1. Asymptomatic Paget's disease with normal alkaline phosphatase requires no treatment at all. A Paget's lesion may be evident by x-ray incidentally when investigating a different site—e.g., standard lumbosacral x-rays may demonstrate Paget's disease in the femoral head and neck of an asymptomatic hip joint. The patient should be told the diagnosis and advised of the fair chance of an excellent prog-

nosis: Most people so afflicted do not develop the generalized disease, and those who do usually take 10–15 years to do so.

2. When localized pain is the only symptom, analgesic anti-inflammatory drugs can give quite satisfactory relief: aspirin grains 10 every 4–6 hours as needed, or indomethacin 25 mg. every 6–8 hours as needed, or ibuprofen 400 mg. every 4–6 hours as needed.

3. When the disease is extensive or is causing radicular symptoms, multiple pathologic fractures, or cardiac failure, an attempt at suppressive treatment is indicated. Calcitonin and Mithramycin have produced symptomatic remissions.

Role of the Primary Practitioner

1. The primary practitioner must keep in mind the possibility that Paget's disease of bone can cause the six syndromes outlined above, and must insure that appropriate x-rays are taken when history and examination suggest one or more bone lesions.

2. When diseased bone is identified, the primary practitioner must insure that qualified physicians interpret the x-rays.

3. When the diagnosis is clear, and the disease inactive, or producing well-localized pain only, the primary practitioner may safely proceed with the measures advised above.

4. When the diagnosis is still in doubt, or the disease is extensive, or causing disabling symptoms, the primary practitioner should refer the patient to an orthopaedist, or an endocrinologist accustomed to evaluating and treating the disease with the newer agents.

Recommended Reading

Classic references, other references of historic interest, and references dealing clearly with the basic principles are noted by an asterisk. Other references are included for those who wish to develop a broader view of matters discussed in the text.

General

Biography

* Watson, F., *Hugh Owen Thomas: A Personal Study*, London, Oxford University Press (1934).

The biography of a singularly dedicated and creative British bonesetter of the last century.

Comprehensive Texts

* Blount, W. P., *Fractures in Children*, Baltimore, Williams and Wilkins Co., 1955.

Though some details of therapy are dated, the text remains of value as a classic which applies the principles of orthopaedic traumatology to the unique characteristics of the developing organism.

Turek, S. L., *Orthopedics, Principles and their Application*, 2nd edition, Philadelphia, J. B. Lippincott Company (1967).

Though out of date, its discussions of pathomechanics are clear and still timely, and its bibliography includes many of the classic writings.

* *Watson-Jones, Fractures and Joint Injuries*, 5th edition, edited by J. N. Wilson, Edinburgh, London, New York, Churchill-Livingstone (1976).

A delightful, unusually clear classic which has been made current by the author's colleagues. Volume I presents the principles of traumatic orthopaedics. We particularly recommend Chapters 1 through 4, 9 through 12, and 17. Volume II presents the injuries in regional chapters and concludes with an inspiring, compassionate biologic chapter concerning musculoskeletal rehabilitation.

Relationship of Bone Architecture to Forces Sustained

* Koch, J. C., *The Laws of Bone Architecture*, American Journal of Anatomy, 21:177 (1917).

Anesthesia and the Elderly Injured Person

Ellison, N. and Mul, T. D., *Unique Anesthetic Problems of the Elderly Patient Coming to Surgery for Fracture of the Hip*, Orthopedic Clinics of North America, Vol. 5, No. 3:493 (1974).

Wyman, J. B., *Symposium on Problems of Fracture in the Aged: Anesthesia*, Proceedings of the Royal Society of Medicine, 46:106 (1953).

Complications of Extremity Injuries

Coleman, S. S., *Aseptic Necrosis of the Bone Due to Trauma*, Orthopedic Clinics of North America, Vol. 5, No. 4:819 (1974).

* Hardy, E. G. and Tibb, D. J., *Acute Ischemia in Limb Injuries*, British Medical Journal 1:1001 (1960).

* Simon, W. H., Friedenburg, S., and Richardson, F., *Joint Congruence*, Journal of Bone and Joint Surgery, 55A:1614 (1973).

Urist, M. R., Mazet, R. and McLean, S. C., *Pathogenesis and Treatment of Delayed Union and Nonunion*, Journal of Bone and Joint Surgery, 36A:931 (1954).

Chapter 1: The Wry Neck

Anatomy

Orofino, C., Sherman, M. S., and Schechter, D., *Luschka's Joint: A Degenerative Phenomenon*, Journal of Bone and Joint Surgery, 42A:853 (1960).

Spondylosis

* Brain, W. R., Northfield, D., and Wilkinson, M., *The Neurologic Manifestations of Cervical Spondylosis*, Brain 75:187 (1952).

Holt, S. and Yates, P. O., *Cervical Spondylosis and Nerve Root Lesions, Incidence at Routine Necropsy*, Journal of Bone and Joint Surgery, 48B:407 (1966).

Terry, P., *Spondylosis of the Cervical Spine with Compression of the Spinal Cord and Nerve Roots*, Journal of Bone and Joint Surgery, 42A:392 (1960).

The Cervical Pain Syndrome

Chrisman, O. D., Gervais, R. S., *Otologic Manifestations of the Cervical Syndrome*, Clinical Orthopaedics, 24:34 (1962).

* Jackson, R., The Cervical Syndrome, third edition, American Lectures in Orthopaedic Surgery Series. Springfield, Illinois, Charles C Thomas (1976).

Steindler, A., *The Cervical Pain Syndrome*, Instructional Course Lectures, The American Academy of Orthopedic Surgeons, Vol. 14, Ann Arbor (1957).

The Cervical Disc Syndrome

* Odom, G. L., Finney, W. and Woodhall, B., *Cervical Disc Lesions*, Journal of the American Medical Association 166:24 (1958).

Cervical Injury

* Frankel, C. J., *Medical-Legal Aspects of Injuries to the Neck,* Journal of the American Medical Association, 169:216 (1959).
* Marar, B. C., *Hyperextension Injuries of the Cervical Spine,* Journal of Bone and Joint Surgery, 56A:1655 (1974).
McKeever, D. C., *The Mechanism of the So-Called Whiplash Injury,* Orthopedics Vol. 2, pp. 3–6, 1960.
* Watson-Jones, R., *Spontaneous Hyperemic Dislocation of the Atlas,* Proceedings of the Royal Society of Medicine, 25:58 (1932).
Wickstrom, J. and Larocca, H., *Management of Patients with Cervical Spine and Head Injuries from Acceleration Forces,* Current Practice in Orthopaedic Surgery, 6:83 (1975).

Chapter 2: Thoracic Outlet Syndrome

* Adson, A. W. and Coffey, J. R., *Cervical Rib,* Annals of Surgery 85:839 (1927).
* Beyer, J. A. and Wright, I. S., *Hyperabduction Syndrome,* Circulation 4:161 (1951).
* Falconer, M. A. and Weddell, G., *Costoclavicular Compression,* Lancet 2:539 (1943).
* Tyson, R. R. and Kaplan, G. T., *Modern Concepts of Diagnosis and Treatment of the Thoracic Outlet Syndrome,* Orthopedic Clinics of North America, 6:507 (1975).

Chapter 3: The Shoulder

Anatomy

Rothman, R. H., Marvel, J. P., Jr. and Heppenstall, B., *Anatomic Considerations of the Glenohumeral Joint,* Orthopedic Clinics of North America, 6:341 (1975).

Tendinous Cuff Disorders

* Codman, E. A., *Rupture of the Supraspinatus Tendon,* Surgery, Gynecology and Obstetrics, 52:579 (1931).
Dimond, B., *The Obstructing Acromion,* Springfield, Illinois, Charles C Thomas (1964).
* Rathbun, J. and McNabb, I., *The Microvascular Pattern of the Rotator Cuff,* Journal of Bone and Joint Surgery, 52B:540 (1970).
Simon, William H., *Soft Tissue Disorders of the Shoulder,* Orthopedic Clinics of North America, 6:521 (1975).
* Sonnenschein, H. D., *Rupture of the Biceps Tendon,* Journal of Bone and Joint Surgery, 14:416 (1932).

Clavicle Injuries

Heppenstall, R. B., *Fractures and Dislocations of the Distal Clavicle,* Orthopedic Clinics of North America, 6:477 (1975).
* Rockwell, C. A., Jr. and Green, D. P., *Fractures,* Philadelphia, J. E. Lippincott Company, Vol. 1, page 756f (1975).

Glenohumeral Dislocations

McLaughlin, H. L., *Posterior Dislocation of the Shoulder,* Journal of Bone and Joint Surgery, 34A:584 (1952).
Rothman, R. H., Marvel, J. P., Jr. and Heppenstall, B., *Recurrent Anterior Dislocation of the Shoulder,* Orthopedic Clinics of North America 6:415 (1975).

Chapter 4: The Shaft of the Upper Arm

The Fractures

Klenerman, L., *Fractures of the Shaft of the Humerus,* Journal of Bone and Joint Surgery, 48B:105 (1966).

The Associated Nerve Injuries

* Sim, F., Kelly, P. J. and Henderson, E. D., *Radial Nerve Palsy Complicating Fractures of the Humeral Shaft,* Journal of Bone and Joint Surgery, 53A:1023 (1971).

Chapter 5: The Elbow

Diagnosis of Humeral Condylar Fractures in Young Children

* Cohn, I., *Observations of the Normally Developing Elbow,* Archives of Surgery, 2:455 (1921).

The Painful Elbow

Bosworth, D. M., *The Role of the Orbicular Ligament in Tennis Elbow,* Journal of Bone and Joint Surgery, 37A:527 (1955).
* Cyriax, J. H., *The Pathology and Treatment of Tennis Elbow,* Journal of Bone and Joint Surgery, 18:921 (1936).
Kerlan, R. K., Jobe, S. W., Blazina, M. E., Carter, V. S., Shields, C. L., Jr., Fox, J. M., Stokesbary, D. L. and Carlson, D. J., *Throwing Injuries of the Shoulder and Elbow in Adults,* Current Practice in Orthopaedic Surgery, 6:41 (1975).
* Mills, G. P., *The Treatment of Tennis Elbow,* British Medical Journal 1:12 (1928).
Newman, J. H. and Goodfellow, J. W., *Fibrillation of the Head of the Radius: One Cause of Tennis Elbow,* Journal of Bone and Joint Surgery, 57B:115 (1975).
* Roberts, R., and Hughes, R., *Osteochondritis Dissecans of the Elbow Joint,* Journal of Bone and Joint Surgery, 32B:348 (1950).

Radiohumeral Subluxation

Magill, H. K. and Aitken, A. P., *Pulled Elbow,* Surgery, Gynecology and Obstetrics, 98:753 (1954).

Chapter 6: The Forearm, Wrist, and Hand

Fractures of the Forearm

* Barton, J. R., *Views and Treatment of an Important Injury of the Wrist*, Medical Examiner, 1:365 (1838).

* Colles, Abraham, *On the Fracture of the Carpal Extremity of the Radius*, Edinburgh, Medical and Surgical Journal, 10:182 (1814).

King, R. E., *Barton's Fracture-Dislocation of the Wrist*, Current Practice in Orthopaedic Surgery, 6:133 (1975).

* Smith, R. W., *A Treatise on Fractures in the Vicinity of Joints and on Certain Accidental and Congenital Dislocations*, Dublin, Hodges and Smith, page 162f (1847).

VanHerpe, L. B., *Fractures of the Forearm and Wrist: Symposium of Fractures and Other Injuries in Childhood*, Orthopedic Clinics of North America, 7:543 (1976).

Carpal Injuries

Linscheid, R. L., Dobyus, J. H., Beabout, J. W. and Bryan, R. S., *Traumatic Instability of the Wrist, Diagnosis, Classification, and Pathomechanics*, Journal of Bone and Joint Surgery, 54A:1612 (1972).

* Squire, M., *Carpal Mechanics and Trauma*, Journal of Bone and Joint Surgery, 41B:210 (1959).

* Taleisnik, J. and Kelly, P. J., *The Extraosseous and Intraosseous Blood Supply of the Scaphoid Bone*, Journal of Bone and Joint Surgery, 48A:1125 (1966).

Bennett's Fracture

* Bennett, E. H., *Fractures of the Metacarpal Bones*, Journal of Medical Science, 73:72 (1882).

Pollen, A. G., *The Conservative Treatment of Bennett's Fracture-Subluxation of the Thumb Metacarpal*, Journal of Bone and Joint Surgery, 50B:91 (1968).

Spanberg, O. and Thóren, L., *Bennett's Fracture. A Method of Treatment with Oblique Traction*, Journal of Bone and Joint Surgery, 45B:732 (1963).

Hand Injuries

* Mikie, Z. and Helal, D., *The Treatment of Mallett Finger by the Oakley Splint*, Hand: Journal of the British Society for Surgery of the Hand, 6:76 (1974).

* Pulvertaft, R. G., *Twenty-Five Years of Hand Surgery*, Journal of Bone and Joint Surgery, 55B:32 (1973).

Wood, V. E., *Fractures of the Hand in Children*, Orthopedic Clinics of North America, 7:527 (1976).

DeQuervain's Stenosing Tenosynovitis

* DeQuervain, F., *Über eine Form von chronischer Tenovaginitis*, Korrespondenzblat für Schweizer Ärzte, 25:389 (1895).

DuPuytren's Contracture

Tubiana, R., *Prognosis and Treatment of Dupuytren's Contracture*, Journal of Bone and Joint Surgery, 37A:1155 (1955).

Volkmann's Ischemic Contracture

Ahstrom, J. P., Jr., *Treatment of Established Volkmann's Ischemic Contracture of the Forearm and Hand*, Current Practice in Orthopaedic Surgery, 6:213 (1975).

Chapter 7: Nerve Injuries of the Upper Extremity Summarized

* Watson-Jones, R., *Primary Nerve Lesions in Injuries of the Elbow and Wrist*, Journal of Bone and Joint Surgery, 12:121 (1930).

Chapter 9: The Back

Adolescent Kyphosis

* Scheuermann, H., *Kyphosis Dorsalis Juvenilis*, Ugeskrift for Laeger, 82:385 (1920).

Disorders of the Low Back

Barr, J. S., *Lumbar Disc Lesions in Retrospect and Prospect*, Clinical Orthopaedics and Related Research, 129:4 (1977).

Caldwell, A. B., and Hase, C. C., *Diagnosis and Treatment of Personality Factors in Chronic Low Back Pain*, Clinical Orthopaedics and Related Research, 129:141 (1977).

Davis, P. R., *Variations of the Human Intra-Abdominal Pressure During Weight Lifting in Various Postures*, Journal of Anatomy, 90:601 (1956).

Davis, P. R., *Pressure in the Trunk Cavities when Pulling, Pushing, and Lifting*, Ergonomics, 7:465 (1964).

Elves, M. P., Bucknell, T. and Sullivan, M. F., *In Vitro Inhibition of Leukocyte Migration in Patients with Intervertebral Disc Lesions*, Orthopedic Clinics of North America, 6:59 (1975).

Fahni, W. H., *Conservative Treatment of Lumbar Disc Degeneration: Our Primary Responsibility*, Orthopedic Clinics of North America, 6:93 (1975).

* Finneson, B. E., *Psychosocial Considerations in Low Back Pain: The Cause "and Cure" of Industry-Related Low Back Pain*, Orthopedic Clinics of North America, 8:23 (1977).

Garvin, P. J., Jennings, R. B. and Stern, I. J., *Enzymatic Digestion of the Nucleus Pulposus: A Review of Experimental Studies with Chymopapain*, Orthopedic Clinics of North America, 8:27 (1977).

Gentzbein, S. D., *Autoimmunity and Degenerative Disc Disease of the Lumbar Spine*, Orthopedic Clinics of North America, 6:67 (1975).

Gentzbein, S. D., *Degenerative Disc Disease of the Lumbar Spine, Immunologic Implications*, Clinical

Orthopaedics and Related Research, 129:68 (1977).

Kazarian, L. E., with comment by Pheasant, H. C., *Creep Characteristics of the Human Spinal Column,* Orthopedic Clinics of North America 6:3 (1975).

* Koreska, J., Robertson, D., Mills, R. H., Gibson, D. A. and Albisser, A. M., *Biomechanics of the Lumbar Spine and its Clinical Significance,* Orthopedic Clinics of North America, 8:121 (1977).

Lindblom, K., Hultquist, G., *Absorption of the Disc Tissue,* Journal of Bone and Joint Surgery, 32A:557 (1950).

Naylor, A., *Enzyme and Immunological Activity in the Intervertebral Disc,* Orthopedic Clinics of North America, 6:51 (1975).

Nordby, E. J. and Brown, M. D., *Present Status of Chymopapain and Chemonucleolysis,* Clinical Orthopaedics and Related Research, 129:79 (1977).

Pritzker, K. P. H., *Aging and Degeneration in the Lumbar Intervertebral Disc,* Orthopedic Clinics of North America, 8:65 (1977).

* Smyth, M. J. and Wright, Z. J., *Sciatica and the Intervertebral Disc, an Experimental Study,* Journal of Bone and Joint Surgery, 40A:1401 (1958). Reprinted in Clincial Orthopaedics and Related Research, 129:9 (1977).

Troupe, J. D. G., *The Etiology of Spondylolysis,* Orthopedic Clinics of North America, 8:57 (1977).

Williams, P. C., *Lesions of the Lumbosacral Spine,* American Academy of Orthopaedic Surgeons, Lectures, Vol. 4 (1947).

Williams, P. C., *Low Back and Neck Pain, Causes and Conservative Treatment,* Springfield, Illinois, Charles C Thomas (1974).

Wiltse, L. L., *Surgery for Intervertebral Disc Disease of the Lumbar Spine,* Clinical Orthopaedics and Related Research, 129:22 (1977).

Scoliosis

* Blount, W. P. and Moe, J. H., *The Milwaukee Brace,* Baltimore, Williams and Wilkins (1973).

We particularly recommend Chapter 2, The Principles of Nonoperative Treatment, Chapter 3, Indications for Nonoperative Treatment, and Chapter 5, Exercises with Brace Treatment.

* Kleinberg, S., *Scoliosis,* Baltimore, Williams and Wilkins (1951).

Chapter 10: Fractures of the Spine

Cervical Spine Fractures

* Beatson, T. R., *Fractures and Dislocations of the Cervical Spine,* Journal of Bone and Joint Surgery, 45B:21 (1963).

Rehabilitation after Spinal Cord Injury

Botterell, E. H., Callaghan, J. C. and Jousse, A. T., *Pain and Paraplegia. Clinical Management and Surgical Treatment,* Proceedings of the Royal Society of Medicine, 47:281 (1954).

* Gowlland, E. L., *The After-Treatment of Para-*

plegic Patients Following Injuries to the Spine, British Medical Journal, 1:814 (1941).

* Guttman, L., *Discussions on Treatment and Prognosis of Traumatic Paraplegia,* Proceedings of the Royal Society of Medicine, 40:219 (1947).

* Hardy, A. G., *Early Management of the Bladder in Traumatic Paraplegia,* Journal of Bone and Joint Surgery, 36B:368 (1954).

* Holmes, G., *The Goulstonian Lectures on Spinal Injuries of Warfare,* British Medical Journal, 2:769, 815, 855 (1915).

* Munro, D., *Rehabilitation of Veterans Paralyzed as a Result of Injury to the Spinal Cord and Cauda Equina,* American Journal of Surgery, 75:3 (1948).

Chapter 11: The Hip

Legg-Calvé-Perthes Disease

* Calvé, F., *Sur une forme particulière de coxalgie Greffée. Sur des désformations charactéristiques des l'extrémité supérieure du fémur,* Revue de Chirurgie, 42:54 (1910).

* Gladhill, H. B., *Transient Synovitis and Legg-Calvé-Perthes Disease,* Canadian Medical Association Journal, 100:311 (1969).

* Legg, A. T., *An Obscure Affection of the Hip Joint,* Boston, Medical and Surgical Journal, 162:202 (1910).

* Miller, O. L., *Acute Transient Epiphysitis of the Hip Joint,* Journal of the American Medical Association, 96:575 (1931).

* O'Hara and Winter, *Long-Term Follow-up of Perthes Disease Treated Nonoperatively,* Clinical Orthopaedics and Related Research, 125:49 (1977).

* Perthes, A. C., *Über Arthritis Desformans Juvenilis,* Deutsche Zeitschrift für Chirurgie, 107:111 (1910).

* Snyder, C. R., *Legg-Perthes Disease in the Young Hip: Does It Necessarily Do Well?* Journal of Bone and Joint Surgery, 57A:751 (1975).

Tachdjian, M. O., *Pediatric Orthopedics,* Philadelphia, W. B. Saunders Co., 1972 (Section concerning Legg-Perthes Disease, in Volume 1, page 384f).

Anteversion of the Femur

* Reynolds, T. G. and Herzer, F. E., *Anteversion of the Femoral Neck,* Clinical Orthopaedics, 14:80 (1959).

* Ryder, C. T. and Craine, L., *Measuring Femoral Anteversion: A Problem and Method,* Journal of Bone and Joint Surgery, 35A:321 (1953).

Slipped Femoral Epiphysis

Harris, W. R., *The Endocrine Basis for Slippage of the Upper Femoral Epiphysis, An Experimental Study,* Journal of Bone and Joint Surgery, 32B:5 (1950).

* Jacobs, P., *A Note on the Diagnosis of Early Adolescent Coxa Vera,* British Journal of Radiology, 35:619 (1962).

Klein, A., Joplin, R. J., Ready, J. A. and Havelin, J., *Roentgenographic Changes in Slipped Femoral Epiphysis,* Journal of Bone and Joint Surgery, 31A:1 (1943).

* Meyer, L., *The Importance of Early Diagnosis in*

the Treatment of Slipping Femoral Epiphysis, Journal of Bone and Joint Surgery, 19:1046 (1937).

Myositis Ossificans

Goodwin, M. A., *Myositis Ossificans in the Region of the Hip Joint*, British Journal of Surgery, 46:547 (1959).

Fractures of the Pelvis

Harris, N. H. and Murray, R. D., *Lesions of the Symphysis Pubis in Adults*, Journal of Bone and Joint Surgery, 56B:563 (1974).

Holdsworth, F., *Injuries to Genitourinary Tract Associated with Fractures of the Pelvis*, Proceedings of the Royal Society of Medicine, 56:1044 (1963).

Patterson, F. P. and Morton, K. S., *On the Cause of Death in Fractures of the Pelvis*, Journal of Bone and Joint Surgery, 55B:660 (1973).

Dislocations of the Hip

Austin, R. T., *Hip Function After Central Fracture Dislocation. A Long Term Review*, Injury 3:114 (1971).

Epstein, H. C., *Posterior Fracture Dislocation of the Hip. Long Term Follow-Up*, Journal of Bone and Joint Surgery, 56A:1103 (1974).

Pennsylvania Orthopaedic Society, *Traumatic Dislocation of the Hip Joint in Children. Final Report by the Scientific Research Committee*, Journal of Bone and Joint Surgery, 50A:79 (1968).

* Scott, J. E. and Thomas, F. B., *Delayed Presentation of Post-Traumatic Posterior Dislocation of the Hip with Acetabular Rim Fracture*, Injury, 5:325 (1974).

* Thompson, V. P. and Epstein, H. C., *Traumatic Dislocation of the Hip: A Survey of 204 Cases, Covering a Period of 21 Years*, Journal of Bone and Joint Surgery, 33A:746 (1951).

Fractures of the Neck of the Femur

Fielding, W. J., Wilson, S. A. and Retzan, S., *A Continuing End-Result Study of Displaced Intracapsular Fractures of the Neck of the Femur Treated with Pugh Nail*, Journal of Bone and Joint Surgery, 56A:1464 (1974).

* Smith-Peterson, M. N., Cove, E. S. and Van Gorder, G. W., *Intracapsular Fractures of the Neck of the Femur*, Archives of Surgery, 23:715 (1931).

* Trueta, J. and Harrison, M. H. M., *The Normal Vascular Anatomy of the Femoral Head in Adult Man*, Journal of Bone and Joint Surgery, 35B:442 (1953).

* Whitman, R., *The Abduction Treatment of Fractures of the Neck of the Femur*, Annals of Surgery, 81:374 (1925).

Chapter 12: The Thigh and Knee

Injuries

Fractures of the Thigh: Two classic discussions by the inventors of the Thomas splint and Russell's traction:

Russell, R. H., *Fractures of the Femur: A Clinical Study*, British Journal of Surgery, 11:491 (1924).

* Thomas, H. D., *Fractures, Dislocations, Deformations, and Diseases of the Lower Extremity*, Part VII of Contributions to Surgery and Medicine, London, H. K. Lewis (1890).

Osgood Schlätter's Disease, Original Papers

Osgood, R. B., *Lesions of the Tibial Tubercle Occurring During Adolescence*, Boston Medical and Surgical Journal, 148:114 (1903).

Schlätter, C., *Verletzungen des schnabelförmigen Vorsätzes der oberen Tibiaepiphyse*, Beitraege zur Klinischen Chirurgie, 38:874 (1903).

Popliteal Cyst: Anatomic Clarification

Wilson, P. D., Eyer-Brook, A. L. and Francis, J. D., *A Clinical and Anatomical Study of the Semimembranosus Bursa in Relation to Popliteal Cyst*, Journal of Bone and Joint Surgery, 20:963 (1938).

Meniscus Injury

* King, E., *The Healing of Semilunar Cartilages*, Journal of Bone and Joint Surgery, 18:333 (1936).

* McMurray, T. P., *The Semilunar Cartilages*, British Journal of Surgery, 29:407 (1942).

A Common Complication of Prepatellar Contusion

Gordon, G. C., *Traumatic Prepatellar Neuralgia*, Journal of Bone and Joint Surgery, 34B:41 (1952).

Chapter 13: Leg, Ankle, and Foot

The Painful Foot

Basmajian, J. V. and Stecko, G., *The Roles of Muscle in Arch Support of the Foot*, Journal of Bone and Joint Surgery, 45A:1184 (1963).

* Betts, L. O., *Morton's Metatarsalgia, Neuritis of Fourth Digital Nerve*, Medical Journal of Australia, 1:514 (1940).

Freeman, M. A., Dean, M. R. and Hanham, I. W., *The Etiology and Prevention of Functional Instability of the Foot*, Journal of Bone and Joint Surgery, 47:678 (1965).

* Freiberg, A. H., *Infraction of the Second Metatarsal Bone*, Surgery, Gynaecology, and Obstetrics, 19:191 (1914).

MacConaill, M. A., *The Postural Mechanism of the Human Foot*, Proceedings of the Royal Irish Academy, 1B:265 (1945).

Mann, R. and Inman, V. T., *Phasic Activity of Intrinsic Muscles of the Foot*, Journal of Bone and Joint Surgery, 46A:469 (1964).

Milgram, J. E., *Office Measures for the Relief of the Painful Foot*, Journal of Bone and Joint Surgery, 46A:1096 (1964).

* Morton, T. G., *A Peculiar and Painful Affection About the Fourth Metatarso-Phalangeal Articulation,* American Journal of Medical Science, NS 71:37 (1876).

Waugh, W., *The Ossification and Vascularization of the Tarsal Navicular and Their Relation to Köhler's Disease,* Journal of Bone and Joint Surgery, 40B:765 (1958).

Congenital Deformities of the Leg and Foot

Bleck, E. E., *Congenital Clubfoot, Pathomechanics, Radiologic Analysis, and results of Surgical Treatment,* Clinical Orthopaedics and Related Research, 125:119 (1977).

Chomley, J. A., *Hallux Valgus in Adolescents,* Proceedings of the Royal Society of Medicine, 51:903 (1958).

Hutter, C. G. and Scott, W., *Tibial Torsion,* Journal of Bone and Joint Surgery, 31A:511 (1949).

Keller, W. L., *Surgical Treatment of Bunions and Hallux Valgus,* New York Medical Journal, 80:741 (1904).

Kite, J. H., *Congenital Metatarsus Varus, Report of 300 Cases,* Journal of Bone and Joint Surgery, 32A:500 (1950).

Leibolt, F. L., *Shoes for Children, Symposium in Pediatric Orthopedics,* Pediatric Clinics of North America, Philadelphia, W. B. Saunders (1955).

McBride, E. D., *A Conservative Operation for Bunions,* Journal of Bone and Joint Surgery, 10:735 (1928).

McCauley, J., Jr., Luskin, R. and Bromley, J., *Recurrence in Congenital Metatarsus Varus,* Journal of Bone and Joint Surgery, 46A:525 (1964).

Injuries in Childhood

Frykman, Gay F., *Peripheral Nerve Injuries in Children (Symposium on Fractures and Other Injuries in Childhood),* Orthopedic Clinics of North America, 7:701 (1976).

Pappas, A. M., *Fractures of the Leg and Ankle (Symposium on Fractures and Other Injuries in Childhood),* Orthopedic Clinics of North America, 7:657 (1976).

Trott, A. W., *Fractures of the Foot in Children (Symposium on Fractures and Other Injuries in Childhood),* Orthopedic Clinics of North America, 7:677 (1976).

Fractures of the Shaft of the Leg

* Ellis, H., *The Speed of Healing After Fractures of the Tibial Shaft,* Journal of Bone and Joint Surgery, 40B:42 (1958).

* Ellis, H., *Disabilities After Tibial Shaft Fractures. With Special Reference to Volkmann's Ischaemic Contracture,* Journal of Bone and Joint Surgery, 40B:190 (1958).

Hamza, K. N., Dunkerley, G. E. and Murray, C. M. M., *Fractures of the Tibia, A Report on 50 Patients Treated by Intramedullary Nailing,* Journal of Bone and Joint Surgery, 53B:696 (1971).

Pinder, I. M., *Refracture of the Shaft of the Adult Tibia,* Journal of Bone and Joint Surgery, 55B:878 (1973).

* Watson-Jones, R. and Coltart, W. D., *Critical Review. Slow Union of Fractures with a Study of 804 Fractures of the Shaft of Tibia and Femur,* British Journal of Surgery, 30:260 (1943).

Ankle Injuries

* Ashurst, A. P. C. and Bromer, R. F., *Classification and Mechanisms of Fracture of the Leg Bones Involving the Ankle,* Archives of Surgery, 4:5 (1922).

* Davis, M. W., *Bilateral Talar Osteochondritis Dissecans with Lax Ankle Ligaments,* Journal of Bone and Joint Surgery, 52A:168 (1970).

Freeman, M. A. R., *Treatment of Ruptures of the Lateral Ligament of the Ankle,* Journal of Bone and Joint Surgery, 47B:661 (1965).

Hughes, J. R., *The Articular Damage in Complete Ruptures of the Lateral Ligaments of the Ankle,* Journal of Bone and Joint Surgery, 37B:723 (1955).

* Lapidus, P. W. and Guidotti, F. P., *Immediate Mobilization and Swimming Pool Exercises in Some Fractures of the Foot and Ankle Bones,* Clinical Orthopaedics, 56:197 (1968).

* Lauge-Hansen, N., *Fractures of the Ankle. II. Combined Experimental-Surgical and Experimental-Roentgenological Investigations,* Archives of Surgery, 60:957 (1950).

* Leonard, A. W. F., *Sprained Ankle May be More Serious Injury than Fracture,* The American Surgeon, 20:660 (1954).

Lettin, A. W. F., *Diagnosis and Treatment of Sprained Ankle,* British Medical Journal, 1:1056 (1963).

Ruben, C. and Witten, M., *The Talar Tilt Angle and the Fibular Collateral Ligaments. A Method for the Determination of Talar Tilt,* Journal of Bone and Joint Surgery, 42A:311 (1960).

Dislocations of Peroneal Tendons

Kelly, R. E., *An Operation for the Chronic Dislocation of the Peroneal Tendons,* British Journal of Surgery, 7:502 (1920).

Fractures of the Foot

Anthonsen, W., *An Oblique Projection for Roentgen Examination of the Talocalcaneal Joint, Particularly Regarding Intra-Articular Fractures of the Calcaneus,* Acta Radiologica, 24:306 (1943).

Gissane, W., *A Dangerous Type of Fracture of the Foot,* Journal of Bone and Joint Surgery, 33B:535 (1951).

Node, S. and Monahan, P. R. W., *Fractures of the Calcaneum. A Study of the Long Term Prognosis,* Injury, 4:201 (1973).

Watson-Jones, R., *Classification of Fractures of the Calcaneum, and Treatment of Fractures of the Calcaneum,* Chapter 31 of Watson-Jones, Fractures and Joint Injuries, 5th edition, edited by J. N. Wilson,

Edinburgh, London, and New York, Churchill-Livingstone, page 1161f (1976).

Chapter 15: Summary of Orthopedic Disorders Unique to Children

The Osteochondroses: An Overview

Jaffe, H. L., *Certain Disorders of the Individual Epiphyses, Apophyses, and Epiphysoid Bones*, Chapter 19 of Metabolic, Degenerative and Inflammatory Diseases of Bones and Joints, Philadelphia, Lea and Febiger, page 565f (1972).

Epiphyseal Injuries

Langerskiold, A., *An Operation for Partial Closure of an Epiphyseal Plate in Children and its Experimental Basis*, Journal of Bone and Joint Surgery, 57B:325 (1975).

* MacFarland, B., *Traumatic Arrest of Epiphyseal Growth at the Lower End of the Tibia*, British Journal of Surgery, 19:78 (1931).

* Salter, R. B. and Harris, W. R., *Injuries Involving the Epiphyseal Plate*, Journal of Bone and Joint Surgery, 45A:587 (1963).

Watson-Jones, R., *Fractures in Children*, Chapter 17 of Watson-Jones, *Fractures and Joint Injuries*, edited by J. N. Wilson, New York, Churchill-Livingstone (1976).

Chapter 16: Regional and Local Anesthesia in the Outpatient Practice

Adriani, J., *Techniques and Procedures of Anesthesia*, 3rd edition, Springfield, Illinois, Charles C Thomas (1972).

Collins, V. J., *Principles of Anesthesiology*, 2nd edition, Philadelphia, Lea and Febiger (1976).

Moore, B. C., *Regional Block, a Handbook for Use in the Clinical Practice of Medicine and Surgery*, 4th edition, Springfield, Illinois, Charles C Thomas (1976).

Winnie, A. P., *Interscalene Brachial Plexus Block*, Anesthesia and Analgesia, Volume 49, No. 3 (May-June 1970).

Winnie, A. P. and Collins, V. J., *The Subclavian Perivascular Technique of Brachial Plexus Anesthesia*, Anesthesiology, 25:353 (May-June 1964).

Chapter 17: Mechanical Therapeutics and Rehabilitation Summarized

Manipulative Reductions

* Watson-Jones, R., *Manipulative Reduction of Fractures*, Chapter 12 from Watson-Jones, *Fractures and Joint Injuries*, 5th edition, edited by J. N. Wilson, New York, Churchill-Livingstone, page 273f (1976).

Traction Techniques

Schmeisser, G., Jr., *A Clinical Manual of Orthopedic Traction Techniques*, Philadelphia, W. B. Saunders Company (1963).

Rehabilitation

Caldwell, A. B., Hase, C. C., *Diagnosis and Treatment of Personality Factors in in Chronic Low Back Pain*, Clinical Orthopaedics and Related Research, 129:141 (1977).

Cotton, F. J. and Peterson, T. H., *Physiotherapy in Fracture Treatment*, Journal of Bone and Joint Surgery, 16:658 (1934).

* Finneson, B. E., *Psychosocial Considerations in Low Back: The Cause "and Cure" of Industrial Related Low Back Pain*, Orthopedic Clinics of North America, 8:23 (1977).

McCann, V. H., Phillips, C. A. and Quigley, T. R., *Preoperative and Postoperative Management. The Role of Allied Health Professionals*, Orthopedic Clinics of North America, 6:881 (1975).

Sternbach, R. A., *Psychological Aspects of Chronic Pain*, Clinical Orthopaedics and Related Research, 129:150 (1977).

* Watson-Jones, R., *Rehabilitation After Fractures and Joint Injuries*, Revised by S. Mattingly, Chapter 34 from Watson-Jones, *Fractures and Joint Injuries*, 5th edition, edited by J. N. Wilson, New York, Churchill-Livingstone, page 1315f (1976).

Chapter 18: Non-Traumatic Arthropathies

Referred Pain

* Keldrin, J. H., *Observations on Referred Pain Arising from Muscle*, Clinical Science, 3:175 (1938).

* Keldrin, J. H., *On the Distribution of Pain Arising from Deep Somatic Structures with Charts of Segmental Pain Areas*, Clinical Science, 4:35 (1939).

Joint Play and Joint Dysfunction

Menell, J. M., *Joint Pain. Diagnosis and Treatment by Manipulative Technique*, Boston, Little, Brown and Company (1964).

Another View of the Myofascial Pain Syndromes

* Watson-Jones, R., *Surgery is Destined to the Practice of Medicine (Hunterian Oration: The Royal College of Surgeons of England)*, Edinburgh and London, E. and S. Livingstone (1961).

The Aseptic Arthritides

American Rheumatism Association, *Primer on the Rheumatic Diseases*, 7th edition, Journal of the American Medical Association, 224 Supplement:661 (1973).

* Bayles, T. B., *A History of the Treatment of Rheumatoid Arthritis (1939-1975)*, Orthopedic Clinics

of North America, 6:603 (1975).

Cheatum, D. E. and Kier, C. M., *Ankylosing Spondylitis and its Variants*, Clinical Orthopaedics and Related Research, 129:196 (1977).

Moskowitz, R. W., *Clinical Rheumatology: A Problem-Oriented Approach to Diagnosis and Management*, Philadelphia, Lea and Febiger (1975).

Murray, W. R., *Juvenile Rheumatoid Arthritis*, Current Practice in Orthopaedic Surgery, 6:171 (1975).

Reynolds, M. D. and Rankin, T. J., *Diagnosis of "Rheumatoid Variants:" Ankylosing Spondylitis, the Arthritides of Gastrointestinal Disease and Psoriasis and Reiter's Syndrome*, Western Journal of Medicine, 120:441 (1974).

Gout

Grahame, R. and Scott, I. T., *Clinical Survey of 354 Patients with Gout*, Annals of the Rheumatic Diseases, 29:461 (1970).

Spelberg, I., *Current Concepts of the Mechanism of Acute Inflammation in Gouty Arthritis*, Arthritis and Rheumatism, 18:129 (1975).

Wallace, S. L., *The Treatment of Gout*, Arthritis and Rheumatism, 15:317 (1972).

Degenerative Joint Disease

Bollet, A. J., *An Essay on the Biology of Osteoarthritis*, Arthritis and Rheumatism, 12:152 (1969).

Chapter 19: Infections of Bones and Joints

Infections in Children

Griffin, P. P., *Bone and Joint Infection in Children*, Pediatric Clinics of North America, 14:533 (1967).

Osteomyelitis

Kelly, T. J., Wikowske, C. J. and Washington, J. A. II, *Chronic Osteomyelitis in the Adult*, Current Practice in Orthopaedic Surgery, 6:120 (1975).

Waldvogel, F. A., Medoff, G. and Swartz, M. N., *Osteomyelitis, A Review of Clinical Features, Therapeutic Considerations, and Unusual Aspects* (Three Parts), New England Journal of Medicine, 282:196, 260, 316 (1970).

Waldvogel, F. A., Medoff, G., Swartz, M. N., *Treatment of Osteomyelitis*, New England Journal of Medicine, 283:822 (1970).

Gonococcal Arthritis

Brandt, K. D., Cathcart, E. S. and Cohen, A. S., *Gonococcal Arthritis: Clinical Features Correlated with Blood, Synovial Fluid, and Genitourinary Cultures*, Arthritis and Rheumatism, 17:503 (1974).

Non-Gonococcal Septic Arthritis

Goldenberg, D. L., Cohen, A. S., *Acute Infectious Arthritis: A Review of Patients with Non-gonococcal Joint Infections*, American Journal of Medicine, 60:369 (1976).

Chapter 20: Diseases of Bone

Jaffe, H. L., *Paget's Disease*, Chapter 10 from Jaffe, H. L., *Metabolic Degenerative and Inflammatory Diseases of Bones and Joints*, Philadelphia, Lea and Febiger, page 240f (1972).

Wallach, S., editor, *Paget's Disease, A Symposium*, Clinical Orthopaedics and Related Research, 127:2 (1977).

Index